CLINICAL CHALLENGES IN DIABETES

CLINICAL CHALLENGES IN DIABETES

Edited by

Anthony H. Barnett
Professor of Medicine
Department of Diabetes and Endocrinology
Heart of England NHS Foundation Trust and University of Birmingham
Birmingham Heartlands Hospital
Birmingham, UK

CLINICAL PUBLISHING

OXFORD

Clinical Publishing
an imprint of Atlas Medical Publishing Ltd

Oxford Centre for Innovation
Mill Street, Oxford OX2 0JX, UK
Tel: +44 1865 811116
Fax: +44 1865 251550
Email: info@clinicalpublishing.co.uk
Web: www.clinicalpublishing.co.uk

Distributed in USA and Canada by:
Clinical Publishing
30 Amberwood Parkway
Ashland OH 44805, USA
Tel: 800-247-6553 (toll free within US and Canada)
Fax: 419-281-6883
Email: order@bookmasters.com

Distributed in UK and Rest of World by:
Marston Book Services Ltd
PO Box 269
Abingdon
Oxon OX14 4YN, UK
Tel: +44 1235 465500
Fax: +44 1235 465555
Email: trade.orders@marston.co.uk

© Atlas Medical Publishing Ltd 2010

First published 2010

Although every effort has been made to ensure that all owners of copyright material have been acknowledged in this publication, we would be glad to acknowledge in subsequent reprints or editions any omissions brought to our attention.

Clinical Publishing and Atlas Medical Publishing Ltd bear no responsibility for the persistence or accuracy of URLs for external or third-party internet websites referred to in this publication, and do not guarantee that any content on such websites is, or will remain, accurate or appropriate.

A catalogue record for this book is available from the British Library.

ISBN 13   978 1 84692 054 7
ISBN e-book   978 1 84692 609 9

The publisher makes no representation, express or implied, that the dosages in this book are correct. Readers must therefore always check the product information and clinical procedures with the most up-to-date published product information and data sheets provided by the manufacturers and the most recent codes of conduct and safety regulations. The authors and the publisher do not accept any liability for any errors in the text or for the misuse or misapplication of material in this work.

Project manager: Gavin Smith, GPS Publishing Solutions, Hertfordshire, UK
Typeset by Mizpah Publishing Services Private Limited, Chennai, India
Printed by Marston Book Services Ltd, Abingdon, Oxon, UK
Cover image reproduced with permission from: Hodgkin MN, Rogers GJ, Squires PE. *Pancreas* 2007; **34**(1):170-1

Contents

Editor

ANTHONY H. BARNETT, Bsc(Hons), MD, FRCP, Professor of Medicine, Department of Diabetes and Endocrinology, Heart of England NHS Foundation Trust and University of Birmingham, Birmingham Heartlands Hospital, Birmingham, UK

Contributors

SRIKANTH BELLARY, MD, MRCP (UK), Senior Lecturer and Consultant Physician, Life and Health Sciences, University of Aston; Department of Diabetes, Heart of England NHS Foundation Trust, Birmingham, UK

BIRGITTE BROCK, MD, PhD, Head of Department, Department of Clinical Pharmacology, Aarhus University Hospital, Aarhus, Denmark

CHRISTOPHE E. DE BLOCK, MD, PhD, Assistant Professor, University of Antwerp, Faculty of Medicine, Department of Endocrinology, Diabetology and Metabolism, Antwerp University Hospital, Antwerp, Belgium

FIDELMA DUNNE, MD, PhD, MMedEd, Consultant Endocrinologist, Head of School of Medicine, School of Medicine, National University of Ireland, Galway and Galway University Hospitals, Galway, Ireland

MARC EVANS, MD, MRCP, Consultant Diabetologist, Department of Diabetes, University Hospital Llandough, Cardiff, UK

MILES FISHER, MD, FRCP (Glas), FRCP (Ed), MB ChB, Consultant Physician, Department of Medicine, Glasgow Royal Infirmary, Glasgow, UK

ROGER GADSBY, MBE, BSc, MB ChB, DCH, DRCOG, FRCGP, General Practitioner and Associate Clinical Professor, Institute of Clinical Education, Warwick Medical School, University of Warwick, Coventry, UK

BAPTIST GALLWITZ, MD, PhD, Consultant Endocrinologist, Department of Medicine IV, Eberhard Karls University Tübingen, Tübingen, Germany

JILL HILL, BSc(Hons), RGN, Diabetes Nurse Consultant, Community Diabetes Team, NHS Birmingham East and North, Birmingham, UK

CRYSTAL M. HOLMES, DPM, CWS, Clinical Instructor, Podiatry, University of Michigan, Department of Internal Medicine, Division of Metabolism, Endocrinology and Diabetes, Ann Arbor, Michigan, USA

FRANKLIN JOSEPH, MRCP, Consultant Physician in Diabetes and Endocrinology, Department of Diabetes and Endocrinology, The Countess of Chester Hospital NHS Foundation Trust, Chester, UK

MICHEL MARRE, MD, PhD, Head of Diabetology Department, Director of INSERM Unit U695, Faculté Xavier Bichat, Université Paris VII; Department of Diabetology, Endocrinology and Nutrition, Hospital Bichat (Assistance Publique - Hôpitaux de Paris), Paris, France

AUNG MON, MBBS, MRCP, Specialist Registrar, Diabetes and Endocrinology, Royal Liverpool University Hospital, Liverpool, UK

RAJ PETER, MD, MRCP, Consultant Diabetologist, Department of Diabetes, Neath Port Talbot Hospital, Port Talbot, UK

RODICA POP-BUSUI, MD, PhD, Assistant Professor of Internal Medicine, Division of Metabolism, Endocrinology and Diabetes, Department of Internal Medicine, University of Michigan, Ann Arbor, Michigan, USA

JØRGEN RUNGBY, MD, DMSc, Head of Department, Department of Endocrinology, Aarhus University Hospital, Aarhus, Denmark

MARTIN J. STEVENS, MD, FRCP, Professor of Medicine, Honorary Consultant Physician, School of Clinical and Experimental Medicine, University of Birmingham and Heart of England NHS Foundation Trust, Birmingham, UK

FLORENCE TRAVERT, MD, PhD, Senior Consultant in Diabetology, Department of Diabetology, Endocrinology and Nutrition, Hospital Bichat (Assistance Publique - Hôpitaux de Paris), Paris, France

LUC F. VAN GAAL, MD, PhD, Professor of Endocrinology and Diabetology, Antwerp University Hospital, Faculty of Medicine, Department of Endocrinology, Diabetology, and Metabolism, Antwerp, Belgium

JITEN VORA, MA, MD, FRCP, Consultant Endocrinologist, Department of Diabetes and Endocrinology, Royal Liverpool University Hospital, Liverpool, UK

JONATHAN WEBBER, DM, FRCP, Consultant Diabetologist, Diabetes Centre, University Hospital Birmingham Foundation Trust, Birmingham, UK

1

Diabetes: early screening costs and benefits

M. Marre, F. Travert

BACKGROUND

Although it is well-recognised that type 2 diabetes has become a huge burden for the general adult worldwide population, there is presently no systematic or structured screening policy for type 2 diabetes in any country or region except for some general guidance recently issued by the UK National Screening Committee [1].

Screening for type 2 diabetes will logically allow for early diagnosis and treatment. This might be important as early diagnosis and treatment could prevent future associated microvascular and macrovascular complications. An estimated 50% of people with diabetes are currently undiagnosed. According to several major studies, around 20–30% of people with type 2 diabetes have already developed complications at diagnosis. The approach could be either to screen for type 2 diabetes alone, or to anticipate the progression to diabetes from pre-diabetic states and therefore to lower the threshold to allow screening for both impaired glucose tolerance (IGT) and type 2 diabetes. In addition, for earlier diagnosis of type 2 diabetes, interventions could be designed for those identified to have IGT in order to attempt to delay the onset of type 2 diabetes and/or to prevent complications.

One major programme has been developed in the US, the Diabetes Prevention Program (DPP), which targeted only individuals with IGT [2]. It clearly demonstrated that behavioural modifications and drug treatments can delay or prevent the development of type 2 diabetes in this population. The DPP randomly assigned subjects with IGT and elevated fasting glucose to three treatment groups: placebo, a lifestyle modification programme with goals of 7% weight loss and 150 min of weekly physical activity, or metformin. The average follow-up was 2.8 years. In comparison with placebo, the lifestyle and metformin interventions reduced the incidence of type 2 diabetes by 58% and 31%, respectively. Versus placebo, the lifestyle and metformin interventions were estimated to delay development of type 2 diabetes by 11 and 3 years, respectively; the corresponding reductions in absolute lifetime incidence of diabetes were 20% and 8%, respectively. Compared with placebo, the cost per quality adjusted life-year (QALY) from a health system perspective was $1100 and $31 300 for the lifestyle and metformin interventions, respectively.

Because this programme focused solely on individuals with known IGT, it concluded only that it is cost-effective to prevent the conversion from pre-diabetes to diabetes. It did not answer a distinct, and important, public health question: is it cost-effective to screen

Michel Marre, MD, PhD, Head of Diabetology Department, Director of INSERM Unit U695, Faculté Xavier Bichat, Université Paris VII; Department of Diabetology, Endocrinology and Nutrition, Hospital Bichat (Assistance Publique - Hôpitaux de Paris), Paris, France.

Florence Travert, MD, PhD, Senior Consultant in Diabetology, Department of Diabetology, Endocrinology and Nutrition, Hospital Bichat (Assistance Publique - Hôpitaux de Paris), Paris, France.

patients to identify individuals with pre-diabetes or even more crucial to detect individuals already with full diabetes status?

Only one other trial (with acarbose) was conducted mostly in middle-aged men (STOP-NIDDM) [3]. Interestingly, a secondary analysis of this trial suggested that those on active treatment to reduce or delay type 2 diabetes were also protected from cardiovascular events. The latter account for most of the reduced life expectancy of people with type 2 diabetes.

No definitive trials have yet examined the effectiveness of screening for type 2 diabetes or IGT: assessment of preventive policies has so far been conducted through simulation studies [4, 5]. A recent systematic review and meta-analysis of intervention trials for prevention of type 2 diabetes, including the DPP, found that both lifestyle and pharmacological interventions significantly reduced the risk of type 2 diabetes in people with IGT [6]. Initial models of screening for type 2 diabetes alone have generally assessed the impact of early treatment on cardiovascular events, though some also included microvascular events such as retinopathy. Several more recent decision models have been compiled that have assessed either the clinical and cost effectiveness of interventions to prevent type 2 diabetes [7–14] or strategies for screening and early detection of diabetes [4, 15–18]. Overall, most of the models produced favourable results for screening, but cost-effectiveness varied with age group screened and the population targeted for screening. Only two studies reported costs for a UK setting [4, 17], one of which had a limited time horizon of five years [17]. Both studies concluded that there was uncertainty concerning the cost-effectiveness of screening for diabetes. Of the eight models assessing cost-effectiveness of interventions for prevention of diabetes, only three included costs of identifying individuals with IGT [8, 10, 14]. The time horizon over which the models were run ranged from just three years after the intervention up to the expected lifetime of the population. Models used data from various sources: published trials, epidemiological studies and national statistics. In general, data were limited to a few sources. All models compared a strategy of intervention against no intervention, rather than screening for IGT followed by intervention compared with no screening. All but one model simulated populations where all individuals had IGT at the start of the model and the end states were development of diabetes or death. Hence, only a limited section of the disease pathway was modelled. Also, the models did not take into account that screening for IGT will at the same time allow individuals with undiagnosed diabetes to be identified, thus allowing for early treatment and possibly reducing rates of complications. Hence, while these studies offer an assessment of the cost-effectiveness of interventions for prevention of diabetes, none assessed the impact of screening followed by intervention on the whole disease pathway.

In this chapter we will consider what early screening means and whether diabetes could be a good candidate for such a process. We will describe how it could be possible to screen for diabetes, and what benefits could be expected from early detection. Finally, we will develop and illustrate our topic and give some idea of the cost by analysing two recently published models of cost-effectiveness in type 2 diabetes.

CONSIDERING THE PURPOSE OF EARLY SCREENING, WHY COULD DIABETES BE A GOOD CANDIDATE FOR SUCH A PROCESS?

The World Health Organization (WHO) defined the minimal criteria to propose a disease for an early detection programme. The five main reasons to recommend a disease for a screening programme are:

1. The disease should represent an important health economic concern.
2. The natural history of the disease and the prognosis when not treated should be known.
3. There should be a latent preclinical time before the occurrence of symptomatic disease during which diagnosis is possible.

4. There should exist reliable and safe diagnostic tests which are acceptable for screening the population.
5. The disease should be able to be efficiently treated when diagnosed; the earlier the treatment is started the more efficient it is.
(Wilson and Jungner, WHO 1968)

So where does type 2 diabetes fit into these five criteria?

CRITERION 1

This is obviously satisfied. Diabetes is a major worldwide and health economic concern. Its prevalence is more than 8% of the worldwide adult population [19]. It is a major cause of morbidity and mortality linked to both microvascular complications (blindness, renal failure, amputation) and macrovascular complications (myocardial infarction and stroke).

CRITERION 2

Regarding the natural history of diabetes, it is known that the duration of diabetes and the level of hyperglycaemia correlate with the occurrence of microvascular, and possibly with macrovascular, complications. Diabetes also often clusters with hypertension and dyslipidaemia and these are powerful risk factors for cardiovascular complications. The co-occurrence of cardiovascular risk factors in the same patient has led to the term 'metabolic syndrome'. Screening for diabetes without screening for hypertension and dyslipidaemia is a crucial issue that we will not address here.

CRITERION 3

Type 2 diabetes is typically a disease characterized by a latent phase before the occurrence of the clinical symptoms. This has been demonstrated by various epidemiological surveys and during detection programmes performed by physicians. Moreover, at the time of clinical diagnosis (commonly because of symptoms of hyperglycaemia), a percentage of these newly diagnosed diabetic patients already have complications, especially retinopathy (2–39%), nephropathy (8–18%) or neuropathy (5–13%). On this basis, various models estimate the preclinical phase as 7 to 12 years [20]. During this preclinical phase we have the possibility of making an earlier diagnosis since hyperglycaemia may remain asymptomatic for years.

CRITERION 4

Performing a blood glucose assessment is relatively easy and acceptable to the people to be screened.

CRITERION 5

This is the most difficult to address: does a treatment started at the phase of screening result in a benefit in terms of prevention of the complications? The evidence is currently weak and there is no large-scale intervention study demonstrating that screening for diabetes provides a true advantage in terms of preventing complications. Some studies are currently underway which aim to evaluate the impact of an early treatment initiated during the pre-diabetes stage (ORIGIN, NAVIGATOR) [21, 22].

HOW WOULD IT BE POSSIBLE TO SCREEN FOR DIABETES?

Fasting venous plasma glucose assessment is the most recommended measure since it matches the definition of diabetes which is two consecutive values >7 mmol/l. What about screening using random glucose values? This is easier because it is not mandatory to give a specific appointment when fasting, but it is less widely used. Is it possible to use a home blood glucose meter? This could be an attractive method if the practitioner is very familiar with the device and its calibration, and as long as the difference between capillary glucose values and venous plasma glucose are taken into account: the venous value being higher than the capillary one (6 mmol capillary corresponds to 7 mmol/l venous plasma). But this method is not considered to be sufficiently standardized to be applicable to a large-scale programme.

What about the oral glucose tolerance test (OGTT)? While this has been considered the 'gold standard' for a long time, it is too difficult and too expensive to be proposed for large-scale screening. HbA1c is often proposed for diagnosis, but is not recommended because of genetic variants that may alter its predictive value and the fact that it is expensive and still remains to be validated diagnostically.

WHAT BENEFITS CAN BE EXPECTED FROM EARLY DETECTION OF TYPE 2 DIABETES?

Benefits from screening are predicted because it is now accepted that microvascular complications are mainly determined by the level and duration of hyperglycaemia. Simulation studies show potential benefits of screening, which would reduce microvascular complications, especially the risk of blindness [23, 24].

From the point of view of macrovascular complications, we can speculate that detecting diabetes would categorize a patient in an 'at risk population' and therefore draw the attention of the physician to providing multifactorial care focused on blood glucose, blood pressure and cholesterol. These are logical arguments but assumptions only. Indeed, one study concluded that public funds would be better spent on treating people with diagnosed diabetes properly rather than on searching for new cases among the whole population [21].

Only serious and recent modelling studies can help with responding to the cost-effectiveness question and these are discussed below.

ARE THE PROPOSED MODELS OF COST-EFFECTIVENESS RECENTLY PUBLISHED IN THE LITERATURE CONCLUSIVE?

In this section we carefully consider the results and the conclusions of two major recent papers in order to provide an opinion on cost-effectiveness of early detection of type 2 diabetes.

(A) THE 'NARROW ANALYSIS'

This takes into account only the detection of pre-diabetes in an obese population [25]. The DPP demonstrated that intensive lifestyle intervention could prevent or delay the onset of type 2 diabetes. However, the intervention was expensive, and some worried that it might not prove cost-effective. To address this issue, some authors have applied a simulation model to estimate lifetime outcomes and costs for subjects known to have IGT and elevated fasting glucose concentrations [26]. The DPP lifestyle intervention had a relatively attractive cost-effectiveness ratio from the perspective of the healthcare system. Other studies [27–30] have examined the cost-effectiveness of lifestyle interventions or drug therapy to prevent type 2 diabetes among subjects with IGT. All studies but one [29] found that the interventions delay or prevent diabetes onset and reported favourable cost-effectiveness ratios. These previous results led to a natural next question: if applying the DPP lifestyle intervention to subjects known to have IGT and impaired fasting glucose (IFG) is cost-effective, would it also be cost-effective to screen for pre-diabetes and then treat subjects identified as having this condition? To answer this question, Hoerger and colleagues studied the cost-effectiveness of screening for pre-diabetes among overweight and obese US adults [25]. To evaluate the screening issue, they performed a new cost-effectiveness analysis to compare screening/treatment strategies for pre-diabetes (defined formally as IGT and/or IFG) among overweight and obese US adults aged 45–74 years. They added screening to the simulation model to compute the possible benefits and costs of screening to identify pre-diabetes in the population. They compared two screening/treatment strategies with a baseline scenario of no screening and no treatment for pre-diabetes to estimate each strategy's cost-effectiveness. This approach was conducted only in terms of pre-diabetes detection in an at risk population. This narrows the spot of interest but gives more chance for such a programme to be cost-effective.

This study proved very informative as an aid to understanding the complexity of all the items we have to consider when building up a model of cost-effectiveness in the field of type 2 diabetes. The authors had chosen to restrict their model to an 'at-risk population' – overweight and obese people – and to screen mainly for pre-diabetes. This strategy gave them the best probability to detect a large number of subjects. They analyzed the effects of screening and treatment in the obese and overweight (body mass index [BMI] ≥ 25 kg/m^2) population aged 45–74 in the US. They created the virtual study cohort using data from the overweight population in the 1999–2000 US National Health and Nutrition Examination Survey [5–7]. Among overweight subjects aged 45–74 years not previously diagnosed with diabetes, estimates of the prevalence was 9.7% for undiagnosed diabetes; 10.4% for both IFG and IGT; 23.2% for IFG only; and 7.0% for IGT only. In their model, overweight subjects without diagnosed diabetes underwent a one-time screening test for pre-diabetes during a scheduled physician visit. Those screened positive underwent diagnostic testing. Subjects who had pre-diabetes entered a pre-diabetes module and received the DPP lifestyle intervention. Some subjects with pre-diabetes eventually developed diabetes; they were assumed to be diagnosed shortly after onset and entered into a diagnosed diabetes module. Screening was performed through a random capillary blood glucose (CBG) test and added 10 minutes to a usual 15-minute office visit, incurring costs of $32.68 per screened patient. The CBG test was selected for screening based on its relatively low cost [4]. Based on previous analysis, they set 100 mg/dl as the screening cut-off point for the random CBG test. The CBG test and physician costs come from Medicare fees schedules [8, 9]. All subjects with a positive screening test received a diagnostic test (either a fasting plasma glucose [FPG] or oral glucose tolerance test). If the first diagnostic test was positive, a second was performed for confirmation. Because two consecutive elevated FPG tests or OGTT define diabetes [11], they assumed that this strategy has 100% sensitivity and 100% specificity for diabetes and for IGT and/or IFG. The cost per diagnostic test totalled $42.92. They considered two different screening-plus-treatment strategies for subjects with pre-diabetes.

In strategy 1, only subjects diagnosed with both IGT and IFG received the DPP lifestyle intervention. In strategy 2, subjects diagnosed with either IFG or IGT (or both) received the lifestyle intervention.

In both strategies, the lifestyle intervention was provided until the subjects developed diabetes. Progression to diabetes depended on whether the subject had both IGT and IFG or only one of the conditions. The progression rate for subjects with both IGT and IFG came directly from the DPP [2], whereas the progression rate for subjects with only one condition was set to half the DPP value, based on the Hoorn Study [12]. They assumed that the lifestyle intervention produced the same relative risk reduction if the subject had both IGT and IFG or only one of these conditions. The cost of the DPP intervention equalled the incremental cost of the DPP lifestyle intervention relative to placebo. The DPP lifestyle intervention had a median follow-up of 3 years. For their analysis, they had to make assumptions about the intervention's costs and effectiveness in subsequent years. They assumed that the intervention year 3 costs and the reduction in risk from participating in the DPP continued in subsequent years as long as the intervention continued. Diabetes subjects with pre-diabetes entered the diabetes module after developing diabetes. The diagnosed diabetes module, which has been described elsewhere [2, 14], models the progression of five complications of type 2 diabetes: nephropathy, neuropathy, retinopathy, coronary heart disease, and stroke. Based on earlier analyses [14, 15], they assumed that subjects with diagnosed diabetes receive intensive glycaemic control once their HbA1c levels reach 6.8% and that subjects with hypertension and diagnosed diabetes receive intensive hypertension control. Transition probabilities for diabetes complications were based primarily on results from the UK Prospective Diabetes Study [31–33]. They applied a multiplicative equation that estimated annual direct medical costs for diabetes according to demographic characteristics, diabetes treatment, risk factors for cardiovascular disease, and microvascular and macrovascular complications [10, 30]. Health utility scores for patients with diabetes were estimated using an additive prediction model [34]. For the main analysis they used the simulation model to assess lifetime progression of disease, costs and QALYs. They calculated cost-effectiveness ratios for the two screening/treatment strategies relative to a baseline of no screening and, consequently, no treatment for pre-diabetes. They adopted a health system perspective that considered only direct medical costs and QALYs. They examined repeated screening, with screening tests performed three times, 3 years apart. For computational purposes, this analysis focused on a single cohort. They evaluated screening followed by applying the DPP metformin intervention (assuming generic metformin costs) for patients diagnosed with pre-diabetes. They also evaluated the lifestyle intervention provided in a group setting, assuming it would produce the same risk reduction but have lower costs. In their main analysis, the intervention continued and had the same cost and relative reduction in risk as during the 3-year DPP trial. To assess this critical assumption, they assumed, for all years, that the relative reduction in risk from the DPP was actually 20% lower than that observed in the trial; costs were the same as in the main analysis. They then assumed that people received the DPP intervention for only 3 years, neither receiving benefits nor paying costs thereafter. Because some subjects diagnosed with pre-diabetes may forego the intervention, they evaluated cost-effectiveness when only 50% of those diagnosed began the intervention. They also performed an analysis where the lifestyle intervention did not directly affect the quality of life for subjects while they had pre-diabetes.

What did they find?

Under strategy 1, 80% of overweight subjects with IFG and IGT were diagnosed and began treatment. Strategy 2 diagnosed and treated these same subjects but also provided DPP treatment to 53% of subjects with only IFG or only IGT. As a result, the total number of subjects receiving treatment tripled.

Relative to no screening, strategy 1 lowered the percentage of subjects with both IFG and IGT who subsequently developed diabetes from 76.4 to 58.6%. Strategy 2 produced the same reduction for subjects with both IFG and IGT. Among subjects with only IFG or only IGT, this strategy lowered cumulative incidence from 57.4 to 45.2%.

In Table 1.1, the cost-effectiveness of strategies 1 and 2 are compared with the alternative of no screening. The first panel presents numbers per person screened, whereas the second panel highlights the costs and benefits per screened person with pre-diabetes – the primary target for the screening/treatment interventions. This alternative presentation does not change the cost-effectiveness ratios.

Strategy 1 produced higher total costs and more QALYs than the no-screening alternative. Per-person screening costs accounted for a relatively small fraction of the overall cost increase. Treatment costs increased because subjects with IFG and IGT received the lifestyle intervention. This treatment reduced the cost of diabetes complications but not enough to generate total cost savings. Strategy 1 had a cost-effectiveness ratio of $8181 per QALY.

Strategy 2 produced higher costs and higher QALYs than strategy 1 because more subjects received the lifestyle intervention. The cost-effectiveness ratio for strategy 2 was $9511 per QALY relative to no screening.

Table 1.1 The cost-effectiveness of strategies 1 and 2 for subjects with pre-diabetes compared with no screening

| | Per screened subject | | | | | | Per screened subject, with pre-diabetes | | | | | |
| | No screening (total) | Strategy 1 | | Strategy 2 | | | No screening (total) | Strategy 1 | | Strategy 2 | |
		Total	Incremental	Total	Incremental			Total	Incremental	Total	Incremental
Screening costs ($)	–	68	68	68	68		–	168	168	168	168
Treatment costs ($)	10 312	10 794	443	11 879	1538		25 440	26 530	1089	29 223	3783
Complication costs ($)	6209	6026	(182)	5724	(484)		15 273	14 825	(448)	14 082	(1192)
Total costs ($)	16 550	16 879	329	17 672	1122		40 714	41 523	809	43 473	2759
Life-years (undiscounted)	NC*	NC	0.043	NC*	0.122		18.705	18 811	0.106	19.005	0.300
QALYs	NC*	NC*	0.040	NC*	0.118		8.910	9.009	0.099	9.200	0.290
Cost-effectiveness ratio relative to no screening ($/QALY)			8181		9511				8181		9511

*Only life-years and QALYs for individuals with pre-diabetes are tracked. Because life-years and QALYs for individuals without pre-diabetes are not affected by the intervention, we can calculate incremental life-years and QALYs. NC, not computed.

For both strategies, the cost-effectiveness ratios increased with age. From the societal cost perspective, the cost-effectiveness ratios were $16 345 and $18 777 per QALY for strategies 1 and 2, respectively. Changing screening parameters produced relatively small changes in the cost-effectiveness ratios. Repeated screening every 3 years, for example, produced small increases in these ratios. Changing the CBG cut-off or using an alternative IFG definition had negligible effects. Changing assumptions about the intervention for subjects diagnosed with pre-diabetes produced relatively large changes in cost-effectiveness ratios. Using a metformin intervention produced much higher cost-effectiveness ratios than the lifestyle intervention. If the lifestyle intervention could be applied in a group setting with lower costs and the same effectiveness, strategy 1 would be cost saving (i.e. higher effectiveness and lower costs) and strategy 2 would have a very low cost-effectiveness ratio.

Conversely, if the effects of the lifestyle intervention were 20% less than that seen in the DPP, the cost-effectiveness ratios would rise by $5000 per QALY. If the DPP lifestyle intervention was implemented for only 3 years and subsequently did not affect progression to diabetes or incur costs, the cost-effectiveness ratios would also rise. If the lifestyle intervention had no direct effect on the quality of life of subjects with pre-diabetes, the cost-effectiveness ratios for strategies 1 and 2 would be $12 773 and $16 149 per QALY, respectively. If 50% of subjects diagnosed with pre-diabetes chose not to participate in the intervention, the strategies would still have nearly the same cost-effectiveness ratios as in the main analysis. Including the costs and benefits of treating subjects diagnosed with diabetes during screening had relatively small effects on cost-effectiveness. Lowering the discount rate reduced cost-effectiveness ratios, and raising this rate increased the ratio.

Finally for strategy 1, they estimated a cost-effectiveness ratio of $8 per QALY, which is generally considered to be relatively attractive. They found that strategy 2 had a higher cost-effectiveness ratio than strategy 1 but even for strategy 2 the ratio is still attractive when compared with many existing healthcare interventions.

(B) THE 'OVERALL' ANALYSIS

Taking into account the detection of pre-diabetes and IGT in the general population what can we conclude on cost-effectiveness [35]?

First of all it is of interest to remember how cost-effectiveness may be assessed. The group of Gillies built a hybrid model combining a decision tree and a Markov model.

The decision tree comprises three main arms, representing no screening, screening for undiagnosed type 2 diabetes, and screening for IGT and undiagnosed diabetes, with either lifestyle or pharmacological interventions applied in those with IGT and type 2 diabetes. The decision tree uses prevalence of IGT and undiagnosed type 2 diabetes to determine how many individuals from the population start in each state of the Markov model.

The Markov model consists of seven states: normal glucose tolerance, undiagnosed impaired glucose tolerance, diagnosed impaired glucose tolerance, death, and three states for people with diabetes (undiagnosed, diagnosed clinically, or diagnosed through screening). Each model cycle represents one year and the model is run for a time horizon of 50 years. Model results include both clinical and cost-effectiveness outcomes, with cost per QALY being the primary outcome. The base case scenario for the model was a one-off screening for a population aged 45 years, in whom type 2 diabetes had not previously been diagnosed. Costs were estimated from various sources: screening costs included the costs of an initial screening test of fasting plasma glucose and a confirmatory OGTT in those who tested positive. They estimated the cost of nurse time of 5 minutes for the screening test and 25 minutes for the OGTT.

People with undiagnosed diabetes incur costs before diagnosis because of increased visits to the general practitioner and prescriptions; with a reported average of three additional visits the year before diagnosis and an average of 1.4 additional visits in the two to five years before diagnosis. For lifestyle interventions they included dietitian costs and costs of twice-weekly group exercise sessions. Costs of pharmacological interventions were based on 250 mg of metformin three times a day, the standard dose used by most intervention studies.

For people with diagnosed diabetes, they took average annual costs of antidiabetic treatment, implementation of treatment, and costs of complications from the UK Prospective Diabetes Study (UKPDS). For the people with diabetes detected at screening, in whom they would expect costs of complications to be lower, they used costs from the intensively treated arm of the UKPDS. For those with clinically diagnosed diabetes, which represents how individuals are diagnosed currently, they used the reported costs of the conventionally treated group. The effects of compliance to both screening and interventions were also important as they assumed 100% compliance to both in the base case model, which could never be achieved in practice.

What did they find?

Costs for each QALY gained, compared with no screening, were £14 150 for type 2 diabetes screening, £6242 for screening for diabetes and IGT with lifestyle interventions, and £7023 for screening for both diabetes and IGT with pharmacological interventions. At a willingness to pay threshold of £20 000 per QALY, the probability of each strategy being cost-effective was 49% for screening for type 2 diabetes only, 93% for screening for both diabetes and IGT with lifestyle interventions, and 85% for screening for both diabetes and IGT with pharmacological intervention. Both intervention strategies showed potential benefits in terms of average years spent without diabetes and cases of diabetes prevented.

Although clinical effects seem small, it must be remembered that they are average gains across a population, in which only 17% had either IGT or undiagnosed type 2 diabetes at the time of screening. The comparisons of the three active screening/intervention strategies compared with no screening remained fairly constant in terms of costs per QALY and probability of cost-effectiveness. When they lowered compliance with screening, the impact on results was minimal. Reducing compliance with interventions, however, had a greater impact in that the total costs and cost per QALY gained increased for both the screening/intervention strategies. The probability that these strategies were cost-effective compared with no screening still remained high, with an estimated probability of 88% for screening with lifestyle interventions and 84% for screening with pharmacological interventions at the willingness to pay threshold of £20 000. The intervention strategies became cost-effective when they considered a time horizon of at least 30 years (probability of being cost-effective of 0.97 for lifestyle and 0.91 for pharmacological interventions at the willingness to pay threshold of £20 000). Overall, the model's conclusions were robust to changes made to the sensitivity analyses, giving strength to the conclusions. When they ran the model for a South Asian cohort, results for QALYs were lower because of a higher prevalence of type 2 diabetes at the start of the model and an increased rate of transition to diabetes.

Table 1.2 shows clinical and cost-effectiveness outcomes for an undiscounted model and a model discounted for both costs and benefits at 3.5% a year.

Finally, the strategies involving interventions for prevention of diabetes seem to be cost-effective compared with no screening in an 'at risk' population.

SUMMARY

Type 2 diabetes is a major challenge for our worldwide healthcare economy system and it is easy to demonstrate how this disease is one of the best candidates for an early detection programme: screening for diabetes and for pre-diabetes is technically and ethically feasible. The presented modelling studies tend to confirm the proposal that it is useful and cost-

Table 1.2 Clinical and cost-effectiveness outcomes for an undiscounted model and a model discounted for both costs and benefits at 3.5% a year

	No screening	Screening for diabetes only	Screening for diabetes and impaired glucose tolerance	
			Lifestyle interventions	Pharmacological interventions
Undiscounted				
Total life-years	30.34 (27.75 to 32.86)	0.06 (0.02 to 0.12)	0.15 (0.08 to 0.22)	0.13 (0.06 to 0.20)
QALYs	28.06 (23.49 to 32.01)	0.07 (−0.03 to 0.18)	0.22 (0.08 to 0.36)	0.17 (0.03 to 0.32)
Years spent without diabetes	20.85 (10.36 to 29.45)	–	0.33 (0.21 to 0.43)	0.20 (0.10 to 0.37)
Lifetime risk of diabetes (%)	64.55 (18.02 to 91.83)	–	−0.98 (−0.50 to −1.42)	−0.54 (−0.21 to −1.17)
Total cost	17 290 (5746 to 39 580)	730 (9 to 2341)	610 (−373 to 2693)	579 (−428 to 2658)
Cost per life-year gained		11 460	4179	4768
Cost per QALY gained		8681	2861	3429
Cost per case prevented			62 810	105 000
Probability of cost-effectiveness at willingness to pay threshold per QALY (%):				
£20 000		68.1	98.6	94.7
£30 000		76.5	99.6	97.3
Discounted at 3.5% a year for both costs and benefits				
Total life-years	18.19 (17.25 to 18.98)	0.02 (−0.01 to 0.05)	0.05 (0.03 to 0.08)	0.05 (0.02 to 0.07)
QALYs	17.13 (15.02 to 18.49)	0.03 (−0.02 to 0.09)	0.09 (0.03 to 0.17)	0.07 (0.01 to 0.15)
Years spent diabetes-free	13.69 (7.99 to 17.08)	–	0.17 (0.11 to 0.23)	0.11 (0.06 to 0.19)
Total cost	7636 (2636 to 19 370)	587 (61 to 1525)	580 (−103 to 1760)	528 (−163 to 1719)
Cost per life-year gained		23 710	10 900	11 690
Cost per QALY gained		14 150	6242	7023
Probability of cost-effectiveness at willingness to pay threshold per QALY (%):				
£20 000		48.6	93.0	85.0
£30 000		60.8	97.4	91.6

Table 1.3 Risk factors for developing type 2 diabetes (adapted with permission from [18, 33, 36])

The presence of two or more among the below factors may lead to a screening procedure: 　■　Age 45 years or more 　■　Body mass index 30 kg/m² or more 　■　History of type 2 diabetes in first-degree relatives The presence of one of these factors or more may lead to a screening procedure: 　■　Age 55 years or more 　■　History of abnormal glycaemic value 　■　History of diabetes during pregnancy 　■　History of newborn >4 kg 　■　Polycystic ovarian syndrome Other risk factors: 　■　Sedentarity 　■　Ethnic origin

effective to perform a programme of screening/treatment for type 2 diabetes and pre-diabetes. These models have been developed because in such situations, clinical trials are extremely expensive and cannot produce timely recommendations; in their absence, simulations can help policy-makers make better informed decisions.

However, such sophisticated analyses have several limitations inherent in efforts to estimate the cost-effectiveness of interventions targeting chronic diseases. Most deal with the use of a simulation model to project the lifetime costs and health outcomes of simulated subjects. All simulation models must make assumptions about the future using the best possible medical, epidemiological and economic data. As an example, the authors assumed in their main analysis that the probability of diabetes progression does not change over time; that adherence to, cost of, and effectiveness of a DPP-like intervention do not change over time. One might argue with some of these assumptions. There is no broadly accepted consensus on the cost-effectiveness ratio that represents the cut-off for deeming an intervention as cost-effective or not cost-effective [36]. Some researchers have proposed a cut-off of $50 000 per QALY, whereas others recommend comparing an intervention's cost-effectiveness ratio to the highest ratios for treatments currently covered by Medicare or other insurers. Against either of these criteria, screening for pre-diabetes followed by the DPP lifestyle intervention seem to have a favourable cost-effectiveness ratio.

Although there are uncertainties due to the structure of the modelling systems and the lack of specific trials, several scientific societies have reached a compromise which suggests systematically screening for diabetes in some narrow at risk populations [19, 37, 38]. It is generally proposed to perform a plasma venous glucose assessment at the occasion of a visit to the physician for another reason. This pragmatic attitude is called 'opportunistic screening'. If screening is negative, it is recommended to re-test within a time interval of 3 to 5 years. Table 1.3 lists the main characteristics of the most at risk population to help physicians target their screening processes.

The American Diabetes Association (ADA) recommends a detection test on every patient aged over 45 years regardless of other risk factors [19] while the Australian guidelines suggest waiting until 55 years old [37]. We have to keep in mind the following key issues before concluding on the topic:

1. The older the patients are when detected, the shorter the time they will have in which to benefit from screening and treatment. Nobody has suggested fixing an upper limit of age, but such screening does not seem logical if life expectancy is below 15 years [39].

2. Another population who might be involved in a screening programme for diabetes are hypertensive and or dyslipidaemic patients and/or those already with evidence of cardiovascular disease with the purpose of multi-intervention care management.

3. Neither model nor trial can reproduce real life, where compliance to guidelines by doctors is very variable, and where patients screened positive are not always well informed or systematically properly treated. We must remember that screening without education and/or without intervention is cost without benefit. Whether now is the time for large-scale screening remains controversial [40].

REFERENCES

1. UK National Screening Committee. *Handbook for vascular risk assessment, risk reduction and risk management.* University of Leicester, Leicester, 2008.

2. Knowler WC, Barrett-Connor E, Fowler SE *et al*, the Diabetes Prevention Program Research Group. Reduction in the incidence of type 2 diabetes with lifestyle intervention or metformin. *N Engl J Med* 2002; 346:393–403.

3. Chiasson JL, Josse RG, Gomis R, Hanefeld M, Karasik A, Laakso M. STOP-NIDDM Trial Research Group. Acarbose for prevention of type 2 diabetes mellitus: the STOP-NIDDM randomised trial. *Lancet* 2002; 359:2072–2077.

4. Waugh N, Scotland G, McNamee P *et al*. Screening for type 2 diabetes: literature review and economic modelling. *Health Techno Assess* 2007; 11:1–125.

5. Davies MJ, Tringham JR, Troughton J, Khunti KK. Prevention of type 2 diabetes mellitus. A review of the evidence and its application in a UK setting. *Diabet Med* 2004; 21:403–414.

6. Gillies CL, Abrams KR, Lambert PC *et al*. Pharmacological and lifestyle interventions to prevent or delay type 2 diabetes in people with impaired glucose tolerance. *BMJ* 2007; 334:299–302.

7. Avenell A, Broom J, Brown TJ *et al*. Systematic review of the long-term effects and economic consequences of treatments for obesity and implications for health improvement. *Health Technol Assess* 2004; 8:1–182.

8. Caro JJ, Getsios D, Caros I, Klittich WS, O'Brien JA. Economic evaluation of therapeutic interventions to prevent type 2 diabetes in Canada. *Diabet Med* 2004; 21:1229–1236.

9. Eddy DM, Schlessinger L, Kahn R. Clinical outcomes and cost-effectiveness of strategies for managing people at high risk for diabetes. *Ann Intern Med* 2005; 143:251–264.

10. Herman WH, Hoerger TJ, Brandle M *et al*. The cost-effectiveness of lifestyle modification or metformin in preventing type 2 diabetes in adults with impaired glucose tolerance. *Ann Intern Med* 2005; 142:323–332.

11. Icks A, Rathmann W, Haastert B *et al*. Clinical and cost-effectiveness of primary prevention of type 2 diabetes in a 'real world' routine healthcare setting: model based on the KORA Survey 2000. *Diabet Med* 2007; 24:473–480.

12. Jacobs-van der Bruggen MA, Bos G, Bemelmans WJ, Hoogenveen RT, Vijgen SM, Baan CA. Lifestyle interventions are cost-effective in people with different levels of diabetes risk. *Diabetes Care* 2007; 30:128–134.

13. Palmer AJ, Roze S, Valentine WJ, Spinas GA, Shaw JE, Zimmet PZ. Intensive lifestyle changes or metformin in patients with impaired glucose tolerance: modelling the long-term health economic implications of the diabetes prevention program in Australia, France, Germany, Switzerland, and the United Kingdom. *Clin Ther* 2004; 26: 304–321.

14. Segal L, Dalton AC, Richardson J. Cost-effectiveness of the primary prevention of non-insulin dependent diabetes mellitus. *Health Promot Int* 1998; 13:197–209.

15. CDC Diabetes Cost-Effectiveness Study Group. The cost-effectiveness of screening for type 2 diabetes. *JAMA* 1998; 280:1757–1763.

16. Chen TH, Yen MF, Tung TH. A computer simulated model for cost-effectiveness analysis of mass screening for type 2 diabetes mellitus. *Diabetes Res Clin Pract* 2001; 54:S37–S42.

17. Glumer C, Yuyun M, Griffin S *et al*. What determines the cost-effectiveness of diabetes screening? *Diabetologia* 2006; 49:1536–1544.

18. Hoerger TJ, Harris R, Hicks KA, Donahue K, Sorensen S, Engelgau M. Screening for type 2 diabetes mellitus: a cost-effectiveness analysis. *Ann Intern Med* 2004; 140:756–758.

19. American Diabetes Association. Screening for type 2 diabetes. *Diabetes Care* 2004; 27:S11–S14.

20. Engelgau MM, Narayan KM, Herman WH. Screening for type 2 diabetes. *Diabetes Care* 2000; 23:1563–1580.
21. Gerstein HC, Yusuf S, Riddle MC, Ryden L, Bosch H. Rationale, design, and baseline characteristics for a large international trial of cardiovascular disease prevention in people with dysglycaemia: The ORIGIN Trial (Outcome Reduction with an Initial Glargine Intervention). *Am Heart J* 2008; 155:26–32.
22. Califf RM, Boolell M, Haffner SM *et al*, for the NAVIGATOR Study Group. Prevention of diabetes and cardiovascular disease in patients with impaired glucose tolerance: Rationale and design of the Nateglinide And Valsartan in Impaired Glucose Tolerance Outcomes Research (NAVIGATOR) Trial. *Am Heart J* 2008; 156:623–632.
23. CDC Diabetes Cost-Effectiveness Study Group, Centers for Disease Control and Prevention.The cost-effectiveness of screening for type 2 diabetes. *JAMA* 1998; 280:1757–1763.
24. Vijan S, Hofer TP, Hayward RA. Estimated benefits of glycemic control in microvascular complications in type 2 diabetes. *Ann Intern Med* 1997; 127:788–795.
25. Hoerger TJ, Hicks KA, Sorensen SW *et al*. Cost-effectiveness of screening for pre-diabetes among overweight and obese U.S. adults. *Diabetes Care* 2007; 30:2874–2879.
26. Zhang P, Engelgau MM, Valdez R, Benjamin SM, Cadwell B, Narayan KM. Costs of screening for pre-diabetes among U.S. adults: a comparison of different screening strategies. *Diabetes Care* 2003; 26:2536–2542.
27. Palmer AJ, Roze S, Valentine WJ, Spinas GA, Shaw JE, Zimmet PZ. Intensive lifestyle changes or metformin in patients with impaired glucose tolerance: modelling the long-term health economic implications of the Diabetes Prevention Program in Australia, France, Germany, Switzerland, and the United Kingdom. *Clin Ther* 2004; 26:304–321.
28. Caro JJ, Getsios D, Caro I, Klittich WS, O'Brien JA. Economic evaluation of therapeutic interventions to prevent type 2 diabetes in Canada. *Diabet Med* 2004; 21:1229–1236.
29. Quilici S, Chancellor J, Maclaine G, McGuire A, Andersson D, Chiasson JL. Cost-effectiveness of acarbose for the management of impaired glucose tolerance in Sweden. *Int J Clin Pract* 2005; 59:1143–1152.
30. Brandle M, Zhou H, Smith BR *et al*. The direct medical cost of type 2 diabetes. *Diabetes Care* 2003; 26:2300–2304.
31. Stevens RJ, Kothari V, Adler AI, Stratton IM. The UKPDS risk engine: a model for the risk of coronary heart disease in type II diabetes (UKPDS 56). *Clin Sci (Lond)* 2001; 101:671–679.
32. Kothari V, Stevens RJ, Adler AI *et al*. UKPDS 60: risk of stroke in type 2 diabetes estimated by the UK Prospective Diabetes Study risk engine. *Stroke* 2002; 33:1776–1781.
33. Adler AI, Stevens RJ, Manley SE, Bilous RW, Cull CA, Holman RR, UKPDS Group: Development and progression of nephropathy in type 2 diabetes: the United Kingdom Prospective Diabetes Study (UKPDS 64). *Kidney Int* 2003; 63:225–232.
34. Coffey JT, Brandle M, Zhou H *et al*. Valuing health related quality of life in diabetes. *Diabetes Care* 2002; 25:2238–2243.
35. Gillies CL, Lambert PC, Abrams KR *et al*. Different strategies for screening and prevention of type 2 diabetes in adults: cost effectiveness analysis. *BMJ* 2008; 336:1180–1185.
36. Gold MR, Siegel JE, Russell LB, Weinstein MC (eds). *Cost-Effectiveness in Health and Medicine*. Oxford University Press, New York, 1996.
37. Colagiuri S, Hussain Z, Zimmet P, Cameron A, Shaw J. Screening for type 2 diabetes and impaired glucose metabolism: The Australian experience. *Diabetes Care* 2004; 27:367–371.
38. Harris R, Donahue K, Rathore SS, Frame P, Woolf SH, Lohr KN. Screening adults for type 2 diabetes: A review of the evidence for the U.S. Preventive Services Task Force. *Ann Intern Med* 2003; 138:215–229.
39. Feig DS, Palda VA, Lipscombe L. Screening for type 2 diabetes mellitus to prevent vascular complications: Updated recommendations from the Canadian Task Force on Preventive Health Care. *CMAJ* 2005; 172:177–180.
40. Borch-Johnsen K, Lauritzen T, Glumer C, Sandbaek A. Screening for Type 2 diabetes—should it be now? *Diabet Med* 2003; 20:175–181.

2

Obesity-related disease: how can we stem the tide?

J. Webber

BACKGROUND

The prevalence of obesity has been increasing dramatically in most parts of the world (Figure 2.1). Sixty-six per cent of adults in North America are obese or overweight [1]. From a European perspective, while obesity rates may not yet have reached those of North America, they are following a similar trend [2]. In rapidly-developing countries such as China, while overall prevalence is low compared to many developed countries, the number of obese subjects is already huge [3].

In England, the 2006 Health Survey for England [4] revealed that 67% of men and 56% of women were either overweight or obese. This is part of a continuing marked increase over the last 20 to 30 years such that the prevalence of obesity has increased four-fold over this time period. In the same report, the figures for obesity in children are equally worrying with 29.7% of children aged 2 to 15 classed as overweight or obese in 2006. The Foresight: Tackling Obesities: Future Choices project predicts that if no action is taken, by 2050, 60% of men, 50% of women and 25% of children in England will be obese [5].

Closely linked with this obesity epidemic is an increase in obesity-related comorbidities, the foremost of these being type 2 diabetes. The total number of people with diabetes in England is expected to rise from 2.5 million today to 4 million in 2025 [6]. Globally, the figures are even more frightening, with the number of people with diabetes rising from 30 million in 1985 to 150 million in 2000 and a projected rise to 380 million by 2025 [7]. Most of the resource currently invested in obesity-related diseases such as type 2 diabetes, is spent on the diabetes rather than the underlying weight problem. Thus, in type 2 diabetes, the approach has been centred on trying to correct blood glucose levels, whether or not this has adverse effects on body weight. There has been great reluctance to champion more weight-focused approaches that may correct more than just glucose. We are just starting to change the emphasis in the treatment of those with obesity and obesity-related disease. Only by tackling obesity at an earlier stage before comorbidities have developed will the tide be turned.

Stemming the tide of obesity is not easy. So far this is a health-related target that it has not been possible for governments or society to meet (in contrast to many other areas where goals have been achieved). In 1992, the English national strategy for public health introduced a target to reduce the proportion of obese men aged 16–64 years in the population from 7% in 1986–1987 to 6% in 2005, and obese women from 12% in 1986–1987 to 8% in 2005 [8]. A

Jonathan Webber, DM, FRCP, Consultant Diabetologist, Diabetes Centre, University Hospital Birmingham Foundation Trust, Birmingham, UK.

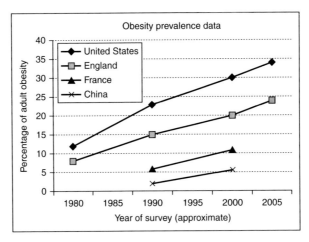

Figure 2.1 Obesity prevalence in North America, France, China and England (data taken from [1–4]).

1996 review of the Health of the Nation by the National Audit Office showed that by 1993, the proportions of obese men and women in the population had risen to 13% and 16%, respectively [9]. By 2003, 22% of men and 23% of women were obese and by 2010, on these trends, obesity will rise to 33% of men and 28% of women [10]. Governments have so far underestimated the difficulties of the task. The present UK government has set itself the task of reversing the rising tide of obesity and overweight in the population. Its initial focus is to be on children, aiming, by 2020, to reduce the proportion of overweight and obese children to 2000 levels.

WHERE DO THE SOLUTIONS LIE?

Whilst it is apparent that there is an epidemic of obesity, the causes of this epidemic and hence the preferred solutions remain hotly debated. In terms of the cause of the problem much research has focused on whether increased energy intake or reduced energy expenditure is more important? The answer to even this deceptively simple question is not clear. In 1995 it was suggested that UK data based on National Food Surveys showed that obesity was rising at a time when actual energy intake had fallen. At the same time, some proxies for reduced physical activity, such as car ownership per household and television viewing, had increased. The conclusion drawn was that low levels of physical activity were playing a predominant role in driving the obesity epidemic [11]. However, recent US surveys have shown that both per capita availability of energy and mean energy intake have increased from the 1970s to around 2000 [12]. Critical to the interpretation of this information on energy intake is the accuracy of the food surveys used in capturing what people actually eat and drink as opposed to what they record and recall doing.

In contrast to the debate on trends in energy intake, there is much more agreement that physical activity has been declining for some time. The reasons for this include increased time spent in sedentary behaviours such as the use of personal computers, televisions, the automation of many household and work processes, and transportation trends [13]. It has been estimated that the average reduction in daily energy expenditure over the past 50 years has been roughly 250–500 kcal per day [14]. This would more than explain the current obesity epidemic. One interesting lesson from recent history is the Cuban economic crisis, which led to both decreased energy intake and an increase in physical activity of the population that was sustained for five years. This was associated with 4–5 kg weight loss and a decline in all-cause mortality and death rates from diabetes and cardiovascular disease [15].

PHYSICAL ACTIVITY AND THE PREVENTION AND TREATMENT OF WEIGHT GAIN

Whilst it is agreed that reduced physical activity is one of the key drivers for weight gain, the question is whether increasing physical activity can prevent weight gain as well as being an effective management strategy for those who are already overweight or obese. Perhaps even more challenging is finding ways to facilitate and maintain increased individual and population activity levels. A number of small trials have shown positive effects of increased physical activity on the prevention of unhealthy weight gain in both children and adults in the short term, but the effect size has been small and it is often unclear which part of the intervention was the most important [16].

One of the simplest interventions to increase physical activity in individuals is the use of a pedometer. These are small, inexpensive devices that count the number of steps walked per day. They have become popular as a tool to motivate and monitor physical activity and some guidelines recommend taking 10 000 steps per day. A recent systemic review of their use has supported their short-term efficacy in increasing activity and in lowering weight and blood pressure [17]. Setting a realistic step goal for the individual was important in success. However, most of the reviewed studies included only small numbers of participants and were of short duration.

The main areas of physical activity are recreational, occupational and domestic, and purposeful walking and cycling [18]. Efforts to increase sport participation in the UK have not proved very effective to date. Research has indicated that part of the reason for the failure of this policy has been the perception by many people that they are not very competent at sports and see sport as too demanding for them. Changing this perception is critical for future policy initiatives on sports participation. Another limiting factor is that access to recreational facilities is socially patterned, with fewer opportunities for people living in the most deprived neighbourhoods. Strategies to make sports participation more attractive and more accessible to these people are needed.

Whereas it does seem at least possible to increase recreational activity, it seems much less likely that we can reverse the trends that have led to reduced domestic and occupational activity. Labour-saving devices are here to stay for the foreseeable future. One might assume that the availability of devices that make many chores easier and less time-consuming would lead to increased opportunities for physical activity. Unfortunately, the extra time that has been generated has been filled with low-energy level activities such as computer use. Trying to persuade people to reduce sedentary activities such as sitting in front of the television is likely to be hard to achieve by public message campaigns alone. Instead, we should look at policies that enhance the availability and appeal of local amenities that involve more physical activity.

How much activity is required to prevent weight gain? In the United Kingdom, at least five sessions a week, each lasting 30 minutes, have been recommended for a general health benefit [19]. To make this more achievable, so-called lifestyle activities that were performed as part of everyday life, such as climbing stairs or brisk walking were included. In order to prevent obesity, a higher target of 45–60 minutes of moderate-intensity physical activity was suggested. Four methods have been proposed to increase physical activity:

1. Brief interventions in primary care.
2. Exercise referral schemes.
3. Pedometers
4. Community-based exercise programmes for walking and cycling [20].

The evidence behind these interventions is variable to say the least. For instance, brief interventions are described as a health professional delivering opportunistic advice on activity levels to patients. Whether provision of information is, on its own, sufficient to change behaviour is a moot point. Similar guidance to improve activity levels in the workplace has also been developed [21].

SOCIETAL APPROACHES TO TACKLING OBESITY

The relative failure of individual approaches to obesity prevention and management has focused attention on societal and social engineering solutions. An influential hypothesis, the obesogenic environment, suggests that it is the external environment more than individual differences in metabolism that is driving the obesity epidemic. The solutions may therefore lie with changing the environment and relying on this approach to change individual behaviour [22]. Environmental influences, such as transport policy, are likely to be at least as strong a determinant of activity as the more easily measured individual-based interventions. A simple example is how to go about measuring the effects of a traffic congestion scheme (aimed at reducing car use, whilst increasing cycling and walking to work) on overall activity levels. Whilst energy expenditure involved in commuting will go up, does this adversely impact on leisure time activity?

Figures from the UK Department of Transport reveal that the average distance walked per year per person for transport fell from 255 miles in 1975 to 192 miles in 2003 [23]. Bicycle distances fell from 51 miles per person to 34 miles over the same period and unsurprisingly the distance travelled by car went up. Further analysis shows the main reasons for different types of trips. Walk-only trips were mainly for shopping and these had decreased from 42% to 30% over the period studied. Only 6% of people now walk to work. Increasing numbers of people now use the car both for getting to work and for shopping. Understanding what lies behind these trends is essential to finding solutions to reverse them. Much attention is now being focused on how the built environment influences activity patterns of those living there. The proximity of frequently used destinations such as shops, schools and employment determines the likelihood of walking and cycling to access them [24]. Ensuring there is convenient access to commonly visited destinations may be one of the most important and achievable ways of increasing physical activity and helping to stem the tide of obesity. Appropriate urban planning to help facilitate more walking, even amongst those people who are less likely to take up recreational opportunities, has the potential to impact on the vast majority of the population.

LEGISLATION AND OBESITY-RELATED POLICY

A number of countries have introduced proposals centred around food legislation in order to try and tackle obesity [25]. A traffic light scheme is being trialled in Europe to try and make it clear to consumers if products have low, medium, or high amounts of fat, saturates, sugar and salt, by labelling them as green, amber and red respectively. This European Union scheme is voluntary at present and has run into much opposition from food manufacturers. Restrictions on the advertising of junk food have been more widely accepted and adopted, although data on their efficacy are lacking.

In many walks of life, monetary rewards influence behaviour. Financial incentives have been utilized in the treatment of obesity and overweight. Whilst potentially attractive, this approach does not appear to be successful at least in terms of weight loss. However, there is some suggestion that rewarding behaviour changes rather than weight loss *per se* may be more effective [26]. At present, financial incentives have not been much studied outside North America, but perhaps they might be employed as part of a package of interventions.

Table 2.1 Obesity policy options derived from The Policy Options for Responding to the Growing Challenge of Obesity Research Project (adapted from [27])

Core options	Desired effects
Change planning and transport policies	Encourage more physical activity Improved facilities for walking and cycling Better public transport
Improve communal sports facilities	Better recreational facilities in schools and communities
Controls on food and drink advertising	Restrict advertising and promotion of obesity-promoting foods
Controlling sales of foods in public institutions	Restrict sale of fatty snacks, confectionery and sweet drinks in schools and hospitals Catering outlets and vending machines based in public institutions to sell only healthy foods
Mandatory nutritional information labelling	Energy density traffic light system Help consumers to make healthy choices
Subsidies on healthy foods	Improve patterns of food consumption
Taxes on obesity-promoting foods	Reduce consumption of unhealthy foods

One attempt to bring together the various initiatives that may help stem the tide of obesity has been The Policy Options for Responding to the Growing Challenge of Obesity Research Project (PorGrow) [27]. This European project has brought together potential policies ranging from those centred around activity levels to those influencing diet (Table 2.1). The question is whether there is the political will to take these initiatives forward.

CHILDHOOD OBESITY

In England, childhood obesity has been prioritized, with a stated ambition to be the first major nation to reverse the rising tide of obesity and overweight in the population by ensuring that everyone is able to achieve and maintain a healthy weight [28] (Table 2.2). Childhood obesity, as with adult obesity, has progressively increased over the last 30 years. Prevalence rates have been increasing by up to 1% per year in many countries with a consequent doubling of childhood obesity [29]. As in adults, as the problem of childhood obesity has emerged, initial solutions have targeted physical activity and diet [30, 31].

The rapid increase in childhood obesity, once again as in adults, is due to a combination of increasing energy intake and decreasing physical activity. Among children, foods that are energy-dense (often high in fat content) have become popular, widely available and cheap [32]. At the same time, massive marketing campaigns have made many such foods very desirable, particularly to children [33]. Children are very receptive to marketing when placed in the context of child-based entertainment. Food advertisements have been shown to influence children's food preferences, requests and consumption [34]. If advertising is so important in guiding food choices in children, should we look to legislate to ban such advertising, or should we look to cooperate in some way with the food industry?

Many parallels have been drawn with the tobacco industry [35]. Both smoking and eating can be pleasurable experiences, and appetite and enjoyment of food persist above intake levels needed to maintain energy balance. Restrictions around tobacco advertising took many years to gain public acceptance and hence governmental approval and subsequent legislation. A number of issues led to gradual reductions in tobacco consumption. These included concern over adverse health effects (enhanced by education campaigns), financial

Table 2.2 Summary, focusing on children from *Healthy Weight, Healthy Lives: A Cross Government Strategy for England, 2008* (with permission from [28])

The healthy growth and development of children	Identify at risk families as early as possible
	Promote breast-feeding as the norm for mothers
	Make cooking compulsory for all 11- to 14-year-olds
	Give better information to parents about their children's health
Promoting healthier food choices	All schools to develop healthy lunchbox policies
	Finalise a Healthy Food Code of Good Practice, in partnership with the food and drink industry, to reduce consumption of saturated fat, sugar and salt
	Help local authorities to manage the proliferation of fast food outlets
	Review restrictions on the advertising of unhealthy foods to children
Building physical activity into people's lives	Develop tailored programmes in schools to increase the participation of obese and overweight pupils in physical education and sporting activities
	A 'walking into health' campaign
	Develop 'healthy towns'
	Invest in improving cycling infrastructure and skills in areas where child weight is a particular problem
	Develop tools that allow parents to manage the time that their children spend on sedentary games

costs of smoking (raised significantly by taxation in many countries) and social disapproval of smoking. In addition, there is strong evidence that smoking causes harm to others. These issues led to a climate where it was possible for legislation to be introduced that placed restrictions on where and when people could smoke.

At present, while there is widespread acceptance that excess intake of many foods is associated with weight gain, there is less enthusiasm to restrict the food supply in any way. Provision of education about the risks of obesity and its links with certain foods does not appear to have had any major effect on consumption so far. It has been proposed that unhealthy products should be taxed at premium rates with the hope that price would deter consumers. Such a policy does not have much public support at this time, but perhaps with increasing public concern about obesity, its time may come. Restricting the availability of certain foodstuffs is more difficult than with similar policies around tobacco, but could be enforced fairly easily in schools (e.g. removal of vending machines containing high-calorie drinks and snacks). There is growing awareness of the obesity issue and it looks likely that a more favourable climate for legislation is emerging. However, perhaps the promotion of healthy food as part of a healthy lifestyle has more chance of succeeding. Punitive measures against what are seen to be unhealthy (but 'nice') foods risk making them even more attractive to many consumers.

In terms of physical activity it is readily apparent that a major change in childhood behaviour in many countries is the increased sedentary time spent in front of televisions and computers. Reducing the time spent viewing televisions and computers can prevent obesity and lower body mass index in young children [36]. However, on closer examination of this study, the positive result appeared more related to reductions in energy intake than increases in physical activity. It seems that whilst other equally sedentary activities may have replaced the television, at least these were not linked to food intake.

Whilst influencing large groups of adults from varied backgrounds is difficult, school-based interventions for children allow a greater and more uniform approach to tackling the problem of preventing and treating obesity. A recent Cochrane review [31] concluded that the results of school-based interventions aimed at reducing obesity were disappointing. These studies targeted a number of different facets of children's behaviour, diet, activity and knowledge. These included decreasing television viewing, reducing consumption of high-fat foods, increasing vegetable intake and activity levels. One recent example of such a study is the Christchurch obesity prevention programme in schools [37]. The intervention focused on persuading children to drink fewer carbonated drinks and consisted of four one-hour educational sessions spread over four school terms. Results at one year were positive, with less consumption of carbonated drinks and a modest reduction in the number of children becoming overweight or obese. However, these results were not sustained at three year follow-up.

In order to try and address the complexity of body weight regulation in real life, newer studies attempt to bundle together a group of interventions rather than focusing on any one aspect of behaviour. A study from Rotterdam describes a school-based intervention that targets both individual behaviour (particularly encouraging activity) and the environmental determinants of behaviour [38]. These interventions include increased physical education sessions at school, organization of more sport and play activities outside school hours, cooperation with local sports clubs and fitness tests with score cards for the children. At the same time there is classroom education on healthy nutrition, active living and healthy life-style choices with the emphasis on practical activities to consolidate knowledge. Finally, there is an attempt to involve the parents in what is going on and to promote similar healthy behaviours in the home. Another complex intervention to reduce childhood obesity is termed Switch® and is based in North America [39]. In this trial community, family and school-based approaches are combined and aimed at modifying physical activity, screen time (internet, television and video games) and nutrition. The results of these studies are awaited.

THE POTENTIAL IMPORTANCE OF THE IN UTERO ENVIRONMENT AND EARLY CHILDHOOD FEEDING PRACTICES IN LATER OBESITY

Is the epidemic of childhood obesity being fuelled by early infancy feeding practices and perhaps even earlier by the *in utero* environment? There is considerable evidence that low birth-weight predicts later obesity, coronary heart disease and type 2 diabetes [40]. If this is the case, strategies to prevent obesity will need to address this early stage of development. Adequate maternal nutrition is important with a link shown between low maternal weight and subsequent increased risk of type 2 diabetes in the offspring [41].

In many parts of the world the concern is now with maternal overnutrition and obesity and the impact this may have on both *in utero* and subsequent childhood development. Obesity during pregnancy is associated with an increased risk of developing gestational diabetes [42]. The prevalence of macrosomia is much greater in those mothers who have diabetes or gestational diabetes. Until recently the rationale for active treatment of patients with gestational diabetes has centred upon the need to reduce the risk of macrosomia and with it the increased risk of birth trauma. There is also some evidence that treatment of gestational diabetes improves other outcomes such as perinatal mortality [43]. Now, emerging evidence suggests that intrauterine exposure to maternal diabetes and obesity predisposes to obesity and type 2 diabetes in children and young adults [44]. This link applies both for women with pre-existing diabetes and those with gestational diabetes. The link between *in utero* exposure to hyperglycaemia and later obesity and diabetes cannot be explained by genetic factors alone [45]. It is thought that fetal overnutrition may have long-term adverse effects on adiposity and pancreatic function.

The prevalence of both type 2 diabetes in women of child-bearing age and gestational diabetes are increasing. If *in utero* exposure to hyperglycaemia is important in mediating the risk of later obesity, this is another factor that will increase childhood and subsequent obesity. Indeed, in Pima Indian children, it has been estimated that the recent epidemic of childhood type 2 diabetes can be almost completely explained by exposure to diabetes during pregnancy and the resultant increase in obesity [46]. Further research is needed to see whether better glycaemic control in pregnancy can reduce the risk of obesity in childhood and beyond.

Whilst there remains debate about the long-term consequences of the *in utero* environment on obesity and metabolism, there is consensus on the link between infant feeding practices and the later risk of obesity. Breast-feeding reduces the risk of later excess adiposity [47]. The mechanisms underlying this protective effect are not clear, but include behavioural factors (breast-feeding is often linked with other healthy dietary and lifestyle habits) and nutritional explanations (the specific content of breast milk with bioactive nutrients absent from formula feeds). It may also be that rapid early growth (more often seen in formula-fed infants) in some way programmes later obesity. This has been termed the 'growth acceleration hypothesis' [48]. It is proposed that the first few weeks of postnatal life may be critical in programming long-term health. Infant feeding practices where supplemental feeding is routine for small infants may not have beneficial effects in the longer term. Breast-fed infants tend to have slower growth than formula-fed ones and this may mediate some of the link to reduced risk of obesity. Consequently, the promotion of breast-feeding has a role to play in reducing later obesity.

Even after weaning, it seems likely that infancy and early childhood is a critical time in determining many later behaviours that favour the development of obesity. There is evidence that dietary habits [49] and sedentary behaviour [50] in children track from childhood to adolescence and adulthood. In infancy, parenting practices are crucial in the subsequent behaviour of children. For example, in 2- to 6-year-old children, the strongest predictor of their fruit and vegetable consumption was that of their parents [51]. Similar links are present between parental activity levels and television viewing and that of their offspring. This evidence has been used to develop a randomized controlled trial using first-time parent groups in Australia [52]. Parenting skills will be developed that support positive diet and physical activity behaviours and reduced sedentary behaviours in infancy.

SUMMARY

We can stem the tide, but it will take a lot more political will and resource to achieve this goal. Targeting individuals has so far proven unsuccessful. More promising are policies that tackle the underlying drivers of obesity such as food access, transport and urban planning. In terms of interventions, larger studies looking at longer-term outcomes of multifactorial approaches to obesity treatment are needed. One example is the Look AHEAD trial for diabetes. This long-term trial is aiming to assess the effects over 11.5 years of an intensive weight loss programme delivered over a four-year period in overweight and obese patients with type 2 diabetes. The primary study outcome is time to incidence of a major cardiovascular event and not just short-term effects on weight [53]. Even this could be criticized as a stand-alone initiative that may not be more widely applicable outside the constraints of a clinical trial.

Much resource and hope continues to be poured into quick fixes. It seems unlikely that effective pharmaceutical solutions will be forthcoming given the extent of the problem. A recent article raises the intriguing possibility of an exercise pill that could mimic some of the effects of aerobic exercise in skeletal muscle [54]. Whilst this is a novel tactic, it is a long way from fruition, and given the track record of many other drugs developed for obesity management, let alone obesity prevention, it is probably unlikely to be successful.

There needs to be a focus on strategies to prevent obesity throughout life. This starts with maternal health, and hence the *in utero* environment, and continues with infant feeding practices. Beyond the family and home surroundings, schools provide an opportunity to influence many behaviours that protect against weight gain. As a backdrop to these influences, town planning and legislative policies need to create an environment that fosters healthy choices rather than making it easy to gain weight.

Parallels have been drawn between the obesity challenge and the climate change debate, with obesity seen as the public health equivalent of climate change [55]. The emphasis here is that simple solutions will not suffice to stem the tide of obesity. Both are problems requiring firm actions however unpopular and difficult many of those actions are likely to be. A better understanding of the wider environmental determinants of obesity is needed so that appropriate policy decisions can be made and a less obesogenic environment created. This may seem a distant utopian dream at present. However, if there is a collective commitment by countries and their leaders that tackling obesity is worthwhile, then perhaps it is an achievable goal.

REFERENCES

1. Ogden CL, Carroll MD, Curtin LR, McDowell MA, Tabak CJ, Flegal KM. Prevalence of overweight and obesity in the United States, 1999–2004. *JAMA* 2006; 295:1549–1555.
2. Berghofer A, Pischon T, Reinhold T, Apovian CM, Sharma AM, Willich SN. Obesity prevalence from a European perspective: a systematic review. *BMC Public Health* 2008; 8:200.
3. Levine JA. Obesity in China: causes and solutions. *Chin Med J (Engl)* 2008; 121:1043–1050.
4. The Information Centre Lifestyles Statistics. *Health Survey for England 2006: Latest Trends 2008*.
5. Government Office for Science. *Foresight. Tackling Obesities: Future Choices 2007*.
6. The Information Centre Lifestyles Statistics. *Statistics on Obesity, Physical Activity and Diet*. England 2008.
7. Wild S, Roglic G, Green A, Sicree R, King H. Global prevalence of diabetes: estimates for the year 2000 and projections for 2030. *Diabetes Care* 2004; 27:1047–1053.
8. Department of Health. *The health of the nation: a strategy for health in England*. London 1992.
9. National Audit Office. *Health of the Nation: A Progress Report*. London 1996.
10. Department of Health. *Health Profile of England 2006*.
11. Prentice AM, Jebb SA. Obesity in Britain: gluttony or sloth? *BMJ* 1995; 311:437–439.
12. Jeffery RW, Harnack LJ. Evidence implicating eating as a primary driver for the obesity epidemic. *Diabetes* 2007; 56:2673–2676.
13. Hamilton MT, Hamilton DG, Zderic TW. Role of low energy expenditure and sitting in obesity, metabolic syndrome, type 2 diabetes, and cardiovascular disease. *Diabetes* 2007; 56:2655–2667.
14. Hayes M, Chustek M, Heshka S, Wang Z, Pietrobelli A, Heymsfield SB. Low physical activity levels of modern Homo sapiens among free-ranging mammals. *Int J Obes (Lond)* 2005; 29:151–156.
15. Franco M, Ordunez P, Caballero B, Cooper RS. Obesity reduction and its possible consequences: what can we learn from Cuba's Special Period? *Can Med Assoc J* 2008; 178:1032–1034.
16. Wareham N. Physical activity and obesity prevention. *Obes Rev* 2007; (suppl 1):109–114.
17. Bravata DM, Smith-Spangler C, Sundaram V *et al*. Using pedometers to increase physical activity and improve health: a systematic review. *JAMA* 2007; 298:2296–2304.
18. Fox KR, Hillsdon M. Physical activity and obesity. *Obes Rev* 2007; (suppl 1):115–121.
19. Department of Health. *At least five a week: Evidence on the impact of physical activity and its relationship to health 2004*.
20. National Institute for Health and Clinical Excellence. *Four commonly used methods to increase physical activity: brief interventions in primary care, exercise referral schemes, pedometers and community-based exercise programmes for walking and cycling 2006*.
21. National Institute for Health and Clinical Excellence. *Workplace health promotion: how to encourage employees to be physically active 2008*.
22. Egger G, Swinburn B. An "ecological" approach to the obesity pandemic. *BMJ* 1997; 315:477–480.
23. Department of Transport. *National Travel Survey 2004*.
24. Transportation Research Board. *Does the built environment influence physical activity? Examining the evidence*. Committee on Physical Activity Health, Transportation, and Land Use 2005. Report No. 282.
25. Hyde R. Europe battles with obesity. *Lancet* 2008; 371:2160–2161.

26. Paul-Ebhohimhen V, Avenell A. Systematic review of the use of financial incentives in treatments for obesity and overweight. *Obes Rev* 2008; 9:355–367.

27. Stirling A, Lobstein T, Millstone E. Methodology for obtaining stakeholder assessments of obesity policy options in the PorGrow project. *Obes Rev* 2007; (suppl 2):17–27.

28. Department of Health. *Healthy Weight, Healthy Lives: A Cross Government Strategy for England 2008.*

29. Lobstein T, Baur L, Uauy R. Obesity in children and young people: a crisis in public health. *Obes Rev* 2004; (suppl 1):4–104.

30. Summerbell CD, Ashton V, Campbell KJ, Edmunds L, Kelly S, Waters E. Interventions for treating obesity in children. *Cochrane Database Syst Rev* 2003; 3:CD001872.

31. Summerbell CD, Waters E, Edmunds LD, Kelly S, Brown T, Campbell KJ. Interventions for preventing obesity in children. *Cochrane Database Syst Rev* 2005; 3:CD001871.

32. Chopra M, Galbraith S, Darnton-Hill I. A global response to a global problem: the epidemic of overnutrition. *Bull World Health Org* 2002; 80:952–958.

33. Chopra M, Darnton-Hill I. Tobacco and obesity epidemics: not so different after all? *BMJ* 2004; 328:1558–1560.

34. Wiecha JL, Peterson KE, Ludwig DS, Kim J, Sobol A, Gortmaker SL. When children eat what they watch: impact of television viewing on dietary intake in youth. *Arch Pediatr Adolesc Med* 2006; 160:436–442.

35. West R. What lessons can be learned from tobacco control for combating the growing prevalence of obesity? *Obes Rev* 2007; (suppl 1):145–150.

36. Epstein LH, Roemmich JN, Robinson JL *et al*. A randomized trial of the effects of reducing television viewing and computer use on body mass index in young children. *Arch Pediatr Adolesc Med* 2008; 162:239–245.

37. James J, Thomas P, Kerr D. Preventing childhood obesity: two year follow-up results from the Christchurch obesity prevention programme in schools (CHOPPS). *BMJ* 2007; 335:762.

38. Jansen W, Raat H, Zwanenburg EJ, Reuvers I, van Walsem R, Brug J. A school-based intervention to reduce overweight and inactivity in children aged 6–12 years: study design of a randomized controlled trial. *BMC Public Health* 2008; 8:257.

39. Eisenmann JC, Gentile DA, Welk GJ *et al*. SWITCH: rationale, design, and implementation of a community, school, and family-based intervention to modify behaviors related to childhood obesity. *BMC Public Health* 2008; 8:223.

40. Barker DJ, Eriksson JG, Forsen T, Osmond C. Fetal origins of adult disease: strength of effects and biological basis. *Int J Epidemiol* 2002; 31:1235–1239.

41. Shiell AW, Campbell DM, Hall MH, Barker DJ. Diet in late pregnancy and glucose-insulin metabolism of the offspring 40 years later. *Br J Obstet Gynaecol* 2000; 107:890–895.

42. Scott DA, Loveman E, McIntyre L, Waugh N. Screening for gestational diabetes: a systematic review and economic evaluation. *Health Technol Assess (Rockv)* 2002; 6:1–161.

43. Crowther CA, Hiller JE, Moss JR, McPhee AJ, Jeffries WS, Robinson JS. Effect of treatment of gestational diabetes mellitus on pregnancy outcomes. *N Engl J Med* 2005; 352:2477–2486.

44. Dabelea D, Mayer-Davis EJ, Lamichhane AP *et al*. Association of intrauterine exposure to maternal diabetes and obesity with type 2 diabetes in youth: the SEARCH Case-Control Study. *Diabetes Care* 2008; 31:1422–1426.

45. Dabelea D. The predisposition to obesity and diabetes in offspring of diabetic mothers. *Diabetes Care* 2007; 30(suppl 2):S169–S174.

46. Dabelea D, Hanson RL, Bennett PH, Roumain J, Knowler WC, Pettitt DJ. Increasing prevalence of Type II diabetes in American Indian children. *Diabetologia* 1998; 41:904–910.

47. Singhal A, Lanigan J. Breastfeeding, early growth and later obesity. *Obes Rev* 2007; (suppl 1):51–54.

48. Singhal A, Lucas A. Early origins of cardiovascular disease: is there a unifying hypothesis? *Lancet* 2004; 363:1642–1645.

49. Mikkila V, Rasanen L, Raitakari OT, Pietinen P, Viikari J. Consistent dietary patterns identified from childhood to adulthood: the cardiovascular risk in Young Finns Study. *Br J Nutr* 2005; 93:923–931.

50. Janz KF, Burns TL, Levy SM. Tracking of activity and sedentary behaviors in childhood: the Iowa Bone Development Study. *Am J Prev Med* 2005; 29:171–178.

51. Cooke LJ, Wardle J, Gibson EL, Sapochnik M, Sheiham A, Lawson M. Demographic, familial and trait predictors of fruit and vegetable consumption by pre-school children. *Public Health Nutr* 2004; 7:295–302.

52. Campbell K, Hesketh K, Crawford D, Salmon J, Ball K, McCallum Z. The Infant Feeding Activity and Nutrition Trial (INFANT) an early intervention to prevent childhood obesity: cluster-randomised controlled trial. *BMC Public Health* 2008; 8:103.

53. Ryan DH, Espeland MA, Foster GD *et al*. Look AHEAD (Action for Health in Diabetes): design and methods for a clinical trial of weight loss for the prevention of cardiovascular disease in type 2 diabetes. *Control Clin Trials* 2003; 24:610–628.
54. Goodyear LJ. The exercise pill – too good to be true? *N Engl J Med* 2008; 359:1842–1844.
55. Lang T, Rayner G. Overcoming policy cacophony on obesity: an ecological public health framework for policymakers. *Obes Rev* 2007; (suppl 1):165–181.

3

Managing the normotensive type 2 diabetic patient with microalbuminuria

F. Joseph, A. Mon, J. Vora

BACKGROUND

Diabetic nephropathy occurs in 20% to 40% of patients with types 1 and 2 diabetes mellitus (DM) and is the leading cause of chronic kidney disease (CKD) and end-stage renal disease (ESRD) [1, 2]. The increasing burden of CKD secondary to the epidemic of type 2 DM has led to extensive investigation and research to understand, prevent and aggressively treat diabetic nephropathy.

The natural history of renal disease in type 2 DM has been evaluated in detail. The earliest clinical evidence of nephropathy is the small but abnormal increase in urinary albumin excretion rate (UAER) into the microalbuminuria range (≥30 mg/24 h; ≥20–200 µg/min usually in timed overnight urine collections; albumin/creatinine ratio (ACR) between 10–30 mg/mmol in an early morning spot urine sample) due to glomerular leakage of the protein, which in certain situations may reflect damage to the renal endothelium. Patients with microalbuminuria are also referred to as having incipient nephropathy. Without intervention, structural injury within the kidney, especially in the glomeruli, increases in severity; glomerular filtration rate (GFR) declines; and nephropathy becomes overt with the emergence of macroalbuminuria (UAER ≥200 µg/min or albumin/creatinine ratio ≥30 mg/mmol) [3]. Serum creatinine levels also increase and eventually CKD and ESRD can ensue. Oxidative stress, increased expression of pro-sclerotic growth factors and associated endothelial dysfunction are important mechanistic factors underlying the pathological events that result in glomerulosclerosis, tubulointerstitial fibrosis and vascular sclerosis [4–6].

Type 2 diabetic nephropathy is also recognized as a heterogeneous disease entity [7]. Some studies have suggested that increasing UAER does not necessarily result in a decline in GFR and that GFR can decline even without significant increase in UAER [8]. It has been suggested that micro-architectural changes in the kidney are better predictors of diabetic renal disease progression. These changes include baseline glomerular basement membrane width and mesangial fractional volume expansion [9]. Definite renal lesions including tubular, interstitial and arteriolar lesions are ultimately present in type 1 DM, as the nephropathy

Franklin Joseph, MRCP, Consultant Physician in Diabetes and Endocrinology, Department of Diabetes and Endocrinology, The Countess of Chester Hospital NHS Foundation Trust, Chester, UK.

Aung Mon, MBBS, MRCP, Specialist Registrar, Diabetes and Endocrinology, Royal Liverpool University Hospital, Liverpool, UK.

Jiten Vora, MA, MD, FRCP, Consultant Endocrinologist, Department of Diabetes and Endocrinology, Royal Liverpool University Hospital, Liverpool, UK.

progresses, but the most important structural changes involve the glomerulus. In contrast, the renal morphology is less uniform in microalbuminuric type 2 diabetic patients. It has been demonstrated that a third of microalbuminuric type 2 DM patients have Kimmelstiel–Wilson lesions, a third have non-specific lesions and a third have normal kidneys by light microscopy. Thus, a proportion of type 2 diabetic patients may have microalbuminuria or proteinuria with normal glomerular structure with or without tubulointerstitial and/or arteriolar abnormalities [10].

A number of factors contribute to the chain of pathophysiological events that constitutes the continuum of renal damage [11–14]. These factors include a genetic predisposition as well as various components of the metabolic syndrome including hypertension and hyperglycaemia [15]. Blood pressure (BP) control is vital for renoprotection, but blood pressure-independent mechanisms are also implicated in the development of microalbuminuria. Intraglomerular hypertension may exist whether or not systemic hypertension is present [16]. Transgenic rats, which over-express the human angiotensin 1 receptor (AT1R), develop significant albuminuria, podocyte effacement, progressive fibrosis and eventually focal segmental glomerulosclerosis independent of blood pressure. These changes can be reversed by blocking the renin–angiotensin system (RAS) [17]. Thus, the RAS plays a key role in the BP-independent mechanisms involved in renal damage and is an important therapeutic target in at risk patients.

In patients at risk of renal damage, early intervention is essential and the goals of treatment and therapeutic measures in the individual affected patient should be tailored dependent on the stage of the continuum of renal damage reached. For incipient nephropathy, therapy is aimed at achieving stability of microalbuminuria or indeed regression to normoalbuminuria. In advanced nephropathy, therapy is aimed at retarding progression to ESRD and the requirement of renal support.

MICROALBUMINURIA, MACROALBUMINURIA AND CARDIOVASCULAR RISK

Epidemiological studies have shown that microalbuminuria is an important risk factor for progression of diabetic nephropathy, arteriosclerosis, coronary heart disease and other vascular diseases in persons with type 2 DM.

Over time, the pattern of progression of proteinuria in type 2 diabetic patients with microalbuminuria is variable, but patients with persistent microalbuminuria have about 20 times the risk of developing diabetic nephropathy [18]. Progression from microalbuminuria to overt nephropathy occurs in 20–40% of patients within a 10-year period, with approximately 20% of those with overt nephropathy progressing to ESRD over a period of 20 years [19]. Higher UAERs, even within the normal range, predict the development of diabetic nephropathy in type 2 diabetic patients. Progression to microalbuminuria and progression from microalbuminuria to macroalbuminuria is more frequent in patients with type 2 diabetes with higher baseline UAERs [20, 21]. After a period of 10 years the risk of diabetic nephropathy has been shown to be 29 times greater in patients with type 2 diabetes with UAE values >10 µg/min [22].

Similar factors contribute to the common pathophysiologies of renal and cardiovascular disease (CVD) [23, 24]. Thus, the incidence of renal dysfunction is high in patients with CVD and patients with CVD often develop renal damage simultaneously [25–27]. The reverse is also true and the incidence of coronary heart disease is higher in patients with increased UAER. The increase in cardiovascular risk occurs early in the development of CKD and even when UAER is within the microalbuminuria range [28, 29]. Various studies have shown that microalbuminuria not only predicts progression of renal disease [30] but is also an independent, continuous risk factor for CVD as well, in various populations of patients with or without diabetes. The Prevention of REnal and Vascular ENd-stage Disease (PREVEND) study, for example, demonstrated the predictive value of albuminuria on all-cause mortality among >40 000 subjects in the general population [31]. Even very low levels of albuminuria, within the normoalbuminuric range (10–20 µg/min), increased the cardiovascular risk in the 961-day median follow-up period of the study. In the MIcroalbuminuria, Cardiovascular and Renal Outcomes (MICRO-HOPE) study, the relative risk of myocardial infarction, stroke, and death due to CVD in patients with microalbuminuria was 1.97 among those with DM and 1.61 among those without. An increase in ACR of 0.4 mg/mmol increased the risk of a cardiovascular event by 5.9% [26, 32]. A recent meta-analysis has shown that proteinuria is independently associated with increased risk of subsequent CVD. The results from this meta-analysis of 26 cohort studies included information on over 7000 CVD events in almost 170 000 individuals. Individuals with proteinuria had a risk of CVD that was approximately 50% greater than those without. The strength of the association was substantially higher among individuals with macroalbuminuria compared with those with microalbuminuria and the relationship was consistent across diverse population subgroups including individuals with and without diabetes [33].

Assessment of UAER in patients with Type 2 diabetes is thus imperative as an early clinical manifestation of diabetic nephropathy so as to initiate interventions to reduce the progression of diabetic nephropathy and also to minimize the otherwise increased cardiovascular risk in the early stages of diabetic nephropathy associated with microalbuminuria [3, 25, 34, 35].

TREATING THE NORMOTENSIVE TYPE 2 DIABETIC PATIENT WITH MICROALBUMINURIA

Blood pressure has been shown to increase progressively as normoalbuminuria progresses to microalbuminuria and further to macroalbuminuria [36]. Patients with microalbuminuria may start and even remain normotensive, although with higher BP than those seen with normoalbuminuria [37]. Given that hypertension and albuminuria are both continuous variables, do type 2 diabetic patients who have microalbuminuria warrant treatment before they become, by definition, hypertensive?

The proposed beneficial effect of RAS blockers in renal disease is dependent on their ability to predominantly alter efferent arteriolar tone and consequently decrease intraglomerular pressure independent of their effect on systemic BP. They also modify other biochemical and micro-structural processes in the nephron early in the continuum of diabetic nephropathy [38]. Thus, the evidence for treating patients with type 2 DM with microalbuminuria that are 'normotensive' is limited and has focused predominantly on the use of RAS blockers in this clinical scenario. Studies dating as far back as 1988 have been conducted in this group of patients with RAS blockers [39]. There are some fundamental drawbacks in applying the results of these studies to clinical practice. The majority of studies were of limited duration and had small sample sizes. In addition to these issues, the very definition of hypertension and targets for BP control have changed over the years and patients that were considered 'normotensive' at the time these studies were conducted would now be considered hypertensive [39–48]. The studies also relied on the use of microalbuminuria and changes in microalbuminuria as surrogate markers of renal disease progression as well as CVD. All of these studies showed the benefit of RAS blockade in lowering albumin excretion either attributable to BP lowering or effects of RAS blockade beyond BP lowering (Table 3.1).

In 2002 and later in 2006, the published Appropriate Blood Pressure Control In Hypertensive and Normotensive DM (Normotensive ABCD) and Appropriate Blood Pressure Control In Hypertensive and Normotensive DM-2-Valsartan (ABCD-2-Valsartan) trials were the first to explore outcomes of renal disease progression as well as CVD in conjunction with proteinuria. In the Normotensive-ABCD trial, the investigators randomly assigned 480 normotensive patients with type 2 DM to achieve intensive (mean BP 128/75 mmHg) and moderate (mean BP 137/81 mmHg) control of BP. The moderate group received placebo, and the intensive

Table 3.1 Summary characteristics of the clinical studies that investigated the benefits of RAS blockade

Author (Year) [Trial name]	n	Duration (months)	Baseline Proteinuria	Baseline Mean BP/ defined normotension	Baseline Comparators	Clinical outcomes Kidney disease progression	Clinical outcomes Proteinuria	Clinical outcomes CVD/ Mortality
Marre (1988)	20	12	30–300 mg/day	<160/90	Enalapril / Placebo		*	
Stornello (1989)					ACE-I / Beta-blocker		*	
Ravid (1994)	94	60	30–300 mg/day	≤140/90	Enalapril / Placebo		*	
Sano (1995)	62	48	30–300 mg/day	<150/90	Enalapril / No treatment		*	
Ahmad (1997)	103	60	20–200 µg/min	≤140/90	Enalapril / Placebo		*	
Vongterapak (1997)	103	3			Ramipril / Placebo		*	
Schrier (2002) [ABCD]	480	60	<300mg/24h	≤140/90 mean 136/84	Enalapril/Nisoldipine mean 128/75 / Placebo mean 137/81	*		*
Viberti (2002) [MARVAL]	332	24	20–200 µg/min	≤140/90 mean 129/79	Valsartan / Amlodipine		*	(Results analyzed in normotensive subgroup, independent of BP lowering) *
	(normotensive and hypertensive)							
Sasso (2002)	60	2	20–200 µg/min	≤140/90 mean 126/81	Irbesartan / Placebo		*	(independent of BP lowering)

Study	n	Duration (months)	Albuminuria	BP	Comparison	Result
Zandbergen (2003)	62	3	20–200 µg/min	140/90–150/90 130/80–140/90	Losartan vs. Placebo	*
	53					*
	32			<130/80		* (independent of BP lowering) *
Kubba (2003)	25	3	20–200 µg/min		Losartan vs. Placebo	*
Makino (2005, 2007) [INNOVATION]	163	12	100–300 mg/g	mean 130/75	Telmisartan vs. Placebo	NS *
Estacio (2006) [ABCD-2]	129 (normoalbuminuric and microalbuminuric)	24	<200 µg/min	<140/90	mean 122/72 Valsartan vs. Placebo	*
Agha (2007)	171 (normo/micro/macroalbuminuric)	8	30–300 mg/day	mean 126/84	mean 118/75 Losartan vs. Placebo	*
Cetinkalp (2008)	40	3			Irbesartan vs. Placebo	*
ADVANCE (2007–9)	11 140 (normotensive+hypertensive)	52			Perindopril+Indapamide vs. Placebo	* * (similar benefits seen in all subgroups) * *
ONTARGET (2008)	25 620 (diabetic+non-diabetic) (1/3 normotensive) (normo/micro/macroalbuminric)	60			Telmisartan vs. Ramipril vs. Telmisartan+Ramipril	* * £ (similar patterns seen in all subgroups) * * £

* statistically significant (P <0.01); NS = not significant.

group received either nisoldipine or enalapril in a double-blind fashion. Metoprolol or hydrochlorothiazide was used as secondary antihypertensive therapy. No difference was noted in creatinine clearance between the two treated groups. A lower percentage in the intensive group progressed from normoalbuminuria to microalbuminuria and from microalbuminuria to overt proteinuria. Creatinine clearance remained stable over 5 years in normoalbuminuric and microalbuminuric patients, but not in those with overt macroalbuminuria. Compared with moderate BP control, intensive treatment was associated with a slower progression of diabetic retinopathy and a lower incidence of stroke. The results were the same whether nisoldipine or enalapril was used as the initial antihypertensive therapy [49].

The data from the Normotensive ABCD trial supported a BP target of 130/80 mmHg in type 2 diabetes. The results of the later published ABCD-2 Valsartan trial, provided some support for a BP goal of 120/75 mmHg. During this study, 129 normotensive patients with type 2 diabetes with a mean baseline BP of 128 mmHg were randomly assigned to receive either placebo or valsartan. After a mean of approximately 2 years, the BP in the placebo arm was 124±11/80±6.5 mmHg. The BP of patients in the valsartan group was significantly lower, at 118±11/75±6 mmHg with no difference in creatinine clearance but a significant decrease in UAE rate. Intensive treatment was apparently well tolerated, because the dropout rates were the same in the two groups. The study did have a small sample size, the duration of follow-up was short and again UAE was only a surrogate marker. Nevertheless, the study did provide some evidence that targeting a diastolic blood pressure of 75 mmHg is practical in normotensive microalbuminuric patients with type 2 diabetes. It also offered some suggestion that such a target might actually prevent renal damage [50].

More recent studies have further provided evidence that treatment with various angiotensin receptor blockers (ARBs) or angiotensin-converting enzyme inhibitors (ACE-Is) results in longer-term stabilization or even normalization of proteinuria in normotensive type 2 diabetic patients with microalbuminuria and incipient nephropathy. In this group of normotensive individuals, the effects of RAS blockade have been shown to be beyond their BP-lowering effect and these effects have been shown to exist in both Caucasian as well as non-Caucasian populations [51–59].

Larger-scale studies looking at hard endpoints for renal disease progression, CVD, renal and cardiovascular mortality have recently provided evidence for intensive therapy but have also prompted debate and caution. The Action in Diabetes and Vascular Disease: PreterAx and DiamicroN MR Controlled Evaluation (ADVANCE) trial [60–64] was the first major large-scale clinical trial to demonstrate the benefits of BP reduction on both microvascular and macrovascular events in both hypertensive and normotensive patients with type 2 DM. To examine whether BP lowering provided renoprotection across a broader range of blood pressures beyond the current guideline targets, the primary outcome for this analysis was defined as a composite of new microalbuminuria (ACR of 30–300 µg/mg), new-onset nephropathy (ACR >300 µg/mg), doubling of serum creatinine >200 µmol/l (2.3 mg/dl), requirement for renal replacement therapy, or renal death. Secondary outcomes included the separate components of the primary outcome, progression or regression of ≥1 albuminuria stage, and restoration of normoalbuminuria (ACR <30 µg/mg). During a median follow-up of 4.3 years, mean BP fell from 145.0/80.6 mmHg at entry to 134.7/74.8 mmHg and 140.3/77.0 mmHg in patients on active and placebo treatment, respectively (P <0.0001). Active treatment with perindopril/indapamide reduced the risk of all renal events by 21% (P <0.0001); reduced progression of albuminuria by 22% (P <0.0001); and increased regression of albuminuria by 16% (P = 0.002). The benefits of active treatment were consistent across subgroups defined by baseline systolic blood pressure (SBP) ranging from <120 to ≥160 mmHg or diastolic blood pressure (DBP), ranging from <70 to ≥90 mmHg. A continuous association was seen between renal events and achieved SBP, with a 6.9% relative risk (RR) reduction per 10 mmHg reduction in SBP (P for trend <0.0001). These findings suggested that administration of a fixed-dose combination of perindopril/indapamide to patients with type 2 diabetes resulted in renoprotection, even among those with initial BP in the normal range of <120/70 mmHg. This association was related to the degree of reduction in SBP and was seen down to achieved SBP levels of 106 mmHg, much lower than the SBP levels recommended in current guidelines, which recommend reducing BP to 130/80 mmHg in patients with diabetes or to 125/75 mmHg in those with nephropathy. Significant reductions were also seen in RR of cardiovascular death (18%), and death from any cause (14%) (Figure 3.1).

The benefits observed in ADVANCE were similar in hypertensive and normotensive patients with varying levels of UAE and suggest that normotensive type 2 diabetic patients with microalbuminuria would benefit from treatment with an ACE-I plus thiazide combination.

In the ONTARGET (ONgoing Telmisartan Alone and in combination with Ramipril Global Endpoint Trial) study, dual blockade of RAS was evaluated in a mixture of 25 620 normotensive, hypertensive, micro- and macro-albuminuric patients with vascular disease or high-risk diabetes (n = 6982), who were followed for 5 years. Patients either received ramipril, telmisartan or both agents. Estimated glomerular filtration rate (eGFR) declined less with ramipril, compared with telmisartan (-2.82 ml/min/1.73 m^2 versus -4.12 ml/min/1.73 m^2; P <0.0001) but the increase in UAE was less with telmisartan (P = 0.004) than with ramipril. The primary renal outcome was, however, a composite of dialysis, doubling of serum creatinine and death. This was similar for both telmisartan (13.4%) and ramipril (13.5%). The secondary renal outcome, dialysis or doubling of serum creatinine, was similar with telmisartan and ramipril as well. Ramipril and telmisartan were also equally effective in reducing the combined primary endpoint consisting of cardiovascular death, myocardial infarction, stroke, and hospitalization from heart failure. The conclusion from ONTARGET was that in people at high vascular risk, the effects of telmisartan on major renal outcomes are similar to ramipril. Given that the study included a population of type 2, normotensive patients with microalbuminuria, ONTARGET provides some further evidence to support the use of an ACE-I or ARB in this group of patients.

Co-administration of an ACE-I and an ARB has been shown to provide a greater degree of blockade of the RAS with additional reductions in BP. These additional reductions in BP have been shown to maintain or even decrease UAER in diabetic patients with microalbuminuria and nephropathy [65–72].

The decrease in proteinuria in diabetic nephropathy and non-diabetic chronic renal failure has also been shown to occur independent of BP reductions [73, 74].The antiproteinuric effect of an ACE-I–ARB combination implies a synergistic action of these agents that is specific to the intrarenal RAS and occurs at plasma concentrations of ACE-I and ARB below levels affecting systemic BP [75]. The role of combination therapy in normotensive type 2 DM patients with microalbuminuria was first explored by Atcama and colleagues in a small study. The study compared the effects of lisinopril, losartan and their combination in 27 patients for 12 months. The 24-h UAE rate decreased significantly in each group but with no significant difference among groups [76].

The much larger ONTARGET trial did not focus specifically on the same group of patients but did have similar patients enrolled. Even though the combination therapy group in this trial achieved greater decreases in proteinuria in association with lower achieved blood pressures, the patients in this arm had higher doubling of serum creatinine, more patients reaching ESRD, more requiring dialysis and higher mortality. Major drawbacks when co-administering ACE-Is and ARBs include the aggravation of CKD, increase in the incidence of acute renal failure in patients with CKD and the increased occurrence of hyperkalaemia. The incidence of these complications was reported to be low in previous meta-analyses [77, 78] but was found to be higher in the ONTARGET study.

The ONTARGET trial raises a number of questions and there are caveats to interpreting its findings. It clearly casts doubt on the use of proteinuria reduction by itself as a definitive

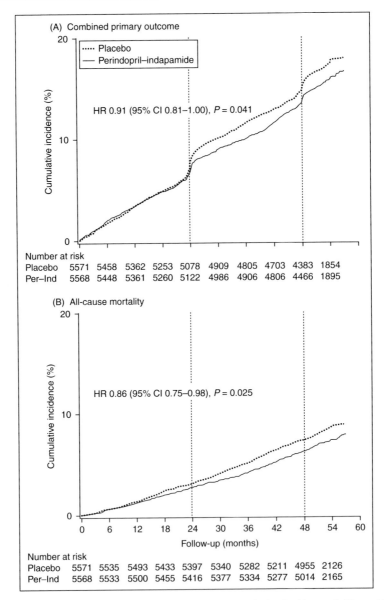

Figure 3.1 For patients assigned active treatment or placebo, cumulative incidence of (A) combined major macrovascular or microvascular outcomes and (B) all-cause mortality. Vertical broken lines indicate 24-month and 48-month study visits, at which additional information on microvascular events (measurement of urinary albumin/creatinine ratio and retinal examination) was obtained. For outcomes relating to these measurements, event times were recorded as the visit date. The curves were truncated at month 57, by which time 99% of events had occurred. The effects of treatment (hazard ratios and P-values) were estimated from unadjusted Cox proportional hazard models that used all available data.

surrogate marker of improved renal function. Type 2 diabetic nephropathy is a heterogeneous disease entity and some individuals have non-persistent albuminuria and some have changes in eGFR discordant with predicted changes in proteinuria. This further complicates the interpretations of proteinuria indices in clinical studies and trials. It must also be borne in mind that the patients included in ONTARGET were high-risk-patients who had CVD but did not have heart failure, a group of patients who have been shown to benefit from the use of dual blockade [79, 80]. The benefits of combination RAS blockade on major renal outcomes in more selected patient groups remain to be demonstrated. Based on the evidence of the ONTARGET trial, dual RAS blockade must only be used in well-selected diabetic patients with proteinuria, without concomitant disease or nephrotoxic medication, who might benefit from a combination treatment strategy. Potassium levels and kidney function should be closely monitored in these patients.

TREATMENT OF THE HYPERTENSIVE TYPE 2 DIABETIC PATIENT WITH ALBUMINURIA

The evidence for the benefit of BP lowering in hypertensive patients with type 2 DM and albuminuria is very strong. Numerous studies have demonstrated that treatment of hypertension, irrespective of the agent used, produces a beneficial effect on albuminuria in both the micro- and macroalbuminuric range [81]. Furthermore, the Modification of Diet in Renal Disease (MDRD) trial demonstrated that the rate of decline in renal function is reduced when BP is lowered to levels below 125/75 mmHg, especially in the presence of significant proteinuria (>1 g over 24 h) [82, 83].

The major progression trials including ADVANCE, ONTARGET, Irbesartan in Diabetic Nephropathy Trial (IDNT), IRbesartan in patients with type 2 diabetes and MicroAlbuminuria (IRMA-2), Reduction in Endpoints in Non-insulin dependent diabetes mellitus with the Angiotensin II Antagonist Losartan (RENAAL), Normotensive ABCD and MICRO-HOPE have provided clear evidence that hypertensive, type 2 diabetic patients with persistent albuminuria, in the micro- as well as macroalbuminuric range, benefit from the renoprotective mechanisms of RAS blockade with ACE-Is and ARBs. The renoprotective effect of RAS blockers occurs independent of their BP-lowering effect and occurs with BP lowered to levels well below current recommended targets [51, 84–88]. In addition to nephroprotection, the use of ACE-Is and ARBs also reduces cardiovascular risk in hypertensive patients with type 2 diabetes and microalbuminuria [28, 29, 89, 90]. The use of these agents is thus recommended in various guidelines [35, 91].

NEWER RAS AGENTS IN THE MANAGEMENT OF MICROALBUMINURIA

The Aliskiren in the Evaluation of Proteinuria in Diabetes (AVOID) study [92] evaluated the renoprotective effects of dual blockade of the RAS by adding aliskiren, the first in the new class of oral direct renin inhibitors, to treatment with 100 mg daily losartan in 599 patients who had hypertension (135/78 mmHg) and type 2 diabetes with nephropathy. Treatment with 300 mg of aliskiren daily, as compared with placebo, reduced the mean urinary ACR by 20% (P <0.001). The benefit of aliskiren appeared to be independent of the small reduction in BP (2/1 mmHg). A reduction in proteinuria of 50% or more was observed in only 25% of the patients receiving the combination of both drugs, suggesting that a number of patients might only have a limited additional benefit from renin inhibition [93]. Other limitations identified were the use of single daytime BP recordings; the limited 6-month study period; and the relatively poor glycaemic control (HbA1c 8.0±1.5%) of the patients included in the AVOID study. The efficacy of these new agents is still to be proven, and after the ONTARGET study, much longer studies over several years and including ESRD, dialysis and death as endpoints are needed to confirm that dual therapy to block the RAS with aliskiren and other agents will provide sustained renal protection and not cause an increased number of adverse events. The role of these agents in normotensive type 2 diabetic patients with microalbuminuria cannot be extrapolated given the inexperience with these agents and requires further investigation.

BEYOND BP LOWERING AND RAS BLOCKADE

Intensive glycaemic control

Intensive diabetes management with the goal of achieving near-normoglycaemia has been shown in large prospective randomized studies to delay the onset of microalbuminuria and the progression of micro- to macroalbuminuria in patients with type 2 diabetes [88, 94, 95], but the effects on CVD have been less clear. The Action to Control Cardiovascular Risk in Diabetes (ACCORD) [96], Veterans Affairs Diabetes Trial (VADT) [97] and ADVANCE [60–64] trials were all designed to clarify this. The patient population and the approach to treatment differed substantially in the three studies but none of the trials showed a reduction in macrovascular or CVD outcomes from intensive glycaemic control (HbA1c <7.0% versus >7.0%). In ACCORD, a greater number of deaths in the intensive glycaemic group caused the trial to be stopped early [96]. The excessive mortality was due to a greater number of deaths from CVD, but the explanation for this finding is not clear – thiazolidinedione usage, hypoglycaemia, heart failure and weight gain all appear *not* to explain the excessive mortality.

Intensive glucose control in the ADVANCE trial [60–64] did result in a significant reduction in renal events, including new or worsening nephropathy (hazard ratio [HR] 0.79; $P = 0.006$) compared with the non-intensive arm (HbA1c levels at study end were 6.4% versus 7.0%). The greatest benefit associated with intensive glucose control was seen for the development of macroalbuminuria (2.9% vs. 4.1% with standard control; HR 0.70; $P <0.001$), with a trend towards a reduction in the need for renal replacement therapy or death from renal causes (0.4% vs. 0.6%; HR 0.64; $P = 0.09$) but no effect on the doubling of serum creatinine level (1.2% vs. 1.1%). The most impressive effect was seen when the joint effect of BP lowering and intensive glucose control was analyzed in ADVANCE [61, 63; new or worsening nephropathy was reduced by a relative risk ratio (RRR) of 33% ($P = 0.005$). It could be argued that given the size of the study population, this effect could be extended to the subset of patients with microalbuminuria who were normotensive at baseline that were included in the study. Furthermore, the patients with microalbuminuria in the intensive BP control group who were rendered 'normotensive' with RAS blockade also did better as a result of intensive glycaemic control.

The ACCORD, ADVANCE and VADT trials compared the effects of glycaemic control and not how that difference in glycaemic control was achieved. The current balance of evidence suggests caution in pursuing intensive glycaemic control in patients with long-standing type 2 diabetes and known or suspected cardiac disease, but such a decision should be individualized [98, 99]. The glycaemic targets for patients with relatively recent-onset type 2 diabetes without CVD are still to be defined. Given the benefits of intensive glycaemic control on microvascular disease, however, it may be beneficial to pursue intensive glycaemic control in normotensive type 2 diabetic patients with microalbuminuria with a view to retarding the progression of diabetic nephropathy in these individuals.

Statin use

Statins have been proposed to have pleiotropic effects, actions independent of their cholesterol-lowering mechanism. These include decreased reactive oxygen species generation via inhibition of nicotinamide adenine dinucleotide phosphate (NADPH) oxidase and therefore statins have a role as renoprotective agents. Statins which are commonly used in patients with type 2 DM for CVD risk reduction have been shown to decrease UAE as well [23].

Dietary protein restriction

High protein intake increases GFR and may induce hyperfiltration, thereby worsening glomerular injury in patients with renal disease. Studies in patients with varying stages of nephropathy have shown that protein restriction helps slow the progression of albuminuria; GFR decline; and occurrence of ESRD [100–103]. Protein restriction should be considered particularly in patients whose nephropathy seems to be progressing despite optimal glucose and blood pressure control with the use of ACE-Is or ARBs [103]. Most experts agree that a high-protein diet may accelerate CKD progression and guidelines recommend that patients with CKD restrict their animal protein intake to less than 0.8 g/kg per day [2].

Smoking cessation

Development of macroalbuminuria decreased in patients with type 2 DM who were former smokers or who had never smoked compared with patients with type 2 DM who were active smokers. This finding suggests that smoking cessation may significantly impact diabetic nephropathy progression in patients with microalbuminuria and that smoking cessation should be promoted for not just nephroprotective effects but also for the added benefits to CVD risk reduction [104, 105].

Obesity

Studies have identified body mass index (BMI) as well as waist circumference as risk factors for albuminuria [106, 107]. Weight loss achieved by various means has been shown to have a positive impact on albuminuria in obese type 2 diabetics with albuminuria and should be actively pursued [108–110].

SUMMARY

Albumin excretion rate is the mainstay of early detection of diabetic kidney disease. It is an important predictive tool in assessing the risk of progression of nephropathy as well as CVD. An approach that identifies other factors which add to its predictive accuracy is also essential. Careful family history, smoking history, consideration of absolute versus categorical UAER values, more frequent UAER measurements, ambulatory BP monitoring, precise GFR measurements, diabetic retinopathy assessments and plasma lipid levels can all add to predictive accuracy for diabetic nephropathy. Comprehensive diabetes care, involving a multifaceted therapeutic approach that targets control of blood pressure and lipids, aspirin use, smoking cessation, weight loss, exercise, and glycaemic control, remains the foundation for the care of the individual with type 2 diabetes. Achievement of recommended goals for these non-glycaemic risk factors should be aggressively pursued in all patients with type 2 diabetes. Such a multifactorial intervention improves the clinical outcome in patients with type 2 DM and microalbuminuria [111]. The evidence to support the management of normotensive type 2 diabetic subjects with microalbuminuria is predominantly based on the use of reduction in microalbuminuria as a surrogate marker. Outcome data in this group have been extrapolated from large trials including this subgroup of patients. Current balance of evidence suggests that BP targets much lower than currently recommended may benefit this group. The early use of an ACE-I or ARB confers benefit. The evidence for the combination of ACE-I and ARB must be restricted to strictly selected patients without concomitant CVD with strict monitoring. As practitioners, we can and should offer our patients an individualized judgment, based on their actual risk profile. We must weigh up the risk and cost benefit assessments in treating normotensive diabetic patients but multifactorial risk reduction should be the cornerstone of the management of these individuals.

REFERENCES

1. KDOQI Clinical Practice Guideline and Clinical Practice Recommendations for anemia in chronic kidney disease: 2007 update of hemoglobin target. *Am J Kidney Dis* 2007; 50:471–530.
2. Standards of medical care in diabetes – 2007. *Diabetes Care* 2007; 30:S4–S41.
3. American Diabetes Association: Diabetic nephropathy (Position Statement). *Diabetes Care* 2002; 25:S85–S89.
4. Becker GJ, Hewitson TD. The role of tubulointerstitial injury in chronic renal failure. *Curr Opin Nephrol Hypertens* 2000; 9:133–138.
5. Ghiadoni L, Cupisti A, Huang Y *et al.* Endothelial dysfunction and oxidative stress in chronic renal failure. *J Nephrol* 2004; 17:512–519.
6. Osto E, Coppolino G, Volpe M, Cosentino F. Restoring the dysfunctional endothelium. *Curr Pharm Des* 2007; 13:1053–1068.
7. Onuigbo MA. Causes of renal failure in patients with type 2 diabetes mellitus. *JAMA* 2003; 290:1855; author reply 1855–1856.
8. Tsalamandris C, Allen TJ, Gilbert RE *et al.* Progressive decline in renal function in diabetic patients with and without albuminuria. *Diabetes* 1994; 43:649–655.
9. Nosadini R, Velussi M, Brocco E *et al.* Course of renal function in type 2 diabetic patients with abnormalities of albumin excretion rate. *Diabetes* 2000; 49:476–484.
10. Fioretto P, Mauer M. Histopathology of diabetic nephropathy. *Semin Nephrol* 2007; 27:195–207.
11. Dzau V, Braunwald E. Resolved and unresolved issues in the prevention and treatment of coronary artery disease: a workshop consensus statement. *Am Heart J* 1991; 121:1244–1263.
12. Dzau V. The cardiovascular continuum and renin-angiotensin-aldosterone system blockade. *J Hypertens Suppl* 2005; 23:S9–S17.
13. Dzau VJ, Antman EM, Black HR *et al.* The cardiovascular disease continuum validated: clinical evidence of improved patient outcomes: part II: Clinical trial evidence (acute coronary syndromes through renal disease) and future directions. *Circulation* 2006; 114:2871–2891.
14. Dzau VJ, Antman EM, Black HR *et al.* The cardiovascular disease continuum validated: clinical evidence of improved patient outcomes: part I: Pathophysiology and clinical trial evidence (risk factors through stable coronary artery disease). *Circulation* 2006; 114:2850–2870.
15. Peralta CA, Kurella M, Lo JC, Chertow GM. The metabolic syndrome and chronic kidney disease. *Curr Opin Nephrol Hypertens* 2006; 15:361–365.
16. Anderson S. Systemic and glomerular hypertension in progressive renal disease. *Kidney Int Suppl* 1988; 25:S119–S121.
17. Hoffmann S, Podlich D, Hahnel B, Kriz W, Gretz N. Angiotensin II type 1 receptor overexpression in podocytes induces glomerulosclerosis in transgenic rats. *J Am Soc Nephrol* 2004; 15:1475–1487.
18. Parving H-H, Østerby R, Anderson PW, Hsueh WA. Diabetic nephropathy. In: *Brenner and Rector's The Kidney*, 5th edition. Saunders, Philadelphia, 1995.
19. Remuzzi G, Schieppati A, Ruggenenti P. Clinical practice. Nephropathy in patients with type 2 diabetes. *N Engl J Med* 2002; 346:1145–1151.
20. Gall MA, Hougaard P, Borch-Johnsen K, Parving HH. Risk factors for development of incipient and overt diabetic nephropathy in patients with non-insulin dependent diabetes mellitus: prospective, observational study. *BMJ* 1997; 314:783–788.
21. Forsblom CM, Groop PH, Ekstrand A *et al.* Predictors of progression from normoalbuminuria to microalbuminuria in NIDDM. *Diabetes Care* 1998; 21:1932–1938.
22. Murussi M, Baglio P, Gross JL, Silveiro SP. Risk factors for microalbuminuria and macroalbuminuria in type 2 diabetic patients: a 9-year follow-up study. *Diabetes Care* 2002; 25:1101–1103.
23. Sandhu S, Wiebe N, Fried LF, Tonelli M. Statins for improving renal outcomes: a meta-analysis. *J Am Soc Nephrol* 2006; 17:2006–2016.
24. Zoccali C. Traditional and emerging cardiovascular and renal risk factors: an epidemiologic perspective. *Kidney Int* 2006; 70:26–33.
25. Klausen K, Borch-Johnsen K, Feldt-Rasmussen B *et al.* Very low levels of microalbuminuria are associated with increased risk of coronary heart disease and death independently of renal function, hypertension, and diabetes. *Circulation* 2004; 110:32–35.
26. Gerstein HC, Mann JF, Yi Q *et al.* Albuminuria and risk of cardiovascular events, death, and heart failure in diabetic and nondiabetic individuals. *JAMA* 2001; 286:421–426.
27. Dinneen SF, Gerstein HC. The association of microalbuminuria and mortality in non-insulin-dependent diabetes mellitus. A systematic overview of the literature. *Arch Intern Med* 1997; 157:1413–1418.

28. Ibsen H, Olsen MH, Wachtell K *et al*. Reduction in albuminuria translates to reduction in cardiovascular events in hypertensive patients: losartan intervention for endpoint reduction in hypertension study. *Hypertension* 2005; 45:198–202.

29. de Zeeuw D, Remuzzi G, Parving HH *et al*. Albuminuria, a therapeutic target for cardiovascular protection in type 2 diabetic patients with nephropathy. *Circulation* 2004; 110:921–927.

30. Mogensen CE, Keane WF, Bennett PH *et al*. Prevention of diabetic renal disease with special reference to microalbuminuria. *Lancet* 1995; 346:1080–1084.

31. Hillege HL, Fidler V, Diercks GF *et al*. Urinary albumin excretion predicts cardiovascular and noncardiovascular mortality in general population. *Circulation* 2002; 106:1777–1782.

32. Mann JF, Gerstein HC, Pogue J, Bosch J, Yusuf S. Renal insufficiency as a predictor of cardiovascular outcomes and the impact of ramipril: the HOPE randomized trial. *Ann Intern Med* 2001; 134:629–636.

33. Perkovic V, Verdon C, Ninomiya T *et al*. The relationship between proteinuria and coronary risk: a systematic review and meta-analysis. *PLoS Med* 2008; 5:e207.

34. Garg JP, Bakris GL. Microalbuminuria: marker of vascular dysfunction, risk factor for cardiovascular disease. *Vasc Med* 2002; 7:35–43.

35. Molitch ME, DeFronzo RA, Franz MJ *et al*. Nephropathy in diabetes. *Diabetes Care* 2004; 27:S79–S83.

36. Mathiesen ER, Hommel E, Giese J, Parving HH. Efficacy of captopril in postponing nephropathy in normotensive insulin dependent diabetic patients with microalbuminuria. *BMJ* 1991; 303:81–87.

37. Viberti GC, Jarrett RJ, Wiseman MJ. Predicting diabetic nephropathy. *N Engl J Med* 1984; 311:1256–1257.

38. Sirmon MD, Kirkpatrick WG. Diabetic nephropathy: new directions in management. *Ren Fail* 1991; 13:51–59.

39. Marre M, Chatellier G, Leblanc H, Guyene TT, Menard J, Passa P. Prevention of diabetic nephropathy with enalapril in normotensive diabetics with microalbuminuria. *BMJ* 1988; 297:1092–1095.

40. Stornello M, Valvo EV, Scapellato L. Angiotensin converting enzyme inhibition in normotensive type II diabetics with persistent mild proteinuria. *J Hypertens Suppl* 1989; 7:S314–S315.

41. Stornello M, Valvo EV, Puglia N, Scapellato L. Angiotensin converting enzyme inhibition with a low dose of enalapril in normotensive diabetics with persistent proteinuria. *J Hypertens Suppl* 1988; 6:S464–S466.

42. Comparison between perindopril and nifedipine in hypertensive and normotensive diabetic patients with microalbuminuria. Melbourne Diabetic Nephropathy Study Group. *BMJ* 1991; 302:210–216.

43. Stornello M, Valvo EV, Scapellato L. Angiotensin converting enzyme inhibition in normotensive type II diabetics with persistent mild proteinuria (Abstract). *J Nephrol* 1989; 2(suppl 1):24.

44. Stornello M, Valvo EV, Scapellato L. Persistent albuminuria in normotensive type 2 diabetics: comparative effects of converting enzyme inhibition and ß-blocker (Abstract). *J Nephrol* 1989; 2(suppl 1):24.

45. Ahmad J, Siddiqui MA, Ahmad H. Effective postponement of diabetic nephropathy with enalapril in normotensive type 2 diabetic patients with microalbuminuria. *Diabetes Care* 1997; 20:1576–1581.

46. Ravid M, Savin H, Jutrin I, Bental T, Lang R, Lishner M. Long-term effect of ACE inhibition on development of nephropathy in diabetes mellitus type II. *Kidney Int Suppl* 1994; 45:S161–S164.

47. Ravid M, Brosh D, Levi Z, Bar-Dayan Y, Ravid D, Rachmani R. Use of enalapril to attenuate decline in renal function in normotensive, normoalbuminuric patients with type 2 diabetes mellitus. A randomized, controlled trial. *Ann Intern Med* 1998; 128:982–988.

48. Sano T, Kawamura T, Matsumae H *et al*. Effects of long-term enalapril treatment on persistent micro-albuminuria in well-controlled hypertensive and normotensive NIDDM patients. *Diabetes Care* 1994; 17:420–424.

49. Schrier RW, Estacio RO, Esler A, Mehler P. Effects of aggressive blood pressure control in normotensive type 2 diabetic patients on albuminuria, retinopathy and strokes. *Kidney Int* 2002; 61:1086–1097.

50. Estacio RO, Coll JR, Tran ZV, Schrier RW. Effect of intensive blood pressure control with valsartan on urinary albumin excretion in normotensive patients with type 2 diabetes. *Am J Hypertens* 2006; 19:1241–1248.

51. Viberti G, Wheeldon NM. Microalbuminuria reduction with valsartan in patients with type 2 diabetes mellitus: a blood pressure-independent effect. *Circulation* 2002; 106:672–678.

52. Sasso FC, Carbonara O, Persico M *et al*. Irbesartan reduces the albumin excretion rate in microalbuminuric type 2 diabetic patients independently of hypertension: a randomized double-blind placebo-controlled crossover study. *Diabetes Care* 2002; 25:1909–1913.

53. Zandbergen AA, Baggen MG, Lamberts SW, Bootsma AH, de Zeeuw D, Ouwendijk RJ. Effect of losartan on microalbuminuria in normotensive patients with type 2 diabetes mellitus. A randomized clinical trial. *Ann Intern Med* 2003; 139:90–96.

54. Makino H, Haneda M, Babazono T *et al*. The telmisartan renoprotective study from incipient nephropathy to overt nephropathy—rationale, study design, treatment plan and baseline characteristics of the incipient to overt: angiotensin II receptor blocker, telmisartan, Investigation on Type 2 Diabetic Nephropathy (INNOVATION) Study. *J Int Med Res* 2005; 33:677–686.

55. Makino H, Haneda M, Babazono T *et al*. Prevention of transition from incipient to overt nephropathy with telmisartan in patients with type 2 diabetes. *Diabetes Care* 2007; 30:1577–1578.

56. Vongterapak S, Dahlan W, Nakasatien S *et al*. Impediment of the progressions of microalbuminuria and hyperlipidemia in normotensive type 2 diabetes by low-dose ramipril. *J Med Assoc Thai* 1998; 81:671–681.

57. Cetinkalp SS, Karadeniz MM, Erdogan MA, Ozgen GA, Yilmaz CO. Short-term effects of irbesartan treatment on microalbuminuria in patients with normotensive type 2 diabetes. *Saudi Med J* 2008; 29:1414–1418.

58. Agha A, Bashir K, Anwar E. Use of losartan in reducing microalbuminuria in normotensive patients with type-2 diabetes mellitus. *Nepal Med Coll J* 2007; 9:79–83.

59. Kubba S, Agarwal SK, Prakash A, Puri V, Babbar R, Anuradha S. Effect of losartan on albuminuria, peripheral and autonomic neuropathy in normotensive microalbuminuric type 2 diabetics. *Neurol India* 2003; 51:355–358.

60. Patel A, Chalmers J, Poulter N. ADVANCE: action in diabetes and vascular disease. *J Hum Hypertens* 2005; 19:S27–S32.

61. Chalmers J, Perkovic V, Joshi R, Patel A. ADVANCE: breaking new ground in type 2 diabetes. *J Hypertens Suppl* 2006; 24:S22–S28.

62. Perkovic V, Joshi R, Patel A, Bompoint S, Chalmers J. ADVANCE: lessons from the run-in phase of a large study in type 2 diabetes. *Blood Press* 2006; 15:340–346.

63. de Galan BE, Perkovic V, Ninomiya T *et al*. Lowering Blood Pressure Reduces Renal Events in Type 2 Diabetes. *J Am Soc Nephrol* 2009; 20:883–892.

64. Patel A, MacMahon S, Chalmers J *et al*. Effects of a fixed combination of perindopril and indapamide on macrovascular and microvascular outcomes in patients with type 2 diabetes mellitus (the ADVANCE trial): a randomised controlled trial. *Lancet* 2007; 370:829–840.

65. Mogensen CE, Neldam S, Tikkanen I *et al*. Randomised controlled trial of dual blockade of renin-angiotensin system in patients with hypertension, microalbuminuria, and non-insulin dependent diabetes: the candesartan and lisinopril microalbuminuria (CALM) study. *BMJ* 2000; 321:1440–1444.

66. Rossing K, Christensen PK, Jensen BR, Parving HH. Dual blockade of the renin-angiotensin system in diabetic nephropathy: a randomized double-blind crossover study. *Diabetes Care* 2002; 25:95–100.

67. Jacobsen P, Andersen S, Rossing K, Hansen BV, Parving HH. Dual blockade of the renin-angiotensin system in type 1 patients with diabetic nephropathy. *Nephrol Dial Transplant* 2002; 17:1019–1024.

68. Jacobsen P, Andersen S, Jensen BR, Parving HH. Additive effect of ACE inhibition and angiotensin II receptor blockade in type I diabetic patients with diabetic nephropathy. *J Am Soc Nephrol* 2003; 14:992–999.

69. Jacobsen P, Andersen S, Rossing K, Jensen BR, Parving HH. Dual blockade of the renin-angiotensin system versus maximal recommended dose of ACE inhibition in diabetic nephropathy. *Kidney Int* 2003; 63:1874–1880.

70. Song JH, Lee SW, Suh JH *et al*. The effects of dual blockade of the renin-angiotensin system on urinary protein and transforming growth factor-beta excretion in 2 groups of patients with IgA and diabetic nephropathy. *Clin Nephrol* 2003; 60:318–326.

71. Rossing K, Jacobsen P, Pietraszek L, Parving HH. Renoprotective effects of adding angiotensin II receptor blocker to maximal recommended doses of ACE inhibitor in diabetic nephropathy: a randomized double-blind crossover trial. *Diabetes Care* 2003; 26:2268–2274.

72. Andersen NH, Poulsen PL, Knudsen ST *et al*. Long-term dual blockade with candesartan and lisinopril in hypertensive patients with diabetes: the CALM II study. *Diabetes Care* 2005; 28:273–277.

73. Toto R, Palmer BF. Rationale for combination angiotensin receptor blocker and angiotensin-converting enzyme inhibitor treatment and end-organ protection in patients with chronic kidney disease. *Am J Nephrol* 2008; 28:372–380.

74. Mori-Takeyama U, Minatoguchi S, Murata I *et al*. Dual blockade of the rennin-angiotensin system versus maximal recommended dose of angiotensin II receptor blockade in chronic glomerulonephritis. *Clin Exp Nephrol* 2008; 12:33–40.

75. Komine N, Khang S, Wead LM, Blantz RC, Gabbai FB. Effect of combining an ACE inhibitor and an angiotensin II receptor blocker on plasma and kidney tissue angiotensin II levels. *Am J Kidney Dis* 2002; 39:159–164.

76. Atmaca A, Gedik O. Effects of angiotensin-converting enzyme inhibitors, angiotensin II receptor blockers, and their combination on microalbuminuria in normotensive patients with type 2 diabetes. *Adv Ther* 2006; 23:615–622.

77. Doulton TW, Macgregor GA. Combination renin-angiotensin system blockade in hypertension. *Kidney Int* 2005; 68:1898.

78. Doulton TW, He FJ, MacGregor GA. Systematic review of combined angiotensin-converting enzyme inhibition and angiotensin receptor blockade in hypertension. *Hypertension* 2005; 45:880–886.

79. Cohn JN. Improving outcomes in congestive heart failure: Val-HeFT. Valsartan in Heart Failure Trial. *Cardiology* 1999; 91(suppl 1):19–22.

80. McMurray JJ, Ostergren J, Swedberg K *et al*. Effects of candesartan in patients with chronic heart failure and reduced left-ventricular systolic function taking angiotensin-converting-enzyme inhibitors: the CHARM-Added trial. *Lancet* 2003; 362:767–771.

81. Mogensen CE. Microalbuminuria and hypertension with focus on type 1 and type 2 diabetes. *J Intern Med* 2003; 254:45–66.

82. Peterson JC, Adler S, Burkart JM *et al*. Blood pressure control, proteinuria, and the progression of renal disease. The Modification of Diet in Renal Disease Study. *Ann Intern Med* 1995; 123:754–762.

83. Bakris GL, Williams M, Dworkin L *et al*. Preserving renal function in adults with hypertension and diabetes: a consensus approach. National Kidney Foundation Hypertension and Diabetes Executive Committees Working Group. *Am J Kidney Dis* 2000; 36:646–661.

84. Jafar TH, Schmid CH, Landa M *et al*. Angiotensin-converting enzyme inhibitors and progression of nondiabetic renal disease. A meta-analysis of patient-level data. *Ann Intern Med* 2001; 135:73–87.

85. Lewis EJ, Hunsicker LG, Clarke WR *et al*. Renoprotective effect of the angiotensin-receptor antagonist irbesartan in patients with nephropathy due to type 2 diabetes. *N Engl J Med* 2001; 345:851–860.

86. Brenner BM, Cooper ME, de Zeeuw D *et al*. Effects of losartan on renal and cardiovascular outcomes in patients with type 2 diabetes and nephropathy. *N Engl J Med* 2001; 345:861–869.

87. Parving HH, Lehnert H, Brochner-Mortensen J, Gomis R, Andersen S, Arner P. The effect of irbesartan on the development of diabetic nephropathy in patients with type 2 diabetes. *N Engl J Med* 2001; 345:870–878.

88. Ohkubo Y, Kishikawa H, Araki E *et al*. Intensive insulin therapy prevents the progression of diabetic microvascular complications in Japanese patients with non-insulin-dependent diabetes mellitus: a randomized prospective 6-year study. *Diabetes Res Clin Pract* 1995; 28:103–117.

89. Yuyun MF, Dinneen SF, Edwards OM, Wood E, Wareham NJ. Absolute level and rate of change of albuminuria over 1 year independently predict mortality and cardiovascular events in patients with diabetic nephropathy. *Diabet Med* 2003; 20:277–282.

90. Ibsen H, Olsen MH, Wachtell K *et al*. Does albuminuria predict cardiovascular outcomes on treatment with losartan versus atenolol in patients with diabetes, hypertension, and left ventricular hypertrophy? The LIFE study. *Diabetes Care* 2006; 29:595–600.

91. Kidney Disease Outcomes Quality Initiative (K/DOQI). *Am J Kidney Dis* 2004; 43(suppl 1):S1–S290.

92. Parving HH, Persson F, Lewis JB, Lewis EJ, Hollenberg NK. Aliskiren combined with losartan in type 2 diabetes and nephropathy. *N Engl J Med* 2008; 358:2433–2446.

93. Schernthaner G. Dual inhibition with losartan and aliskiren: a promising therapeutic option for type 2 diabetic nephropathy? *Nat Clin Pract Nephrol* 2008; 4:656–657.

94. Effect of intensive blood-glucose control with metformin on complications in overweight patients with type 2 diabetes (UKPDS 34). UK Prospective Diabetes Study (UKPDS) Group. *Lancet* 1998; 352:854–865.

95. Intensive blood-glucose control with sulphonylureas or insulin compared with conventional treatment and risk of complications in patients with type 2 diabetes (UKPDS 33). UK Prospective Diabetes Study (UKPDS) Group. *Lancet* 1998; 352:837–853.

96. Gerstein HC, Miller ME, Byington RP *et al*. Effects of intensive glucose lowering in type 2 diabetes. *N Engl J Med* 2008; 358:2545–2559.

97. Duckworth W, Abraira C, Moritz T *et al*. Glucose control and vascular complications in veterans with type 2 diabetes. *N Engl J Med* 2009; 360:129–139.

98. Cefalu WT. Glycemic targets and cardiovascular disease. *N Engl J Med* 2008; 358:2633–2635.

99. Dluhy RG, McMahon GT. Intensive glycemic control in the ACCORD and ADVANCE trials. *N Engl J Med* 2008; 358:2630–2633.

100. Pijls LT, de Vries H, Donker AJ, van Eijk JT. The effect of protein restriction on albuminuria in patients with type 2 diabetes mellitus: a randomized trial. *Nephrol Dial Transplant* 1999; 14:1445–1453.

101. Pedrini MT, Levey AS, Lau J, Chalmers TC, Wang PH. The effect of dietary protein restriction on the progression of diabetic and nondiabetic renal diseases: a meta-analysis. *Ann Intern Med* 1996; 124:627–632.
102. Hansen HP, Tauber-Lassen E, Jensen BR, Parving HH. Effect of dietary protein restriction on prognosis in patients with diabetic nephropathy. *Kidney Int* 2002; 62:220–228.
103. Kasiske BL, Lakatua JD, Ma JZ, Louis TA. A meta-analysis of the effects of dietary protein restriction on the rate of decline in renal function. *Am J Kidney Dis* 1998; 31:954–961.
104. Phisitkul K, Hegazy K, Chuahirun T *et al.* Continued smoking exacerbates but cessation ameliorates progression of early type 2 diabetic nephropathy. *Am J Med Sci* 2008; 335:284–291.
105. Gambaro G, Bax G, Fusaro M *et al.* Cigarette smoking is a risk factor for nephropathy and its progression in type 2 diabetes mellitus. *Diabetes Nutr Metab* 2001; 14:337–342.
106. Tapp RJ, Shaw JE, Zimmet PZ *et al.* Albuminuria is evident in the early stages of diabetes onset: results from the Australian Diabetes, Obesity, and Lifestyle Study (AusDiab). *Am J Kidney Dis* 2004; 44:792–798.
107. Meisinger C, Heier M, Landgraf R, Happich M, Wichmann HE, Piehlmeier W. Albuminuria, cardiovascular risk factors and disease management in subjects with type 2 diabetes: a cross sectional study. *BMC Health Serv Res* 2008; 8:226.
108. Agrawal V, Khan I, Rai B *et al.* The effect of weight loss after bariatric surgery on albuminuria. *Clin Nephrol* 2008; 70:194–202.
109. Woo J, Sea MM, Tong P *et al.* Effectiveness of a lifestyle modification programme in weight maintenance in obese subjects after cessation of treatment with Orlistat. *J Eval Clin Pract* 2007; 13:853–859.
110. Saiki A, Nagayama D, Ohhira M *et al.* Effect of weight loss using formula diet on renal function in obese patients with diabetic nephropathy. *Int J Obes (Lond)* 2005; 29:1115–1120.
111. Gaede P, Valentine WJ, Palmer AJ *et al.* Cost-effectiveness of intensified versus conventional multifactorial intervention in type 2 diabetes: results and projections from the Steno-2 study. *Diabetes Care* 2008; 31:1510–1515.

4

Should south Asians with type 2 diabetes have lower treatment targets?

S. Bellary

BACKGROUND

It is estimated that by 2025 there will be 330 million people globally with diabetes [1]. Nearly a quarter of these will be in the Indian subcontinent alone and there is growing concern that even this figure may be an underestimation. Diabetes is the leading cause of end-stage renal disease (ESRD), blindness, and lower limb amputations [2]. Diabetes also significantly increases the risk of macrovascular complications and is a major risk factor for coronary artery disease and stroke [3]. The cost of diabetes and its complications is therefore huge [3, 4].

Diabetes often tends to co-exist with other metabolic abnormalities such as visceral obesity, dyslipidaemia and hypertension [5]. These risk factors have all been shown to increase the risk of complications in people with diabetes. The overall burden of these risk factors, however, varies between populations, and people of certain ethnicities, such as south Asians, appear to more susceptible than others to complications [6, 7]. While there is little doubt that aggressive management of these risk factors is essential to reduce the burden of the long-term complications, it is not clear if the targets for intervention determined from studies in one ethnic group apply to people of all ethnicities equally [6].

ETHNIC DIFFERENCES IN DIABETES AND CARDIOVASCULAR DISEASE

There is considerable variation in the prevalence of diabetes among different ethnic groups. Studies in migrants of south Asian origin in the United Kingdom and North America suggest that the prevalence rates are particularly high among people of south Asian origin compared to those of white European ethnicity [8, 9]. In the UK, south Asians constitute about 4% of the population. The overall prevalence of diabetes in this ethnic group is around 20%, which is four to six times that observed in the local white European population [9] (Figure 4.1). There is also considerable heterogeneity within the south Asian population, with the prevalence being highest among Bangladeshis, followed by those of Pakistani and Indian origin [10]. Migration, increased life expectancy, and westernized lifestyle have been important contributors to this increased prevalence. A similar trend is emerging in the native countries following recent economic growth, plus increasing urbanization and more sedentary lifestyles. The prevalence of diabetes in the urban Indian population is now estimated to be around 15% with rates in the rural population also increasing [11, 12].

Srikanth Bellary, MD, MRCP (UK), Senior Lecturer and Consultant Physician, Life and Health Sciences, University of Aston; Department of Diabetes, Heart of England NHS Foundation Trust, Birmingham, UK.

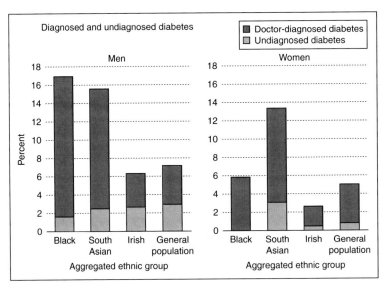

Figure 4.1 Prevalence of diagnosed and undiagnosed diabetes in different ethnic groups in the United Kingdom Health Survey for England, Health of Ethnic Minorities, 2004 (with permission from [10]).

The increased susceptibility to diabetes in south Asians appears to be determined by both environmental and genetic influences. Definitive characterization of genetic susceptibility in south Asians, however, has been difficult largely due to the paucity of genetic studies and the heterogeneity within the population itself. Although the search for genetic differences is ongoing, so far data from published studies have not identified any significant genetic differences between south Asians and other Asian groups [13]. There is, however, indirect evidence that increased susceptibility to insulin resistance and diabetes in south Asians may be genetically determined. Diabetes in south Asians tends to occur early and there is often a strong family history with more than one first-degree relative affected with diabetes, suggesting a strong genetic component. Studies in south Asian children have shown that features such as insulin resistance and visceral obesity present as early as infancy [14]. Recent studies in south Asian pregnant women have shown that maternal malnutrition is associated with development of insulin resistance in babies – an adaptive response to the adverse intrauterine environment [15]. The gene–environment interaction therefore appears to starts very early in south Asians.

Genetic predisposition alone, however, does not fully explain the excess susceptibility to diabetes in south Asians. There is now sufficient evidence to suggest that environmental factors play a much more significant role. A classic example is the relatively higher prevalence of diabetes among migrant south Asians compared to those living in native countries, following exposure to a high-calorie diet and sedentary lifestyle [16]. Studies in migrant Asians have shown that physical activity levels are typically low in south Asians compared to those of white European or afro-Caribbean origins [10, 17]. A report from the Health Survey of England on the health of ethnic minorities identified that less than a third of the people of south Asian origin participated in exercise such as walking for 30 minutes four times a week [10]. Similarly low levels of exercise have been reported by other groups [17]. Although average consumption of fresh fruit and vegetables is higher in migrant south Asians, much of the nutrient value is lost due to excessive cooking [10]. In addition, unhealthy cooking practices such as the use of 'ghee', poor of knowledge of disease, cultural practices and economic deprivation also contribute to the increased risk of diabetes.

Table 4.1 Numbers of deaths and IHD (ICD–10, I20–I25) SMRs by sex and country of birth for people aged ≥20 years (with permission from [20])

Country of birth	Men		Women	
	No. of deaths	SMR (95% CI)	No. of deaths	SMR (95% CI)
England and Wales	149 950	96 (96–97)	125 289	97 (96–97)
Scotland	3813	104 (100–107)	2767	107 (103–111)
Bangladesh	409	175 (158–193)	97	167 (136–204)
India	2528	131 (126–137)	1672	149 (142–157)
Pakistan	1044	162 (152–172)	454	174 (159–192)

CI = confidence interval; IHD = ischaemic heart disease; SMR = standardized mortality rate.

Prevalence of cardiovascular disease (CVD) in south Asians is much higher compared to that observed in white Europeans [18]. The standardized mortality rate in people of south Asian origin living in the UK is 1.5 to 2 times greater than in the local white population [19] (Table 4.1). Diabetes is a major risk factor for CVD and increases the risk of CHD death by up to three times compared to those without diabetes [7, 20]. Although there is a paucity of data from south Asian countries, CVD is thought to be responsible for nearly a quarter of the deaths in this population [21]. A Canadian study comparing CVD in different racial groups showed that south Asians were particularly prone to CVD despite having less atherosclerosis [22]. A popular theory for this excess risk of CVD in south Asians is the coexistence of multiple risk factors in the same individual. Features of metabolic syndrome (presence of visceral obesity, impaired glucose tolerance, hypertension, raised triglycerides, and low high-density lipoprotein [HDL] in the same individual) are more common in people of south Asian ethnicity [23]. Data from the International Diabetes Federation suggest that up to 40% of urban Indians have metabolic syndrome and that this figure rises to over 70% in those with diabetes. The presence of metabolic syndrome has been associated with increased risk of both diabetes and CVD, suggesting that these two diseases may in fact share a common aetiology [24].

The pattern of dyslipidaemia is also very distinct in south Asians. Despite the reportedly lower levels of total cholesterol, lipid profiles of south Asians are typically characterized by high triglycerides, low HDL levels and elevated apolipoprotein (apo)B/apoA ratios [25]. In fact, in the INTERHEART study the elevated apoB/apoA ratio was the most significant contributor to the increased cardiovascular risk in south Asians [26] (Table 4.2). Recently, several novel risk factors such as plasminogen activator inhibitor-1 (PAI-1), fibrinogen, homocysteine and high-sensitivity C-reactive protein (CRP) have been identified as independent markers of cardiovascular risk [27]. Cross-sectional studies have found that these factors are elevated in south Asians [28]. The role of these factors, however, has not been validated in prospective studies and the benefits of modifying these risk factors are at present not clear.

Microvascular complications in south Asians
Among the microvascular complications, nephropathy is the most studied in south Asians with diabetes. This probably reflects the disproportionately higher prevalence of end-stage renal disease in this population, which is not explained merely by the excess prevalence of diabetes [29, 30]. Various studies have estimated the prevalence of microalbuminuria in south Asians to be between 30–40% [31–35] (Table 4.3). A study comparing prevalence of microalbuminuria in different ethnic groups in the UK found that microalbuminuria was present in up to 40% of south Asians [34]. In a study from south India, the crude prevalence

Table 4.2 Comparison of the nine major risk factors for acute myocardial infarction in individuals from South Asia and other countries – the INTERHEART study (adapted with permission from [28])

Risk factor	Cases (%)	Controls (%)	Odds ratio (95% CI)
Diabetes			
Other countries	18.2	7.2	3.20 (2.93–3.50)
South Asia	20.2	9.5	2.52 (2.07–3.07)
Hypertension			
Other countries	40.5	23.6	2.44 (2.30–2.60)
South Asia	29.6	12.7	2.92 (2.46–3.48)
ApoB/ApoA			
Other countries	48.3	31.8	3.01 (2.77–3.26)
South Asia	61.5	43.8	2.57 (2.03–3.26)
High waist-to-hip ratio			
Other countries	46.7	34.0	2.21 (2.06–2.38)
South Asia	44.0	29.6	2.44 (2.05–2.91)
Exercise (moderate or high intensity)			
Other countries	15.8	21.6	0.70 (0.65–0.76)
South Asia	4.6	6.1	0.72 (0.53–0.97)
Smoking (current and former)			
Other countries	65.7	49.4	2.22 (2.09–2.36)
South Asia	61.6	40.8	2.57 (2.22–2.96)
Psychosocial factors			
Other countries	84.2	82.0	1.83 (1.58–2.13)
South Asia	86.0	82.6	2.62 (1.76–3.90)
Alcohol consumption >once/week			
Other countries	25.7	26.9	0.79 (0.74–0.85)
South Asia	13.3	10.7	1.06 (0.85–1.30)
Consumption of fruit and vegetables			
Other countries	38.3	45.2	0.70 (0.65–0.76)
South Asia	20.0	26.5	0.65 (0.53–0.81)

of microalbuminuria was 36% [36]. Interestingly, in another study, microalbuminuria was present in up to a quarter of the subjects with newly diagnosed diabetes [37]. Similarly, higher rates of microalbuminuria in people of south Asian origin have been reported in studies from other countries [38]. Not all studies, however, have reported higher prevalence. In the United Kingdom Prospective Diabetes Study (UKPDS), no differences in the prevalence of microalbuminuria were observed and another study reported prevalence to be the same in south Asians and white Europeans [39]. These disparities in quoted prevalence may have arisen due to the differences in duration of diabetes and the sizes of populations studied. There is also some inconsistency in the reported rates of decline in glomerular filtration rate (GFR). While one study reported faster progression in south Asians with diabetes, no significant difference was found in another study [38, 40]. Despite these inconsistencies, however, it is generally accepted that south Asians have a greater risk of diabetic renal disease.

It is not entirely clear why south Asians should have an increased susceptibility to renal disease. South Asians have much higher rates of ESRD than white Europeans and diabetes accounts for the majority of these cases. Although ethnicity itself may be an independent risk factor, however, traditional risk factors such as hypertension, diabetes duration and glycaemic control are all strong predictors for development of microalbuminuria and nephropathy [37]. While blood pressure (BP) is acknowledged as an important risk factor for

Table 4.3 Studies showing the prevalence of microalbuminuria in south Asians versus white Europeans

Author(s) [Ref]	Study population	Comparison groups	% with microalbuminuria
Mather et al [34]	Diabetes	South Asian vs. white European	40 vs. 33 (Men) 33 vs. 19 (Women)
UKPDS Group [39]	Diabetes	South Asian vs. white European	18 vs. 19 (Men) 17 vs. 23 (Women)
Varghese et al [36]	Diabetes	South Asian (south Indian only)	32.1 (Men) 39.9 (Women)
Fischbacher et al [32]	Non-diabetic and diabetic	South Asian vs. white European	12.7 vs. 6.6
Dixon et al [31]	Diabetes	South Asian vs. white European	31 vs. 20

progression of nephropathy, the ideal BP threshold below which this risk decreases is not known. Data from the pilot phase of the United Kingdom Asian Diabetes Study (UKADS) certainly suggest that this threshold is probably lower in south Asians [31]. Lower targets for BP in these individuals may therefore be needed in order to limit the progression of nephropathy.

In contrast to nephropathy, data on other microvascular complications in south Asians are limited. Differences in methodology and the population screened make it difficult to estimate the true prevalence but reports from various studies suggest that the prevalence of diabetic retinopathy is between 20–27% [41]. This figure is lower than that reported in those of white European origin [42]. However, a recent report from the UKADS suggested the prevalence of retinopathy in south Asians to be as high as 40% [43]. Duration of diabetes, BP and glycaemic control appear to be the main factors that influence the severity of diabetic retinopathy [44]. Aggressive risk factor control therefore appears to be the mainstay for the management of these patients.

Application of treatment targets to south Asians

Susceptibility to disease is determined by several factors including genetic, environmental, cultural and economic factors. As these vary between ethnic groups, there is much difficulty in applying targets based on studies in people from one ethnic group to others. In south Asians, this has proven more difficult due to the lack of large randomized controlled trials and poor representation in clinical trials. As more data emerge and the differences between ethnic groups become more apparent, the need for ethnic-specific targets is being recognized. A typical example is the cut-off values for body mass index (BMI) used to define obesity. Comparative studies in south Asians and other racial groups have shown that even at lower BMIs, south Asians have greater visceral obesity and insulin resistance. Applying the same cut-off values for BMI used in Europeans would significantly underestimate obesity in south Asians. Ethnic-specific cut-offs are therefore required to correct this anomaly [45].

Many studies comparing the risk factors between south Asians and white Europeans have identified important differences between these two groups. A meta-analysis of the studies comparing prevalence of hypertension showed that south Asians had a lower systolic blood pressure and similar or higher diastolic blood pressure than in white Europeans [46]. Comparison of risk factors among patients recruited to the UKPDS showed that south Asians had lower blood pressures compared with Afro-Caribbeans but similar values to those observed in white Europeans [39]. The average systolic blood pressure reported in most studies in south Asians is lower than the recommended target in UK general practice

[47]. It is clear that even at lower BP values the risk of cardiovascular events and nephropathy is much higher in south Asians. Given that even a small reduction in BP offers significant protection from cardiovascular events, a lower target in this population could well be justified. Similarly, studies comparing lipid profiles have shown that south Asians have lower total cholesterol levels. Despite the low levels of total cholesterol, south Asians typically have elevated triglycerides, low HDL levels and raised apoB/apoA ratios [28]. Using total cholesterol level as a target would therefore fail to identify most patients with adverse lipid profiles. Interestingly, despite many guidelines stating that all patients with diabetes should be on statins, only a small proportion of south Asians appear to be prescribed them [47, 48]. Thus, a target-driven approach might result in under-treatment, particularly if it does not adequately reflect the needs of a population.

Many studies have compared the accuracy of risk engines in estimating the cardiovascular risk among different ethnic groups [49]. In a study comparing predicted mortality rates with standardized mortality in south Asians, the risk engines were shown to underestimate the risk. Another study concluded that both the Framingham equation and FINRISK predicted observed mortality rates correctly [50]. The validity of these risk engines in south Asians can only be established by prospective studies, but in the interim, adding 10 years to the age may be a simple option to correct these differences.

A consistent observation in most studies involving south Asians has been the younger age of onset of both diabetes and CVD in south Asians. As the disease process may begin well before diabetes is diagnosed, these individuals are exposed to the risk factors for longer. Furthermore, some of the complications may be well-established even at diagnosis and could explain the excess morbidity and mortality observed in this ethnic group. It is essential that treatment targets should reflect this excess risk from long-term exposure. There are no exclusive trials in south Asians to assess the benefits of intensive glycaemic control. In the UKPDS and ADVANCE studies, however, south Asians treated intensively had similar reductions in microvascular complications to other ethnic groups [51, 52].

NEW APPROACHES TO MANAGEMENT

While the genetic mechanisms of type 2 diabetes and CVD are yet to be unravelled, there is ample evidence now to suggest that disease modification through control of risk factors is associated with significant reduction in long-term complications. Known risk factors still account for more than 80% of risk for CVD and this is true regardless of ethnicity [26]. However, as risk profiles and risk burden differ between ethnic groups, management strategies should be tailored to the needs of each ethnic group.

Two main approaches can be considered in tackling the problem of excess risk of diabetes and CVD in south Asians – early intervention and lower targets.

Primary prevention

As discussed earlier in the chapter, both diabetes and CVD occur 5–10 years earlier in south Asians. It is now well known that insulin resistance can be present very early and most individuals have features of metabolic syndrome even before the diagnosis of diabetes is made. Normal glucose tolerance, impaired glucose tolerance (IGT) and diabetes represent different states in a continuum and it is likely that the risks of CVD and death increase progressively during the transition from one stage to the other [53]. Epidemiological studies have shown a linear relationship between blood glucose and the risk of macrovascular disease, and there is no threshold identified at which this risk becomes non-existent [53]. This is supported by the presence of varying degrees of glucose intolerance in patients with myocardial infarction [54]. It can be argued, therefore, that aggressive management of risk factors at this early stage could protect against future cardiovascular events.

In contrast, the relationship between microvascular complications and glycaemia is less linear. The risk of microvascular complications is known to increase significantly once blood sugars are within the diabetic range [53]. However, the presence of microvascular complications in patients with IGT and in newly diagnosed diabetes patients would strongly support that this threshold is probably much lower than previously thought.

The prevalence of microvascular complications in south Asians is high, suggesting that the diagnosis of diabetes is often delayed and earlier diagnosis would facilitate aggressive treatment of hyperglycaemia in these individuals. Treatment of hyperglycaemia to near-normal levels of HbA1c is associated with substantial reductions in the risk of microvascular complications and this appears to be regardless of ethnicity [51, 52]. Moreover, recent evidence from the UKPDS trial suggests that the benefits of intensive treatment in the early years are associated with long-term benefits for both microvascular and macrovascular complications – the so-called metabolic memory effect [55]. The case for early detection and management could therefore not be more persuasive.

Early detection of disease depends on effective screening strategies. With diabetes this has proven very difficult. Mass screening is clearly not cost-effective and targeted screening has its own limitations [56]. Although several population-based risk scores have been proposed to increase rates of detection, these are specific to populations studied and cannot be universally applied. Moreover, the rates of progression from normal glucose tolerance to IGT and diabetes vary considerably between populations and it is not clear how often individuals have to be re-screened. There are no clear data to suggest the ideal age to screen for diabetes in south Asians [56]. High prevalence of glucose abnormalities and earlier onset would suggest screening in high-risk individuals should begin as early as 30 years of age. Controversy remains as to how these patients are then best managed and whether there is a role for pharmacological intervention, but hopefully this will be answered by some of the ongoing trials [57, 58]. Despite these limitations, early screening offers the best chance of detecting individuals with a risk of diabetes and macrovascular disease and a lower threshold must therefore be applied to screen south Asians for diabetes.

Secondary prevention

While screening and early intervention are appropriate primary prevention strategies, risk factor control still appears to be the most effective strategy for secondary prevention. Many clinical trials have shown that effective risk factor control reduces risk of complications significantly. Evidence from the BP and statin trials suggests that even a modest reduction in these risk factors could offer substantial protection from CVD [59–62]. Similarly, data from the UKPDS and other diabetes studies have shown that even a small decrease in HbA1c is associated with significant reduction in microvascular complications [59, 62]. As a result, there has been a greater emphasis on multiple risk factor interventions. The targets derived from these studies are often used to make treatment decisions. Risk factors, however, operate in a continuum and it is often difficult to identify precisely a point below which the risk becomes negligible. A target-driven approach may therefore fail to identify those with modest risk.

A significant proportion of south Asians have BP and lipid levels lower than the recommended targets. Even at these lower levels they appear to have greater susceptibility to diabetes and its complications. Applying lower targets specific to south Asians will have two major benefits. Firstly, it will increase the proportion of those with modest risk receiving treatment. Secondly, it will allow those individuals who are at greater risk, and who may have already been receiving treatment, to be treated more aggressively. Such an approach would ensure that south Asians who are at a modest risk receive important treatments such as statins and ACE inhibitors [58, 63]. As BP is a major risk factor for CVD and microvascular disease, these lower targets, if achieved, can be hoped to significantly reduce the mortality and morbidity in this group. Recent evidence shows that treating to tighter glycaemic targets can lower the risk of microvascular complications [52]. Given the increased susceptibility of south Asians to microvascular complications there is a greater need to achieve these targets. Aiming for lower glycaemic targets will also help intensification of treatments and early use of insulin in patients with diabetes.

Recommendations

The paucity of large randomized controlled trials in south Asians makes it difficult to set definitive treatment targets for this ethnic group. Indirect evidence from studies in the healthy rural Indian population, however, would suggest that the targets for BP, lipids and glycaemic control should be lower than currently recommended. Accordingly, a BP of 125/75 mmHg, total cholesterol of 4 mmol/l and HbA1c of 6.5% might be considered appropriate. These lower targets can also be justified on the basis of hypertension and lipid trials which have shown continued benefit in individuals treated to lower targets compared to those treated to higher targets. There is no doubt a great need for more randomized studies in south Asians to establish the benefits of intensive risk factor treatment but the decision to treat those at risk must not be delayed for want of such studies.

Intensive treatment strategies obviously raise concerns about safety. Achieving the recommended BP and cholesterol levels would often require the use of two or more agents. As the number of medications increases there is also an increased risk of adverse effects and drug interactions. Similarly, intensive treatments to achieve tighter glycaemic control can be associated with increased risk of hypoglycaemia. Fortunately, however, data from the major trials show that most available agents are well-tolerated and that availability of new therapies should hopefully overcome some of the other problems in the future.

SUMMARY

The disproportionately higher rates of diabetes and cardiovascular disease in the south Asian population remains a major concern. Although ethnicity itself may be an important contributor, a greater proportion of this excess risk can be attributed to known risk factors. At present there is insufficient evidence to advocate lower treatment targets for south Asians but there is little doubt that a more aggressive approach towards control of risk factors is needed if better clinical outcomes are to be achieved. Whilst risk factor management remains the mainstay in those with established disease, there is also a need for effective preventative strategies.

REFERENCES

1. King H, Aubert RE, Herman WH. Global burden of diabetes, 1995–2025: prevalence, numerical estimates, and projections. *Diabetes Care* 1998; 21:1414–1431.
2. Boulton AJ, Vileikyte L, Ragnarson-Tennvall G, Apelqvist J. The global burden of diabetic foot disease. *Lancet* 2005; 366:1719–1724.
3. Klein R. Hyperglycemia and microvascular and macrovascular disease in diabetes. *Diabetes Care* 1995; 18:258–268.
4. Economic costs of diabetes in the U.S. in 2007. *Diabetes Care* 2008; 31:596–615.
5. International Diabetes Federation. The IDF Consensus worldwide definition of the metabolic syndrome. 2007. 10–8–2007. Ref type: internet communication.
6. Barnett AH, Dixon AN, Bellary S et al. Type 2 diabetes and cardiovascular risk in the UK south Asian community. *Diabetologia* 2006; 49:2234–2246.
7. Chaturvedi N, Fuller JH. Ethnic differences in mortality from cardiovascular disease in the UK: do they persist in people with diabetes? *J Epidemiol Community Health* 1996; 50:137–139.
8. Lipscombe LL, Hux JE. Trends in diabetes prevalence, incidence, and mortality in Ontario, Canada 1995–2005: a population-based study. *Lancet* 2007; 369:750–756.

9. Mather HM, Keen H. The Southall Diabetes Survey: prevalence of known diabetes in Asians and Europeans. *Br Med J (Clin Res Ed)* 1985; 291:1081–1084.
10. Health Survey for England 2004: Health of Ethnic Minorities – Full Report. 21–2–2008. Ref type: internet communication.
11. Ramachandran A, Snehalatha C, Latha E, Vijay V, Viswanathan M. Rising prevalence of NIDDM in an urban population in India. *Diabetologia* 1997; 40:232–237.
12. Mohan V, Deepa M, Deepa R *et al*. Secular trends in the prevalence of diabetes and impaired glucose tolerance in urban South India—the Chennai Urban Rural Epidemiology Study (CURES-17). *Diabetologia* 2006; 49:1175–1178.
13. Radha V, Mohan V. Genetic predisposition to type 2 diabetes among Asian Indians. *Indian J Med Res* 2007; 125:259–274.
14. Krishnaveni GV, Hill JC, Veena SR *et al*. Truncal adiposity is present at birth and in early childhood in South Indian children. *Indian Pediatr* 2005; 42:527–538.
15. Yajnik CS, Deshpande SS, Jackson AA *et al*. Vitamin B12 and folate concentrations during pregnancy and insulin resistance in the offspring: the Pune Maternal Nutrition Study. *Diabetologia* 2008; 51:29–38.
16. Mather HM, Verma NP, Mehta SP, Madhu S, Keen H. The prevalence of known diabetes in Indians in New Delhi and London. *J Med Assoc Thai* 1987; 70(suppl 2):54–58.
17. Fischbacher CM, Hunt S, Alexander L. How physically active are South Asians in the United Kingdom? A literature review. *J Public Health (Oxf)* 2004; 26:250–258.
18. Reddy KS, Yusuf S. Emerging epidemic of cardiovascular disease in developing countries. *Circulation* 1998; 97:596–601.
19. Wild SH, Fischbacher C, Brock A, Griffiths C, Bhopal R. Mortality from all causes and circulatory disease by country of birth in England and Wales 2001–2003. *J Public Health (Oxf)* 2007; 29:191–198.
20. Forouhi NG, Sattar N, Tillin T, McKeigue PM, Chaturvedi N. Do known risk factors explain the higher coronary heart disease mortality in South Asian compared with European men? Prospective follow-up of the Southall and Brent studies, UK. *Diabetologia* 2006; 49:2580–2588.
21. Yusuf S, Reddy S, Ounpuu S, Anand S. Global burden of cardiovascular diseases: Part II: variations in cardiovascular disease by specific ethnic groups and geographic regions and prevention strategies. *Circulation* 2001; 104:2855–2864.
22. Anand SS, Yusuf S, Vuksan V *et al*. Differences in risk factors, atherosclerosis, and cardiovascular disease between ethnic groups in Canada: the Study of Health Assessment and Risk in Ethnic groups (SHARE). *Lancet* 2000; 356:279–284.
23. Tillin T, Forouhi N, Johnston DG, McKeigue PM, Chaturvedi N, Godsland IF. Metabolic syndrome and coronary heart disease in South Asians, African-Caribbeans and white Europeans: a UK population-based cross-sectional study. *Diabetologia* 2005; 48:649–656.
24. Lebovitz HE. Insulin resistance—a common link between type 2 diabetes and cardiovascular disease. *Diabetes Obes Metab* 2006; 8:237–249.
25. Kulkarni KR, Markovitz JH, Nanda NC, Segrest JP. Increased prevalence of smaller and denser LDL particles in Asian Indians. *Arterioscler Thromb Vasc Biol* 1999; 19:2749–2755.
26. Yusuf S, Hawken S, Ounpuu S *et al*. Effect of potentially modifiable risk factors associated with myocardial infarction in 52 countries (the INTERHEART study): case-control study. *Lancet* 2004; 364:937–952.
27. Anand SS, Razak F, Yi Q *et al*. C-reactive protein as a screening test for cardiovascular risk in a multiethnic population. *Arterioscler Thromb Vasc Biol* 2004; 24:1509–1515.
28. Joshi P, Islam S, Pais P *et al*. Risk factors for early myocardial infarction in South Asians compared with individuals in other countries. *JAMA* 2007; 297:286–294.
29. Burden AC, McNally PG, Feehally J, Walls J. Increased incidence of end-stage renal failure secondary to diabetes mellitus in Asian ethnic groups in the United Kingdom. *Diabet Med* 1992; 9:641–645.
30. Chandie Shaw PK, Vandenbroucke JP, Tjandra YI *et al*. Increased end-stage diabetic nephropathy in Indo-Asian immigrants living in the Netherlands. *Diabetologia* 2002; 45:337–341.
31. Dixon AN, Raymond NT, Mughal S *et al*. Prevalence of microalbuminuria and hypertension in South Asians and white Europeans with type 2 diabetes: a report from the United Kingdom Asian Diabetes Study (UKADS). *Diab Vasc Dis Res* 2006; 3:22–25.
32. Fischbacher CM, Bhopal R, Rutter MK *et al*. Microalbuminuria is more frequent in South Asian than in European origin populations: a comparative study in Newcastle, UK. *Diabet Med* 2003; 20:31–36.
33. Marshall SM. Recent advances in diabetic nephropathy. *Postgrad Med J* 2004; 80:624–633.

34. Mather HM, Chaturvedi N, Kehely AM. Comparison of prevalence and risk factors for microalbuminuria in South Asians and Europeans with type 2 diabetes mellitus. *Diabet Med* 1998; 15:672–677.

35. Wu AY, Kong NC, de Leon FA *et al*. An alarmingly high prevalence of diabetic nephropathy in Asian type 2 diabetic patients: the MicroAlbuminuria Prevalence (MAP) Study. *Diabetologia* 2005; 48:17–26.

36. Varghese A, Deepa R, Rema M, Mohan V. Prevalence of microalbuminuria in type 2 diabetes mellitus at a diabetes centre in southern India. *Postgrad Med J* 2001; 77:399–402.

37. Unnikrishnan RI, Rema M, Pradeepa R *et al*. Prevalence and risk factors of diabetic nephropathy in an urban South Indian population: the Chennai Urban Rural Epidemiology Study (CURES 45). *Diabetes Care* 2007; 30:2019–2024.

38. Chandie Shaw PK, Baboe F, van Es LA *et al*. South-Asian type 2 diabetic patients have higher incidence and faster progression of renal disease compared with Dutch-European diabetic patients. *Diabetes Care* 2006; 29:1383–1385.

39. UK Prospective Diabetes Study Group. UK Prospective Diabetes Study. XII: Differences between Asian, Afro-Caribbean and white Caucasian type 2 diabetic patients at diagnosis of diabetes. *Diabet Med* 1994; 11:670–677.

40. Koppiker N, Feehally J, Raymond N, Abrams KR, Burden AC. Rate of decline in renal function in Indo-Asians and Whites with diabetic nephropathy. *Diabet Med* 1998; 15:60–65.

41. Rema M, Premkumar S, Anitha B, Deepa R, Pradeepa R, Mohan V. Prevalence of diabetic retinopathy in urban India: the Chennai Urban Rural Epidemiology Study (CURES) eye study I. *Invest Ophthalmol Vis Sci* 2005; 46:2328–2333.

42. Stratton IM, Kohner EM, Aldington SJ *et al*. UKPDS 50: risk factors for incidence and progression of retinopathy in Type II diabetes over 6 years from diagnosis. *Diabetologia* 2001; 44:156–163.

43. Raymond NT, Varadhan L, Reynold DR *et al*. Higher prevalence of retinopathy in diabetic patients of South Asian ethnicity compared with white Europeans in the community: a cross-sectional study. *Diabetes Care* 2009; 32:410–415.

44. Pradeepa R, Anitha B, Mohan V, Ganesan A, Rema M. Risk factors for diabetic retinopathy in a South Indian Type 2 diabetic population—the Chennai Urban Rural Epidemiology Study (CURES) Eye Study 4. *Diabet Med* 2008; 25:536–542.

45. WHO Expert Consultation. Appropriate body-mass index for Asian populations and its implications for policy and intervention strategies. *Lancet* 2004; 363:157–163.

46. Agyemang C, Bhopal RS. Is the blood pressure of South Asian adults in the UK higher or lower than that in European white adults? A review of cross-sectional data. *J Hum Hypertens* 2002; 16:739–751.

47. Khunti K, Gadsby R, Millett C, Majeed A, Davies M. Quality of diabetes care in the UK: comparison of published quality-of-care reports with results of the Quality and Outcomes Framework for Diabetes. *Diabet Med* 2007; 24:1436–1441.

48. Bellary S, O'Hare JP, Raymond NT *et al*. Enhanced diabetes care to patients of south Asian ethnic origin (the United Kingdom Asian Diabetes Study): a cluster randomised controlled trial. *Lancet* 2008; 371:1769–1776.

49. Aarabi M, Jackson PR. Predicting coronary risk in UK South Asians: an adjustment method for Framingham-based tools. *Eur J Cardiovasc Prev Rehabil* 2005; 12:46–51.

50. Bhopal R, Fischbacher C, Vartiainen E, Unwin N, White M, Alberti G. Predicted and observed cardiovascular disease in South Asians: application of FINRISK, Framingham and SCORE models to Newcastle Heart Project data. *J Public Health (Oxf)* 2005; 27:93–100.

51. UK Prospective Diabetes Study (UKPDS) Group. Intensive blood-glucose control with sulphonylureas or insulin compared with conventional treatment and risk of complications in patients with type 2 diabetes (UKPDS 33). *Lancet* 1998; 352:837–853.

52. Patel A, MacMahon S, Chalmers J *et al*. Intensive blood glucose control and vascular outcomes in patients with type 2 diabetes. *N Engl J Med* 2008; 358:2560–2572.

53. Unwin N, Shaw J, Zimmet P, Alberti KG. Impaired glucose tolerance and impaired fasting glycaemia: the current status on definition and intervention. *Diabet Med* 2002; 19:708–723.

54. Norhammar A, Tenerz A, Nilsson G *et al*. Glucose metabolism in patients with acute myocardial infarction and no previous diagnosis of diabetes mellitus: a prospective study. *Lancet* 2002; 359: 2140–2144.

55. Holman RR, Paul SK, Bethel MA, Matthews DR, Neil HA. 10-year follow-up of intensive glucose control in type 2 diabetes. *N Engl J Med* 2008; 359:1577–1589.

56. Waugh N, Scotland G, McNamee P *et al*. Screening for type 2 diabetes: literature review and economic modelling. *Health Technol Assess* 2007; 11:iii-xi, 1.
57. Lauritzen T, Griffin S, Borch-Johnsen K, Wareham NJ, Wolffenbuttel BH, Rutten G. The ADDITION study: proposed trial of the cost-effectiveness of an intensive multifactorial intervention on morbidity and mortality among people with Type 2 diabetes detected by screening. *Int J Obes Relat Metab Disord* 2000; 24:S6–S11.
58. Sandbaek A, Griffin SJ, Rutten G *et al*. Stepwise screening for diabetes identifies people with high but modifiable coronary heart disease risk. The ADDITION study. *Diabetologia* 2008; 51:1127–1134.
59. MRC/BHF Heart Protection Study of cholesterol lowering with simvastatin in 20,536 high-risk individuals: a randomised placebo-controlled trial. *Lancet* 2002; 360:7–22.
60. Dahlof B, Sever PS, Poulter NR *et al*. Prevention of cardiovascular events with an antihypertensive regimen of amlodipine adding perindopril as required versus atenolol adding bendroflumethiazide as required, in the Anglo-Scandinavian Cardiac Outcomes Trial – Blood Pressure Lowering Arm (ASCOT-BPLA): a multicentre randomised controlled trial. *Lancet* 2005; 366:895–906.
61. Gueyffier F, Boutitie F, Boissel JP *et al*. Effect of antihypertensive drug treatment on cardiovascular outcomes in women and men. A meta-analysis of individual patient data from randomized, controlled trials. The INDANA Investigators. *Ann Intern Med* 1997; 126:761–767.
62. Heart Outcomes Prevention Evaluation Study Investigators. Effects of ramipril on cardiovascular and microvascular outcomes in people with diabetes mellitus: results of the HOPE study and MICRO-HOPE substudy. *Lancet* 2000; 355:253–259.
63. UK Prospective Diabetes Study Group. Tight blood pressure control and risk of macrovascular and microvascular complications in type 2 diabetes: UKPDS 38. *BMJ* 1998; 317:703–713.

5

Does pharmacotherapy have a place in the weight management of patients with type 2 diabetes?

L. F. Van Gaal, C. E. De Block

BACKGROUND

Obesity and type 2 diabetes are reaching epidemic proportions worldwide [1, 2]. Type 2 diabetes affects approximately 5% of the Western population, and this number continues to increase. Obesity increases the risks of type 2 diabetes, metabolic syndrome (visceral obesity, dyslipidaemia, hyperglycaemia, and hypertension), cardiovascular disease (CVD) (including stroke, congestive heart failure, myocardial infarction), obstructive sleep apnoea, non-alcoholic fatty liver disease, certain forms of cancer and premature death [3–5]. Diabetes is associated with a very high risk of CVD and is the sixth leading cause of death worldwide. Early identification and treatment of patients at risk for developing type 2 diabetes and CVD is therefore of paramount importance. Indeed, the DECODE study clearly showed that impaired glucose tolerance (IGT) already increased the risk for CVD mortality [6], and a recent population-based retrospective cohort study revealed that diabetes confers an equivalent cardiovascular risk to ageing 15 years in people aged 40 years or older [7]. Correspondingly, the health consequences and associated costs of both obesity and diabetes provide major incentives to reverse this continuing diabesity epidemic. The treatment of multiple cardiovascular risk factors is thus central to the management of type 2 diabetes.

Both obesity and type 2 diabetes are preventable. Lifestyle changes, use of metformin, acarbose and orlistat are partially effective to prevent or slow the development of diabetes. Bariatric surgery has a much more profound and sustained impact on weight, lipids, blood pressure (BP) and glucose metabolism compared with pharmacotherapy. However, do antidiabetes and anti-obesity drugs still have a place in the weight management of patients with type 2 diabetes?

The goals of obesity treatment include sustained weight loss with a preferential reduction of abdominal (visceral) fat, amelioration of obesity-related health risks and reduced quality of life, and reduction in mortality. Intentional weight loss in diabetic patients is associated with reduced mortality, and improved BP, lipid profile, mental health and quality of life [8].

Luc F. Van Gaal, MD, PhD, Professor of Endocrinology and Diabetology, Antwerp University Hospital, Faculty of Medicine, Department of Endocrinology, Diabetology, and Metabolism, Antwerp, Belgium.

Christophe E. De Block, MD, PhD, Assistant Professor, University of Antwerp, Faculty of Medicine, Department of Endocrinology, Diabetology and Metabolism, Antwerp University Hospital, Antwerp, Belgium.

Lifestyle management is recommended as the first-line treatment for obesity and its metabolic consequences. Pharmacotherapy may be useful in patients for whom non-pharmacological approaches alone are ineffective or insufficient. Weight reduction by means of dietary interventions and exercise are beyond the scope of this chapter. Before assigning an individual to a pharmacological treatment, a thorough assessment of the patient should be performed, including the history of weight gain, the maximum body weight, consideration of medications that may contribute to weight gain (such as corticosteroids and antipsychotic drugs), previous attempts at weight reduction, patterns of food intake (quality and quantity), and physical activity [9]. In addition, a thorough endocrine evaluation including laboratory tests (e.g. cytology, biochemistry, hormonology) and measurement of basal metabolic rate are important.

A modest weight loss of 5–10% significantly reduces obesity-related health risks [10, 11]. Regular physical activity, cognitive behavioural modification of lifestyle, including dietary habits, and administration of anti-obesity drugs facilitate weight loss and improve weight loss maintenance. However, weight reduction is hard to achieve in type 2 diabetes since most antidiabetes drugs increase weight [12], with metformin, acarbose, and the recently developed incretin mimetics and dipeptidyl peptidase-4 inhibitors as exceptions. Weight gain is important since the risk of diabetes is increased by 9% for every 1 kg increase in body weight [2].

BENEFITS OF PHARMACOLOGICAL TREATMENT IN THE PRIMARY PREVENTION OF DIABETES AND IN SECONDARY PREVENTION OF CHRONIC VASCULAR COMPLICATIONS

In primary prevention, weight reduction may reduce the risk of developing diabetes in subjects with IGT, as shown by lifestyle interventions [13–16], and by use of drugs such as metformin [15], acarbose [17, 18] and orlistat [18].

The Finnish Diabetes Prevention Study (DPS) included 522 subjects with IGT [13]. After 1 and 3 years, weight reduction was 4.5 and 3.5 kg in the lifestyle intervention group versus 1.0 and 0.9 kg in the control group. Lifestyle intervention included changes in food intake and composition, and increased physical activity. Glycaemic parameters improved more in the intervention group, with a 58% reduction in the incidence of diabetes (4.3 per 100 person-years in the intervention group and 7.4 per 100 person-years in the control group) [14].

In the Diabetes Prevention Program (DPP), enrolling 3234 overweight and obese subjects with elevated fasting and postprandial glucose, lifestyle modification was almost twice as effective as metformin in preventing diabetes (relative reduction 58% vs. 31%) [15]. The lifestyle modification programme resulted in a weight loss of 6.7 kg at 1 year follow-up, compared with weight losses of 2.7 kg and 0.4 kg in the metformin and placebo groups, respectively. After 4 years of follow-up, lifestyle, metformin and placebo groups maintained weight losses of 3.5 kg, 1.3 kg and 0.2 kg, respectively. Lifestyle intervention reduced the incidence of diabetes by 58% and metformin by 31% as compared with placebo [15].

The Study TO Prevent Non-Insulin-Dependent Diabetes Mellitus (STOP-NIDDM), a double-blind, placebo-controlled, randomized trial, assessed the effects of acarbose in 1429 overweight and obese subjects with IGT. Acarbose was associated with a mean weight loss of −1.15 kg compared with 0.26 kg weight gain in the placebo group at 3 years. Acarbose significantly reduced weight, waist circumference, body mass index (BMI), systolic and diastolic blood pressure, 2-h plasma glucose levels and triglycerides compared with placebo. Acarbose treatment was associated with a 36% reduction in the incidence of type 2 diabetes [17] and a 49% relative risk reduction in the development of cardiovascular events [18].

In the XENDOS study, a 4-year double-blind prospective study, 3305 individuals were randomized to lifestyle changes plus either 120 mg of orlistat or placebo, three times daily. Subjects had a BMI ≥30 kg/m^2 and normal (79%) or impaired glucose tolerance (21%). After 4 years, mean weight loss was greater with orlistat (5.8 vs. 3.0 kg with placebo). The incidence of diabetes was 6.2% in the orlistat group compared to 9.0% in the placebo group, corresponding to a 37% risk reduction. This beneficial effect was primarily due to prevention of diabetes in subjects with IGT where a 52% reduction was noted [19]. The XENDOS study is the first study to demonstrate that a weight loss agent in combination with lifestyle changes over 4 years is of greater benefit than lifestyle changes alone for producing long-term weight loss, improvements in cardiovascular risk factors, and prevention of diabetes in high-risk subjects.

However, in secondary prevention, convincing data that weight reduction in patients with type 2 diabetes may beneficially impact chronic complications or outcome are only partially available. Indeed, the feasibility and benefits of weight reduction in established type 2 diabetes are less well documented. Ongoing studies addressing this topic include the Swedish Obese Subjects (SOS) surgery study, the Look AHEAD (Action for Health in Diabetes) study in obese type 2 diabetic subjects in the USA, and the Comprehensive Rimonabant Evaluation Study of Cardiovascular ENDpoints and Outcomes (CRESCENDO) placebo-controlled trial. The Look AHEAD study is an 11-year prospective multicentre clinical trial that will examine whether long-term weight loss is achievable and beneficial in overweight individuals with type 2 diabetes (www.niddk.nih.gov/patients/SHOW/lookahead.htm). The SCOUT trial (Sibutramine Cardiovascular OUTcome trial), including over 8000 patients with type 2 diabetes, was the first study to elucidate to what extent moderate weight loss – partially induced by drug therapy – may have beneficial effects on cardiovascular endpoints [20]. Unfortunately, results have been disappointing (see also page 60).

PHARMACOTHERAPY FOR WEIGHT LOSS

Improving diet combined with reinforced physical exercise constitutes first-line management for overweight patients, but adherence to lifestyle measures is difficult to achieve. Patients who do not lose weight by lifestyle changes alone may benefit from agents that promote weight loss such as orlistat, sibutramine (its licence has recently been withdrawn by the European Medicines Agency because of safety concerns), rimonabant, metformin and the glucagon-like peptide-1 (GLP-1) analogue exenatide. Orlistat and sibutramine are indicated in obese patients (BMI ≥30 kg/m^2) or overweight people (BMI ≥28 kg/m^2 for orlistat) with an additional cardiovascular risk factor. These risk factors include diabetes, hypertension, sleep apnoea or another factor that warrants weight loss. Rimonabant, although withdrawn from the market, is discussed for the sake of completeness and in view of the interesting physiology behind the molecule.

Anti-obesity agents affect different targets in the central nervous system or peripheral tissues and can be divided according to their primary mode of action:

1. Drugs involved in appetite behaviour (nutrient intake), mainly appetite suppression and satiety enhancement.
2. Drugs involved in increasing energy expenditure, mainly thermogenic properties.
3. Drugs affecting metabolism or nutrient partitioning.

Characteristics aimed for by an ideal anti-obesity agent include:

1. Reducing weight and preferentially visceral and/or ectopic fat, in a dose-dependent manner.
2. Safe without major side-effects.
3. Effects should be long-lasting.
4. Activity through oral administration.
5. No addictive properties and/or toxicity.
6. Inexpensive.

However, pharmacotherapy for overweight is sometimes surrounded by a 'negative halo', particularly appetite suppressants, because of concerns about addiction. In addition, the plateau of body weight that is reached (−5 to −10% body weight) when homeostatic

Table 5.1 Characteristics of some anti-obesity agents

	Orlistat	Sibutramine*	Rimonabant*
Commercial name	Xenical	Reductil, Meridia	Acomplia
Mechanism	Pancreatic lipase inhibitor	Monoamine reuptake inhibitor (NE and 5-HT)	Endocannabinoid receptor-1 blocker
Mode of action	Reduces fat absorption	Increases satiety	Central and peripheral effects
Dosage	120 mg 3/day	10 or 15 mg daily	20 mg daily
Time to peak concentration	8 h	1.2 h (3 h for metabolites)	2 h
Elimination half-life	14–19 h	1.1 h (14–16 h for metabolites)	6–9 days (16 days in obese subjects)
Elimination	Faeces (over 96% of total drug ingested; 83% unchanged)	Urine (77%)	Biliary excretion and faecal elimination (86%)
Placebo-subtracted weight loss	3% (or 2.9 kg)	4.6% (or 4.2 kg)	5% (or 4.6 kg)
Lipids			
LDL-cholesterol	−0.27 mmol/l	NS	NS
HDL-cholesterol	NS	Conflicting data	7–9% increase
Triglycerides	NS	Conflicting data	12–16% decrease
Glucose metabolism			
HbA1c (%)	Not reported	−0.3%	−0.7%
Blood pressure			
Systolic (mmHg)	−1.8	1.7	NS
Diastolic (mmHg)	−1.6	2.4	NS
Attrition rate	33%	48%	
Side-effects	Oily spotting, flatulence, faecal urgency	Increase in blood pressure and heart rate	Depression, anxiety, nausea, diarrhoea

*Sibutramine and rimonabant have both been withdrawn from the market because of safety concerns.

mechanisms in the body come into play and stop further weight loss seems somewhat limited. Finally, there are concerns about toxicity associated with some anti-obesity agents.

Orlistat

Orlistat is a potent and selective inhibitor of gastric and pancreatic lipase that reduces the absorption of lipids across the gastrointestinal tract by about 30%. These lipases are responsible for the hydrolysis of ingested triglycerides into fatty acids and monoglycerides, which are absorbed by the enterocytes. Absorption of ingested fat is reduced by one-third and the non-absorbed triglycerides and fat are eliminated in the faeces. Because of low systemic absorption and first-pass metabolism, the bioavailability of orlistat is less than 1%. Most of the drug is excreted unchanged in faeces (Table 5.1).

A meta-analysis of clinical trials showed that treatment with orlistat resulted in a 2.9 kg greater weight loss compared to placebo [21, 22]. Modest positive effects on glycaemic control (fasting glucose and HbA1c), BP (systolic −1.8 mmHg and diastolic −1.6 mmHg), and low-density lipoprotein (LDL)-, high-density lipoprotein (HDL)-cholesterol and triglyceride concentrations have also been observed with its use. Orlistat has a direct cholesterol-lowering effect independent of weight loss, probably due to its inhibitory effect on the absorption of dietary fat and cholesterol from the gastrointestinal tract [23]. Orlistat partially offsets the excess cardiovascular risk in subjects with the metabolic syndrome [24].

There are a limited number of studies performed in patients with diabetes [25–33]. Type 2 diabetic patients treated with orlistat 120 mg three times daily for 1 year lost more weight (between 1.3 and 3.8 kg) than the placebo-controlled group [25–29, 31]. Orlistat-treated patients also showed a greater decrease in HbA1c, ranging from −0.3% to −1.7% absolute reduction. The extent of improvement depends on baseline factors (weight, HbA1c), concomitant antidiabetes treatment, and duration of therapy. There is also a beneficial effect of orlistat on LDL-cholesterol (with reductions up to 12.8%) and on BP.

In a pooled 2-year study including 675 obese subjects, 6.6% of the patients taking orlistat converted from normal to impaired glucose tolerance, compared to 10.8% in placebo-treated individuals. Moreover, in the subjects with IGT at baseline, those assigned to orlistat developed less diabetes (3%) compared to those in the placebo group (7.6%). Furthermore, considering individuals with IGT at baseline, glucose tolerance normalized in more orlistat-treated than placebo-treated subjects (72 vs. 49%) [34]. This report was however a retrospective analysis.

As indicated, the XENDOS study, a 4-year double-blind prospective trial, randomized 3305 individuals to lifestyle changes plus either 120 mg of orlistat or placebo, three times daily. One-fifth of the subjects had IGT (21%). There was a 37% reduction in the incidence of diabetes in the orlistat group (6.2%) compared to the placebo group (9.0%). The overall effect of orlistat in preventing diabetes was primarily due to the beneficial effect in IGT patients. XENDOS illustrates clearly that orlistat plus lifestyle changes is able to reduce incident type 2 diabetes above the result achieved with implementation of lifestyle modifications over 4 years. However, only 43% of the patients completed the study [19]. Although not yet studied in MODY (maturity onset diabetes of the young) or youngsters with classical type 2 diabetes, the effect of orlistat may be of importance in view of the beneficial effects in non-diabetic obese adolescents [35].

Since orlistat is not absorbed, its side-effects are thus related to the blockade of triglyceride digestion in the intestine. Indeed, in 15–30% of subjects, orlistat has gastrointestinal side-effects, including fatty stool, faecal urgency and oily spotting, which are typically short-lived. Orlistat may cause small decreases in fat-soluble vitamins. Orlistat does not seem to influence the absorption of other drugs except acyclovir [36, 37].

The beneficial effect of orlistat on glucose tolerance and metabolic control could be associated with weight loss itself; to the limited absorption of lipids and reduction of plasma free fatty acids (FFA); to increased production of incretins; or to modulation of secretion of adipokines [38]. Orlistat, when given before a relatively high fat content meal in obese type 2 diabetic patients is associated with lower postprandial levels of plasma free fatty acids compared with placebo [39, 40]. This is beneficial since FFA can modulate the severity of insulin resistance in type 2 diabetes, inhibiting whole body glucose utilization and oxidation [41]. In addition, lipotoxicity may impair β-cell function [42].

Another possibility is an incretin response to orlistat treatment. The reduced absorption of fat and the increase in intestinal fat content may lead to increased secretion of GLP-1. Orlistat increases GLP-1 levels, enhancing the insulin secretory response to a meal and blunting the postprandial rise in glycaemia. The increased GLP-1 levels, which lead to diminished food intake, may also contribute to the weight loss that is associated with the use of orlistat [43].

Reductions in inflammatory mediators tumour necrosis factor alpha (TNF-α) and interleukin (IL)-6, in high-sensitivity C-reactive protein (hsCRP) are more pronounced in subjects assigned to orlistat as compared to placebo-treated individuals [44, 45]. Also, significant reductions in leptin and increases in adiponectin have been observed with the use of orlistat [44].

Sibutramine

Sibutramine is a serotonin and norepinephrine reuptake inhibitor that works centrally to produce a feeling of satiety. Its structure and mode of action differ from those of the fenfluramines, which stimulate serotonin release. Sibutramine also stimulates thermogenesis and prevents diet-induced decline in metabolic rate. Serotonin 5-HT$_{2c}$ receptors modulate fat and caloric intake. Sibutramine undergoes extensive first-pass metabolism, mainly by hepatic cytochrome P450 3A4 enzymes to active primary (M1) and secondary (M2) amine metabolites, which are more potent than the parent compound [46]. Most of the drug and its active compounds are renally excreted (Table 5.1).

In clinical trials, subjects receiving sibutramine experienced a 4.2 kg (or 4.6%) greater than placebo weight loss [21, 22]. Sibutramine has been shown to positively influence glycaemic control, reducing HbA1c by 0.3% on average, but has little effect on LDL-cholesterol levels, and the effects on HDL-cholesterol and triglycerides are variable. Sibutramine also improves insulin sensitivity [47]. The recently completed SCOUT study assessed the efficacy of sibutramine in reducing myocardial infarction, stroke and cardiovascular mortality in >10 000 obese and overweight subjects [20]. The results have recently been announced, reporting an increase in mortality in the group taking sibutramine. This has resulted in licence withdrawal by the European Medicines Agency. For completeness, the literature on sibutramine is reviewed below.

The effect of sibutramine in diabetic patients has been examined in a few studies [48–58]. Placebo-substracted weight loss ranged between −1.8 to −8.5 kg, depending on the type of intervention protocol, the baseline antidiabetes treatment and the duration of the trial. HbA1c remained stable or decreased with up to −2.7% unit reduction, also depending on baseline HbA1c level. The results on lipids and BP are variable. Only a few trials that reported on fasting glucose and HbA1c levels provided a detailed assessment of the types of, doses of, and changes in antidiabetes medications that were administered to trial participants.

A meta-analysis of studies in diabetic patients receiving sibutramine showed positive effects on body weight, waist circumference, glucose, HbA1c, triglycerides, and HDL-cholesterol [59, 60]. The mean weight loss was 5.5 kg for those treated with sibutramine and 0.9 kg for placebo-treated patients. There was no significant change in systolic blood pressure, but diastolic blood pressure was higher in sibutramine-treated patients [60]. However, the tendency to increase BP is offset by the weight loss. Hypertension is of particular concern in type 2 diabetes: in the United Kingdom Prospective Diabetes Study (UKPDS), improved BP control (144/82 mmHg vs. routine: 154/87 mmHg) reduced cardiovascular events by 25% [61]. The risk–benefit ratio must therefore be carefully evaluated. In the 6-week run-in period of SCOUT, baseline BP appeared to determine the effect on BP; in patients with diabetes a reduction in systolic blood pressure was observed in those with a baseline tension >130/85 mmHg [20].

Side-effects associated with sibutramine include an increase in BP (+1.7 mmHg in systolic and +2.4 mmHg in diastolic blood pressure) and pulse rate (4–5 beats/min) which are related to its adrenergic properties [22]. In 7–20% of the patients receiving sibutramine, insomnia, nausea, dry mouth and constipation occurred. Sibutramine is contraindicated in patients with a history of uncontrolled hypertension, coronary artery disease, congestive heart failure, cardiac arrhythmias or stroke. Sibutramine should also not be used in subjects using selective serotonin reuptake inhibitors (SSRI) or monoamine oxidase (MAO) blockers, and there should be at least a 2-week interval between stopping MAO-inhibitors and beginning sibutramine. By contrast with fenfluramine and dexfenfluramine, sibutramine does not increase the release of serotonin and has not been associated with valvular heart disease of pulmonary hypertension. Sibutramine is metabolized by the cytochrome P-450 enzyme system (isoenzyme CYP3A4) and may therefore interfere with the metabolism of erythromycin and ketoconazole, and it has a small effect (7% increase in area under the curve) on the metabolism of simvastatin, but not other statins [36].

Rimonabant

Rimonabant, being a selective blocker of the cannabinoid receptor-1 (CB-1), reduces food intake and tobacco dependence by blocking endocannabinoid receptors in the central nervous system. The endocannabinoid system has a key role in energy homeostasis, food intake and body weight. The two endogenous endocannabinoids, anandamine and 2-arachidonoylglycerol, increase food intake by acting on the CB-1 receptor. Rimonabant also affects the metabolic profile by targeting the endocannabinoid system in adipocytes, hepatocytes, and potentially β-cells. Potential peripheral effects include enhanced thermogenesis via increased oxygen consumption in skeletal muscle, diminished hepatic and adipocyte lipogenesis, augmentation of adiponectin concentrations, promotion of vagally mediated cholecystokinin-induced satiety, inhibition of pre-adipocyte proliferation, and increased adipocyte maturation without lipid accumulation [46]. Rimonabant is hepatically metabolized and excreted in bile. Patients with obesity or type 2 diabetes exhibit higher concentrations of endocannabinoids in visceral fat or serum, respectively, than the corresponding controls [62].

In clinical trials, rimonabant reduced weight by 3.9–5.4 kg more than placebo [63–66]. It also had a beneficial effect on the lipid profile, lowering triglycerides and increasing HDL-cholesterol levels and LDL-cholesterol particle size. Approximately half of the observed effect of rimonabant on the lipid levels was reported to be independent of weight loss, which may be explained by direct effects of rimonabant on adipocytes, including increasing adiponectin [65] and reducing leptin concentrations. Positive effects on systolic and diastolic blood pressure have also been observed.

In 1047 overweight or obese type 2 diabetic patients who were already on metformin or sulphonylurea monotherapy, rimonabant (RIO-Diabetes study) reduced weight by 3.9 kg more than placebo-treated patients, and reduced HbA1c by 0.7% from a baseline of 7.5% [66]. This is clinically relevant since every 1% reduction in HbA1c has been shown to be associated with a reduction in risk of 21% for any diabetes-related endpoint [67]. HDL-cholesterol (+15.4%), triglycerides (–9.1%), non-HDL-cholesterol (–1.8%), and systolic blood pressure (–0.8 mmHg) were also beneficially affected in patients treated with rimonabant 20 mg/day. Also, self-esteem and measures of quality of control increased in rimonabant-treated individuals. However, the retention rate of about 66% in all treatment groups might be considered as rather low. A second 6-month study in 278 drug-naive diabetic patients (SERENADE) confirmed the above-mentioned findings [68]. The beneficial metabolic effects obtained in diabetic patients with use of rimonabant can be explained by weight loss and by reduced lipogenesis and free fatty acid synthesis preventing hepatic fat accumulation, by increased adiponectin release, and by improved skeletal muscle glucose uptake.

Common side-effects of rimonabant include nausea, dizziness, diarrhoea and insomnia, each occurring 1–9% more frequently than with placebo. Patients given rimonabant were 2.5 times more likely to discontinue the treatment because of depressive mood disorders than were those given placebo [69, 70]. Moreover, the Food and Drug Administration (FDA) did not approve rimonabant because of concerns over depression (with suicidality risk) and anxiety, which occurred in 6% of rimonabant-treated subjects and in 3% of the placebo group. In late 2008, after the EMEA (European Medicines Agency) advised a temporary halt to the marketing of rimonabant in Europe because of concerns over the risk–benefit analysis, the company decided to withdraw the drug from the market worldwide. Consequently, the CRESCENDO study (Comprehensive Rimonabant Evaluation Study of Cardiovascular ENDpoints and Outcomes) investigating the outcome effect of rimonabant on myocardial infarction, stroke, and cardiovascular death in 17 000 obese subjects was stopped.

Depression has been associated with obesity, especially in women and in severely obese men, and obese subjects who are seeking treatment for obesity are especially prone to depression.

Phentermine
Phentermine is an adrenergic stimulant that enhances the release of norepinephrine in certain brain regions and reduces food intake.

The efficacy and safety of this drug are limited [9]. In randomized controlled trials of phentermine, weight reduction was 3–4% greater than in the placebo group.

However, BP must be closely monitored, and there are concerns over dependency. Limited data suggest that phentermine may be effective for more than 10 years, but it has only been approved for short-term use [9]. No randomized controlled trials of this agent have been performed in diabetic subjects.

Fluoxetine

Fluoxetine is a selective serotonin reuptake inhibitor that blocks the transporters that remove serotonin from the neuronal cleft into the presynaptic space for metabolism by monoamine oxidase or storage in granules. It reduces food intake. Fluoxetine is approved by the FDA for treatment of depression.

Fluoxetine results in short-term weight loss in the first 6 months of treatment, but in the next 6 months usually 50% of the weight lost is regained. Therefore, fluoxetine is an inappropriate choice for chronic treatment. Modest reductions in weight are observed with fluoxetine, with a placebo-substracted weight loss of approximately 5–6 kg at 1 year. A few studies have been performed in diabetic subjects [71–75]. Placebo-substracted weight loss ranged between 1.8 and 8.0 kg. Fluoxetine also produces a significant decrease in HbA1c levels, ranging between −0.8% and −1.8% unit reduction. No data on lipid levels or BP have been reported. Side-effects commonly reported with the use of fluoxetine include tremor, somnolence, and sweating.

Combination therapy

Combination therapy with sibutramine and orlistat did not influence weight loss as compared to either agent alone [76, 77]. The combination of phentermine and fenfluramine, two agents that act by separate mechanisms, showed a highly significant weight loss of nearly 15%, but due to reports of aortic valvular regurgitation associated with fenfluramine, this drug was withdrawn from the market worldwide in 1997 [78]. No studies are available in patients with diabetes.

ANTIDIABETIC AGENTS THAT PRODUCE WEIGHT LOSS

Metformin

Several studies have reported beneficial effects of metformin on insulin resistance, metabolic parameters and weight loss in obese subjects with type 2 diabetes [79, 80]. Evidence for a modest satiety-promoting effect of metformin has been noted. Metformin has also been shown to significantly increase GLP-1 levels after an oral glucose load [81].

A randomized prospective clinical trial in obese type 2 diabetic patients that were not treated with antidiabetic agents examined the efficacy of sibutramine (2 x 10 mg/d) versus orlistat (3 x 120 mg/d) versus metformin over a 6-month treatment period [82]. At 6 months, all treatment groups experienced significant reductions in BMI: −13.6% with sibutramine, −9.1% with orlistat and −9.9% with metformin. BP, lipid profile and fasting and postprandial glucose levels also improved in all three groups. A limitation of this study was the lack of a placebo group. The DPP, studying subjects with IGT, showed a 2.1 kg weight loss and a 31% decrease in the incidence of diabetes with metformin use. Also, the incidence of the metabolic syndrome was reduced by 17% in the metformin group [15].

Acarbose

Acarbose is an α-glucosidase inhibitor, an antihyperglycaemic agent that reduces postprandial glucose excursions by delaying and reducing carbohydrate absorption. Acarbose binds with high affinity and specificity to α-glucosidases found in the brush border of the small intestine. These enzymes are responsible for the hydrolysis of complex carbohydrates (starch and oligosaccharides) to absorbable simple sugars (monosaccharides such as glucose). Acarbose may also increase GLP-1 levels [83].

In the STOP-NIDDM study, performed in 1429 overweight and obese subjects with IGT, the risk of progression to type 2 diabetes over 3.3 years was reduced by 25% (32% in the acarbose group and 42% in the placebo group) [17]. Furthermore, acarbose increased the likelihood that IGT reverted to normal glucose tolerance. The study also demonstrated that acarbose was associated with a mean weight loss of −1.15 kg compared with 0.26 kg weight gain in the placebo group at 3 years. Acarbose significantly reduced weight, waist circumference, BMI, systolic and diastolic blood pressure, 2-h plasma glucose levels and triglycerides compared with placebo. Acarbose treatment was associated with a 34% relative risk reduction in the incidence of hypertension, and a 49% relative risk reduction in the development of cardiovascular events [18]. A meta-analysis of seven long-term studies of acarbose in type 2 diabetes found that treatment with acarbose led to a small but significant weight loss (−1.1 kg) compared with placebo, improvements in glycaemic control, triglyceride levels, and systolic blood pressure [84]. In addition, a 64% relative risk reduction for myocardial infarction was achieved with acarbose use [84]. When one realizes that CVD is the leading cause of mortality among patients with type 2 diabetes, accounting for 40–50% of all deaths, and that the mortality risk for cardio- and cerebrovascular disease is 2- to 10-fold higher than in the non-diabetic population, the above-mentioned findings are very important.

Side-effects reported with the use of acarbose include flatulence, diarrhoea and abdominal pain. Acarbose is poorly absorbed into the bloodstream, and has a low systemic availability of less than 2%. As a result, the risk of any toxic reaction is very low.

Exenatide

Exenatide is a new injectable treatment for type 2 diabetes. It is a synthetic agonist of receptors of GLP-1, that is resistant to the rapid inactivation by dipeptidyl peptidase-4 (DPP-4) and acts as an incretin mimetic. GLP-1 is an incretin hormone that is released by the enteroendocrine L-cells of the ileum and colon in response to meal intake and that helps to maintain glucose homeostasis. It stimulates insulin release from pancreatic β-cells and inhibits glucagon output from the α-cells in a glucose-dependent manner. Biological effects of GLP-1 include slowing gastric emptying and decreasing appetite.

Exenatide lowers haemoglobin A1c levels, and postprandial glucose excursions, without being directly responsible for hypoglycaemia. This novel incretin-mimetic offers the potential to reduce body weight or prevent weight gain that is typically associated with improved metabolic control. In a meta-analysis, the HbA1c decreased on average by 1% unit and weight decreased by 1.4 kg [85]. In two longer-term observational studies, the weight loss achieved with the use of exenatide was 5.3 kg at 3 years [86, 87]. However, the durability of these effects and the potential long-term benefits remain to be proven. In addition, nearly 40% of patients in clinical studies reported gastrointestinal side-effects, mainly nausea, although only 4% had to stop their treatment due to side-effects [88].

Pramlintide

Pramlintide is a synthetic analogue of amylin, a pancreatic islet cell hormone colocalized within the β-cells and co-secreted with insulin. Amylin complements the influence of insulin on the regulation of the postprandial glucose excursions, contributes to the suppression of glucagon secretion, and slows down gastric emptying. Due to the β-cell dysfunction that occurs in the progression of type 2 diabetes, amylin availability may be compromised [89]. Administration of pramlintide in patients with type 2 diabetes has significantly improved postprandial glycaemia [90–92], abated hyperglucagonaemia [93], and decreased the rate of gastric emptying [94]. This compound may also decrease 24-h caloric intake and binge eating [95]. Studies with longer treatment periods found even greater weight losses, significant reductions in waist circumference, improvements in appetite control [96–98] and a proportionate decline in daily insulin requirements [96]. Patients with a BMI >40 kg/m^2 or those treated with metformin experienced the greatest reduction in body weight [96].

In a 52-week, double-blind, placebo-controlled, parallel-group, multicentre study, 656 patients with type 2 diabetes treated with insulin, were randomized to receive additional preprandial subcutaneous injections of either placebo or pramlintide (60 µg t.i.d., 90 µg b.i.d., or 120 µg b.i.d.). Treatment with pramlintide 120 µg b.i.d. led to a sustained reduction from baseline in HbA1c (–0.6%) and a weight loss of –1.4 kg [99]. In a study of 651 subjects with type 1 diabetes randomized to placebo or subcutaneous pramlintide, 60 µg three or four times a day along with an insulin injection, HbA1c decreased 0.29% to 0.34%, respectively. Weight decreased by 0.4 kg in the pramlintide group, compared to a weight gain of 0.8 kg in the placebo group [100]. In a pooled analysis of two 1-year studies in insulin-treated type 2 diabetic patients randomized to pramlintide 120 µg twice a day or 150 µg three times a day, weight decreased by –2.6 kg and HbA1c by –0.5% [101]. The improvement in diabetes correlated with the weight loss. The most common side-effect was nausea, which was present in 25% of individuals but was mild and confined to the first 4 weeks of treatment. In another pooled *post hoc* analysis of two trials in overweight type 2 diabetic subjects randomized to pramlintide 120 µg b.i.d. or placebo, pramlintide treatment resulted in significant reductions from baseline to week 26 in HbA1c and weight, for placebo-corrected reductions of –0.4% and –1.8 kg, respectively [96]. The potential of pramlintide as an anti-obesity agent was assessed in a 16-week randomized, placebo-controlled study in 204 obese subjects. Individuals completing 16 weeks of pramlintide treatment (maximum of 240 µg daily) experienced placebo-corrected reductions in body weight of 3.6 kg, and waist circumference of 3.6 cm. Appetite control and overall well-being improved significantly more in pramlintide-treated subjects [97].

Liraglutide
Liraglutide is a human GLP-1 analogue with 97% homology to native GLP-1. The addition of a fatty acid side chain and a single amino acid substitution produces self-association of the molecule that prolongs absorption from the subcutaneous depot. The fatty acid side chain also promotes albumin binding that renders the molecule resistant to degradation by DPP-4. The resultant plasma half-life of liraglutide is 13 h. The pharmacokinetic profile makes liraglutide suitable for once-daily injection, in contrast to exenatide, which needs to be administered twice a day.

Depending upon dose, duration of treatment and concomitant therapy, type 2 diabetic patients receiving liraglutide had mean reductions in HbA1c of 0.8–1.5%, and reductions in body weight of 1.2 to 3.0 kg [102–104]. Nausea was reported by 10–20% of patients.

NEW AND FUTURE TREATMENT OPTIONS

Leptin
Leptin is an adipocytokine that acts on the gp130 family of cytokine receptors in the hypothalamus to activate the Janus kinase signal transduction and translation system (JAK-STAT). The lack of leptin, a hormone derived from the adipocyte, causes massive overweight. The discovery of leptin generated hope that leptin administration would be an effective treatment for obesity. In one study, obese subjects were treated with 0.3 mg/kg leptin subcutaneously for 24 weeks. They lost circa 7 kg of body weight [105]. However, pegylated leptin at 20 and 60 mg/week in obese individuals over 8–12 weeks did not produce more weight loss than placebo [106].

Tesofensine

Tesofensine is an inhibitor of the presynaptic uptake of noradrenaline, dopamine, and serotonin. In a 24-week phase II, randomized, double-blind, placebo-controlled trial of 203 obese subjects, tesofensine 0.25 mg, 0.5 mg and 1 mg produced a mean weight loss of 4.5%, 9.2%, and 10.6% respectively, greater than diet and placebo [107]. The most common adverse effects caused by tesofensine were dry mouth, nausea, constipation, hard stools, diarrhoea and insomnia. There was no significant increase in systolic or diastolic blood pressure, but heart rate was increased by 7.4 beats per minute in the tesofensine 0.5 mg group. The efficacy still needs to be validated in phase III and IV studies, and in diabetic patients.

SUMMARY

Weight loss induced by currently available anti-obesity drugs is only modest, reaching 5–10% of initial body weight. The average weight loss is 3–5% greater in the drug-treated than in the control group. However, combination therapy might be more efficacious. Special attention should then be paid to the potential drug interaction and safety.

It has been consistently shown that obese subjects with type 2 diabetes have greater difficulty in achieving and maintaining weight loss than matched non-diabetic overweight subjects [12, 26], probably because of the underlying disease state or because medications used to treat diabetes tend to increase weight. Weight loss may be especially difficult for those patients receiving sulphonylurea, glinides, thiazolidinediones or insulin. Type 2 diabetes requires a holistic approach, including weight reduction, glycaemic control, and adequate treatment of dyslipidaemia and hypertension.

Treatment of a patient with a particular anti-obesity agent should respect its licensed indications and contraindications; sibutramine should not be used in patients with uncontrolled hypertension; orlistat should not be administered to patients with cholestasis; and centrally-acting agents should not be prescribed in patients with a history of depression. Anti-obesity agents should also only be used in patients with an adequate response to the initial phase of treatment over a 1.5- to 3-month period. Non-responders lose less than 1–2 kg after 6 weeks of treatment.

Other important points to be aware of include:

- Nearly all studies performed with anti-obesity agents received funding from the drug manufacturers.
- Two-thirds of participants were women.
- About 90% of participants were white.
- Mean age was 45–50 years.
- Mean weight was 100 kg.
- Mean BMI was 35–36 kg/m^2 [22].
- Attrition rates were high in obesity studies, averaging 30% for orlistat studies and 40% for sibutramine and rimonabant studies, which compromises the validity of the results.

For all the above-mentioned reasons, extrapolation of the results of clinical trials to regular clinical practice must be done with caution. Effects of anti-obesity agents on surrogate endpoints such as lipids, glucose tolerance and BP (except for sibutramine) are positive. However, so far no data on mortality or cardiovascular morbidity are available.

Current anti-obesity agents are costly, ranging between 45–80 Euro for 28 days' treatment.

In the absence of data showing that one particular drug is more effective than another, initial pharmacotherapy can be guided by physician and patient preference, local drug costs and availability.

Future goals for the drug treatment of obesity include:

1. Evaluation of predictors of drug-induced weight loss and its maintenance, which include metabolic, nutritional, psychobehavioural and genetic factors.
2. Primary drug effects on health risks.
3. Efficacy and safety of combined drug treatment.
4. Anti-obesity drugs in children, adolescents and elderly patients.

Since the prevalence of obesity continues to increase, reaching epidemic proportions, the need for effective and safe anti-obesity agents that produce and maintain weight loss and improve morbidity and mortality is evident.

CONCLUSION

Cardiovascular risk factors, including hypertension, dyslipidaemia, and hyperglycaemia commonly cluster, particularly in subjects with type 2 diabetes and abdominal obesity. Obesity and type 2 diabetes significantly affect quality of life and reduce average life expectancy. Excess body weight is the most modifiable risk factor for type 2 diabetes and it is estimated that up to 90% of all type 2 diabetic patients are overweight or obese. Intentional weight loss has proven to reduce cardiovascular risk factors in type 2 diabetic subjects and slows progression of (prevents?) diabetes mellitus in subjects with IGT.

Even modest pharmacologically facilitated weight loss (5–10%) produces important metabolic benefits, including improving glucose metabolism, and reducing LDL-cholesterol and BP. Anti-obesity agents reduce HbA1c levels on average by 0.5%. This decrease should result in reduced risk of vascular complications.

Anti-obesity treatment should be individually tailored according to the following criteria: sex, age, the degree of obesity, individual health risks, psycho-behavioural and metabolic characteristics, and the outcome of previous weight loss attempts [108]. The patient can best be treated in a centre of excellence where a multidisciplinary team including an expert endocrinologist, dietician, psychiatrist, exercise physiologist and experienced surgeon provide comprehensive programmes for the treatment of obesity based upon evidence-based medicine [108].

REFERENCES

1. James PT, Rigby N, Leach R. International Obesity Task Force. The obesity epidemic, metabolic syndrome and future prevention strategies. *Eur J Cardiovasc Prev Rehabil* 2004; 11:3–8.
2. Mokdad AH, Ford ES, Bowman BA. Diabetes trends in the U.S. *Diabetes Care* 2000; 23:1278–1283.
3. Van Gaal LF, Mertens IL, De Block CE. Mechanisms linking obesity with cardiovascular disease. *Nature* 2006; 444:875–880.
4. Adams KF, Schatzkin A, Harris TB *et al.* Overweight, obesity, and mortality in a large prospective cohort of persons 50 to 71 years old. *N Engl J Med* 2006; 355:763–778.
5. Haffner SM, Letho S, Ronnemaa T, Pyorala K, Laakso M. Mortality from coronary heart disease in subjects with type 2 diabetes and in nondiabetic subjects with and without prior myocardial infarction. *N Engl J Med* 1998; 339:229–234.
6. The DECODE study group on behalf of the European Diabetes Epidemiology Group. Glucose tolerance and mortality: comparison of WHO and American Diabetes Association diagnostic criteria. *Lancet* 1999; 354:617–621.
7. Booth Gl, Kapral MK, Fung K, Tu JV. Relation between age and cardiovascular disease in men and women with diabetes compared with non-diabetic people: a population-based retrospective cohort study. *Lancet* 2006; 368:29–36.
8. Wing RR, Koeske R, Epstein LH, Nowalk MP, Gooding W, Becker D. Long-term effects of modest weight loss in type II diabetic patients. *Arch Intern Med* 1987; 147:1749–1753.
9. Eckel RH. Nonsurgical management of obesity in adults. *N Engl J Med* 2008; 358:1941–1950.
10. Van Gaal LF, Wauters MA, De Leeuw IH. The beneficial effects of modest weight loss on cardiovascular risk factors. *Int J Obes Relat Metab Disord* 1997; 21:S5–S9.

11. Mertens IL, Van Gaal LF. Overweight, obesity, and blood pressure: the effects of modest weight reduction. *Obes Res* 2000; 8:270–278.

12. Wing RR, Marcus MD, Epstein LH, Salata R. Type II diabetic subjects lose less weight than their overweight nondiabetic spouses. *Diabetes Care* 1987; 10:563–566.

13. Tuomilehto J, Lindstro J, Eriksson JG *et al*, for the Finnish Diabetes Prevention Study Group. Prevention of type 2 diabetes mellitus by changes in lifestyle among subjects with impaired glucose tolerance. *N Engl J Med* 2001; 344:1343–1350.

14. Linderstrom J, Ilanne-Perikka P, Peltonen M *et al*. Sustained reduction in the incidence of type 2 diabetes by lifestyle intervention: follow-up of the Finnish Diabetes Prevention Study. *Lancet* 2006; 368:1673–1679.

15. Knowler WC, Barrett-Connor E, Fowler SE *et al*, for the Diabetes Prevention Program Research Group. Reduction in the incidence of type 2 diabetes with lifestyle intervention or metformin. *N Engl J Med* 2002; 346:393–403.

16. Pan XR, Li GW, Hu YH *et al*. Effects of diet and exercise in preventing NIDDM in people with impaired glucose tolerance: the Da Qing IGT and Diabetes Study. *Diabetes Care* 1997; 20:537–544.

17. Chiasson JL, Josse RG, Gomis R, Hanefeld M, Karasik A, Laakso M. STOP-NIDDM Trial Research Group. Acarbose for the prevention of type 2 diabetes mellitus: the STOP-NIDDM randomised trial. *Lancet* 2002; 359:2072–2077.

18. Chiasson JL, Josse RG, Gomis R *et al*. Acarbose treatment and the risk of cardiovascular disease and hypertension in patients with impaired glucose tolerance: the STOP-NIDDM trial. *JAMA* 2003; 290:486–494.

19. Torgerson JS, Hauptman J, Boldrin MN, Sjöström L. XENical in the prevention of diabetes in obese subjects (XENDOS) study: a randomized study of orlistat as an adjunct to lifestyle changes for the prevention of type 2 diabetes in obese patients. *Diabetes Care* 2004; 27:155–161.

20. Torp-Pedersen C, Caterson I, Coutinho W *et al*. SCOUT Investigators. Cardiovascular responses to weight management and sibutramine in high-risk subjects: an analysis from the SCOUT trial. *Eur Heart J* 2007; 28:2915–2923.

21. Padwal R, Li SK, Lau DC. Long-term pharmacotherapy for obesity and overweight. *Cochrane Database Syst Rev* 2004: CD004094.

22. Rucker D, Padwal R, Li SK, Curioni C, Lau DC. Long term pharmacotherapy for obesity and overweight: updated meta-analysis. *BMJ* 2007; 335:1194–1199.

23. Muls E, Kolanowski J, Scheen A, Van Gaal L, ObelHyx Study Group. The effects of orlistat on weight and on serum lipids in obese patients with hypercholesterolemia: a randomized, double-blind, placebo-controlled, multicentre study. *Int J Obes Relat Metab Disord* 2001; 25:1713–1721.

24. Didangelos TP, Thanapoulou AK, Bousboulas SH *et al*. The ORLIstat and CARdiovascular risk profile in patients with the metabolic syndrome and type 2 DIAbetes (ORLICARDIA) study. *Curr Med Res Opin* 2004; 20:1393–1401.

25. Hollander PA, Elbein SC, Hirsch IB *et al*. Role of orlistat in the treatment of obese patients with type 2 diabetes: a 1-year randomized double-blind study. *Diabetes Care* 1998; 21:1288–1294.

26. Lindgärde F, on behalf of the Orlistat Swedish Multimorbidity Study Group. The effect of orlistat on body weight and coronary heart disease risk profile in obese patients: the Swedish Multimorbidity Study. *J Intern Med* 2000; 248:245–254.

27. Kelley DE, Bray GA, Pi-Sunyer FX *et al*. Clinical efficacy of orlistat therapy for overweight and obese patients with insulin-treated type 2 diabetes: a 1-year randomized controlled trial. *Diabetes Care* 2002; 25:1033–1041.

28. Miles JM, Leiter L, Hollander P *et al*. Effect of orlistat in overweight and obese patients with type 2 diabetes treated with metformin. *Diabetes Care* 2002; 25:1123–1128.

29. Hanefeld M, Sachse G. The effects of orlistat on body weight and glycaemic control in overweight patients with type 2 diabetes: a randomized, placebo-controlled trial. *Diabetes Obes Metab* 2002; 4:415–423.

30. Halpern A, Mancini MC, Suplicy H *et al*. Latin-American trial of orlistat for weight loss and improvement in glycaemic profile in obese diabetic patients. *Diabetes Obes Metab* 2003; 5:180–188.

31. Berne C, on behalf of the Orlistat Swedish Type 2 Diabetes Study Group. A randomized study of orlistat in combination with a weight management programme in obese patients with Type 2 diabetes treated with metformin. *Diabet Med* 2005; 22:612–618.

32. Shi YF, Pan CY, Hill J, Gao Y. Orlistat in the treatment of overweight or obese Chinese patients with newly diagnosed type 2 diabetes. *Diabet Med* 2005; 22:1737–1743.

33. Kuo CS, Pei D, Yao CY, Hsieh MC, Kuo SW. Effect of orlistat in overweight poorly controlled Chinese female type 2 diabetic patients: a randomised, double-blind, placebo-controlled study. *Int J Clin Pract* 2006; 60:906–910.

34. Heymsfield SB, Segal KR, Hauptman J *et al*. Effects of weight loss with orlistat on glucose tolerance and progression to type 2 diabetes in obese adults. *Arch Intern Med* 2000; 160:1321–1326.

35. Chanoine JP, Hampl S, Jensen C, Boldrin M, Hauptman J. Effect of orlistat on weight and body composition in obese adolescents: a randomized controlled trial. *JAMA* 2005; 293:2873–2883.

36. Bray GA. Lifestyle and pharmacological approaches to weight loss: efficacy and safety. *J Clin Endocrinol Metab* 2008; 93:S81–S88.

37. Van Gaal L, Bray GA. Drugs that modify fat absorption and alter metabolism. In: Bray GA, Bouchard C (eds). *Handbook of Obesity*. Marcel Dekker, New York, 2004.

38. Mancini MC, Halpern A. Orlistat in the prevention of diabetes in the obese patient. *Vasc Health Risk Manag* 2008; 4:325–336.

39. Kelley DE, Kuller LH, McKolanis TM *et al*. Effects of moderate weight loss and orlistat on insulin resistance, regional adiposity, and fatty acids in type 2 diabetes. *Diabetes Care* 2004; 27:33–40.

40. Tan K, Tso A, Tam S *et al*. Acute effect of orlistat on post-prandial lipaemia and free fatty acids in overweight patients with type 2 diabetes. *Diabet Med* 2002; 19:944–948.

41. Randle PJ, Garland PB, Hales CN *et al*. The glucose fatty-acid cycle. Its role in insulin sensitivity and the metabolic disturbances of diabetes mellitus. *Lancet* 1963; 13:785–789.

42. Cnop M. Fatty acids and glucolipotoxicity in the pathogenesis of type 2 diabetes. *Biochem Soc Trans* 2008; 36:348–352.

43. Damci T, Yalin S, Balci H *et al*. Orlistat augments postprandial increases in glucagon-like peptide-1 in obese type 2 diabetic patients. *Diabetes Care* 2004; 27:1077–1080.

44. Hsieh CJ, Wang PW, Liu RT *et al*. Orlistat for obesity: benefits beyond weight loss. *Diabetes Res Clin Pract* 2005; 67:78–83.

45. Samuelsson L, Gottsater A, Lindgärde F. Decreasing levels of tumour necrosis factor alpha and interleukin 6 during lowering of body mass index with orlistat or placebo in obese subjects with cardiovascular risk factors. *Diabetes Obes Metab* 2003; 5:195–201.

46. Padwal RS, Majumdar SR. Drug treatments for obesity: orlistat, sibutramine, and rimonabant. *Lancet* 2007; 369:71–77.

47. Hung YJ, Chen YC, Pei D *et al*. Sibutramine improves insulin sensitivity without alteration of serum adiponectin in obese subjects with type 2 diabetes. *Diabet Med* 2005; 22:1024–1030.

48. Finer N, Bloom SR, Frost GS, Banks LM, Griffiths J. Sibutramine is effective for weight loss and diabetic control in obesity with type 2 diabetes: a randomized, double-blind, placebo-controlled study. *Diabetes Obes Metab* 2000; 2:105–112.

49. Fujioka K, Seaton TB, Rowe E *et al*. Weight loss with sibutramine improves glycaemic control and other metabolic parameters in obese patients with type 2 diabetes mellitus. *Diabetes Obes Metab* 2000; 2:175–187.

50. Gokcel A, Karakose H, Ertorer EM, Tanaci N, Tutuncu NB, Guvener N. Effects of sibutramine in obese female subjects with type 2 diabetes and poor blood glucose control. *Diabetes Care* 2001; 24:1957–1960.

51. Serrano-Rios M, Melchionda N, Moreno-Carretero E. Role of sibutramine in the treatment of obese type 2 diabetic subjects receiving sulphonylurea therapy. *Diabet Med* 2002; 19:119–124.

52. McNulty SJ, Ur E, Williams G. A randomized trial of sibutramine in the management of obese type 2 diabetic subjects treated with metformin. *Diabetes Care* 2003; 26:125–131.

53. Redmon JB, Raatz SK, Reck KP *et al*. One-year outcome of a combination of weight loss therapies for subjects with type 2 diabetes. *Diabetes Care* 2003; 26:2505–2511.

54. Kaukua JK, Pekkarinen TA, Rissanen AM. Health-related quality of life in a randomised placebo-controlled trial of sibutramine in obese patients with type II diabetes. *Int J Obes Relat Metab Disord* 2004; 28:600–605.

55. Sanchez-Reyes L, Fangh G, Yamamoto J, Martinez-Rivas LN, Campos-Franco E, Berber A. Use of sibutramine in overweight Hispanic patients with type 2 diabets mellitus: a 12-month, randomized, double-blind, placebo-controlled clinical trial. *Clin Ther* 2004; 26:1427–1435.

56. Redmon JB, Reck KP, Raatz SK *et al*. Two-year outcome of a combination of weight loss therapies for type 2 diabetes. *Diabetes Care* 2005; 28:1311–1315.

57. Wang TF, Pei D, Li JC *et al*. Effects of sibutramine in overweight, poorly controlled Chinese female type 2 diabetic patients: a randomized, double-blind, placebo-controlled study. *Int J Clin Pract* 2005; 59:746–750.

58. Derosa G, D'Angelo A, Salvadeo SAT *et al*. Sibutramine effect on metabolic control of obese patients with type 2 diabetes mellitus treated with pioglitazone. *Metabolism* 2008; 57:1552–1557.
59. Norris SL, Zhangs X, Avenell A *et al*. Efficacy of pharmacotherapy for weight loss in adults with type 2 diabetes mellitus: a meta-analysis. *Arch Intern Med* 2004; 164:1395–1404.
60. Vettor R, Serra R, Fabris R, Pagano C, Federspil G. Effect of sibutramine on weight management and metabolic control in type 2 diabetes: a meta-analysis of clinical studies. *Diabetes Care* 2005; 28:942–949.
61. UK Prospective Diabetes Study Group: Tight blood pressure and risk of macrovascular and microvascular complications in type 2 diabetes: UKPDS 38. *BMJ* 1998; 317:703–713.
62. Matias I, Gonthier MP, Orlando P *et al*. Regulation, function, and dysregulation of endocannabinoids in models of adipose and β-pancreatic cells and in obesity and hyperglycaemia. *J Clin Endocrinol Metab* 2006; 91:3171–3180.
63. Van Gaal LF, Rissanen AM, Scheen AJ *et al*. Effects of the cannabinoid-1 receptor blocker rimonabant on weight reduction and cardiovascular risk factors in overweight patients: 1-year experience from the RIO-Europe study. *Lancet* 2005; 365:1389–1397.
64. Pi-Sunyer FX, Aronne LJ, Heshmati HM *et al*. Effect of rimonabant, a cannabinoid-1 receptor blocker, on weight and cardiometabolic risk factors in overweight or obese patients: RIO-North America: a randomized controlled trial. *JAMA* 2006; 295:761–775.
65. Després JP, Golay A, Sjostrom L. Effects of rimonabant on metabolic risk factors in overweight patients with dyslipidemia. *N Engl J Med* 2005; 353:2121–2134.
66. Scheen AJ, Finer N, Hollander P, Jensen MD, Van Gaal LF, for the RIO-Diabetes Study Group. Efficacy and tolerability of rimonabant in overweight or obese patients with type 2 diabetes: a randomised controlled study. *Lancet* 2006; 368:1660–1672.
67. Stratton IM, Adler AI, Neil HA *et al*. Association of glycaemia with macrovascular and microvascular complications of type 2 diabetes (UKPDS 35): prospective observational study. *BMJ* 2000; 321:405–412.
68. Rosenstock J, Hollander P, Chevalier S, Iranmanesh A, for the SERENADE Study Group. SERENADE: The study evaluating rimonabant efficacy in drug-naïve diabetic patients. Effects of monotherapy with rimonabant, the first selective CB1-receptor antagonist, on glycemic control, body weight, and lipid profile in drug-naïve type 2 diabetes. *Diabetes Care* 2008; 31:2169–2176.
69. Christensen R, Kristensen PK, Bartels EM, Bliddal H, Astrup A. Efficacy and safety of the weight-loss drug rimonabant: a meta-analysis of randomised trials. *Lancet* 2007; 370:1706–1713.
70. Van Gaal L, Pi-Sunyer X, Després JP, McCarthy C, Scheen A. Efficacy and safety of rimonabant for improvement of multiple cardiometabolic risk factors in overweight/obese patients: pooled 1-year data from the Rimonabant in Obesity (RIO) program. *Diabetes Care* 2008; 31:S229–S240.
71. Kutnowski M, Daubresse JC, Friedman H *et al*. Fluoxetine therapy in obese diabetic and glucose intolerant patients. *Int J Obes Relat Metab Disord* 1992; 16(suppl 4):S63–S66.
72. Gray DS, Fujioka K, Devine W, Bray GA. A randomized double-blind clinical trial of fluoxetine in obese diabetics. *Int J Obes Relat Metab Disord* 1992; 16:S67–S72.
73. O'Kane M, Wiles PG, Wales JK. Fluoxetine in the treatment of obese type 2 diabetic patients. *Diabet Med* 1994; 11:105–110.
74. Connolly VM, Gallagher A, Kesson CM. A study of fluoxetine in obese elderly patients with type 2 diabetes. *Diabet Med* 1995; 12:416–418.
75. Daubresse JC, Kolanowski J, Krzentowski G, Kutnowski M, Scheen A, Van Gaal L. Usefulness of fluoxetine in obese non-insulin-dependent diabetics: a multi-center study. *Obes Res* 1996; 4:391–396.
76. Sari R, Balci MK, Cakir M, Altunbas H, Karayalcin U. Comparison of efficacy of sibutramine or orlistat versus their combination in obese women. *Endocr Res* 2004; 30:159–167.
77. Wadden TA, Berkowitz RI, Womble LG *et al*. Effects of sibutramine plus orlistat in obese women following 1 year of treatment by sibutramine alone: a placebo-controlled trial. *Obes Res* 2000; 8:431–437.
78. Connolly HM, Crary JL, McGoon MD *et al*. Valvular heart disease associated with fenfluramine-phentermine. *N Engl J Med* 1997; 337:581–588.
79. Després JP. Potential contribution of metformin to the management of cardiovascular disease risk in patients with abdominal obesity, the metabolic syndrome and type 2 diabetes. *Diabetes Metab* 2003; 29:6S53–6S61.
80. Lee M, Aronne LJ. Weight management for type 2 diabetes mellitus: global cardiovascular risk reduction. *Am J Cardiol* 2007; 99:68B–79B.
81. Mannucci E, Ognibene A, Cremasco F *et al*. Effect of metformin on glucagon-like peptide 1 (GLP-1) and leptin levels in obese nondiabetic subjects. *Diabetes Care* 2001; 24:489–494.

82. Gokcel A, Gumurdulu Y, Karakose H *et al.* Evaluation of the safety and efficacy of sibutramine, orlistat, and metformin in the treatment of obesity. *Diabetes Obes Metab* 2002; 4:49–55.

83. Qualmann C, Nauck MA, Holst JJ, Orskov C, Creutzfeldt W. Glucagon-like peptide-1 (7–36 amide) secretion in response to luminal sucrose from the upper and lower gut. A study using alpha-glucosidase inhibition (acarbose). *Scand J Gastroenterol* 1995; 30:892–896.

84. Hanefeld M, Cagatay M, Petrowitsch T, Neuser D, Petzinna D, Rupp M. Acarbose reduces the risk for myocardial infarction in type 2 diabetic patients: meta-analysis of seven long-term studies. *Eur Heart J* 2004; 25:10–16.

85. Amori RE, Lau J, Pittas AG. Efficacy and safety of incretin therapy in type 2 diabetes: systematic review and meta-analysis. *JAMA* 2007; 298:194–206.

86. Klonoff DC, Buse JB, Nielsen LL *et al.* Exenatide effects on diabetes, obesity, cardiovascular risk factors and hepatic biomarkers in patients with type 2 diabetes treated for at least 3 years. *Curr Med Res Opin* 2008; 24:275–286.

87. Ratner RE, Maggs D, Nielsen LL *et al.* Long-term effects of exenatide therapy over 82 weeks on glycaemic control and weight in over-weight metformin-treated patients with type 2 diabetes mellitus. *Diabetes Obes Metab* 2006; 8:419–428.

88. Van Gaal LF, Gutkin SW, Nauck MA. Exploiting the antidiabetic properties of incretins to treat type 2 diabetes mellitus: glucagon-like peptide 1 receptor agonists or insulin for patients with inadequate glycemic control. *Eur J Endocrinol* 2008; 158:773–784.

89. Hays NP, Galassetti PR, Coker RH. Prevention and treatment of type 2 diabetes: current role of lifestyle, natural product, and pharmacological interventions. *Pharmacol Therap* 2008; 118:181–191.

90. Weyer C, Maggs DG, Young AA, Kolterman OG. Amylin replacement with pramlintide as an adjunct to insulin therapy in type 1 and type 2 diabetes mellitus: a physiological approach toward improved metabolic control. *Curr Pharm Des* 2001; 7:1353–1373.

91. Buse JB, Weyer C, Maggs DG. Amylin replacement with pramlintide in type 1 and type 2 diabetes: a physiological approach to overcome barriers with insulin therapy. *Clin Diabetes* 2002; 20:137–144.

92. Edelman SV, Weyer C. Unresolved challenges with insulin therapy in type 1 and type 2 diabetes: a potential benefit of replacing amylin, a second β-cell hormone. *Diabetes Technol Ther* 2002; 4:175–189.

93. Fineman M, Weyer C, Maggs DG, Strobel S, Kolterman OG. The human amylin analog, pramlintide, reduces postprandial hyperglucagonemia in patients with type 2 diabetes mellitus. *Horm Metab Res* 2002; 34:504–508.

94. Vella A, Lee JS, Camilleri M *et al.* Effects of pramlintide, an amylin analogue, on gastric emptying in type 1 and type 2 diabetes mellitus. *Neurogastroenterol Motil* 2002; 14:123–131.

95. Smith SR, Blundell JE, Burns C *et al.* Pramlintide treatment reduces 24-h caloric intake and meal sizes and improves control of eating in obese subjects: a 6 week translational study. *Am J Physiol Endocrinol Metab* 2007; 293:E620–E627.

96. Hollander P, Maggs DG, Ruggles JA *et al.* Effect of pramlintide on weight in overweight and obese insulin-treated type 2 diabetes patients. *Obes Res* 2004; 12:661–668.

97. Aronne L, Fujioka K, Aroda V *et al.* Progressive reduction in body weight after treatment with the amylin analog pramlintide in obese subjects: a phase 2, randomized, placebo-controlled, dose-escalation study. *J Clin Endocrinol Metab* 2007; 92:2977–2983.

98. Chapman I, Parker B, Doran S *et al.* Effect of pramlintide on satiety and food intake in obese subjects and subjects with type 2 diabetes. *Diabetologia* 2005; 48:838–848.

99. Hollander PA, Levy P, Fineman MS *et al.* Pramlintide as an adjunct to insulin therapy improves long-term glycemic and weight control in patients with type 2 diabetes. A 1-year randomized controlled trial. *Diabetes Care* 2003; 26:784–790.

100. Ratner RE, Dickey R, Fineman M *et al.* Amylin replacement with pramlintide as an adjunct to insulin therapy improves long-term glycaemic and weight control in type 1 diabetes mellitus: a 1-year, randomized controlled trial. *Diabet Med* 2004; 21:1204–1212.

101. Maggs D, Shen L, Strobel S, Brown D, Kolterman O, Weyer C. Effect of pramlintide on A1c and body weight in insulin-treated African Americans and Hispanics with type 2 diabetes: a pooled post-hoc analysis. *Metabolism* 2003; 52:1638–1642.

102. Nauck M, Frid A, Hermansen K *et al.* Efficacy and safety comparison of liraglutide, glimepiride, and placebo, all in combination with metformin, in type 2 diabetes: the LEAD (liraglutide effect and action in diabetes)-2 study. *Diabetes Care* 2009; 32:84–90.

103. Garber A, Henry R, Ratner R *et al*. Liraglutide versus glimepiride monotherapy for type 2 diabetes (LEAD-3 Mono): a randomised, 52-week, phase III, double-blind, parallel-treatment trial. *Lancet* 2009; 373:473–481.
104. Visbøll T, Zdravkovic M, Le-Thi T *et al*. Liraglutide, a long-acting human glucagon-like peptide-1 analog, given as monotherapy significantly improves glycemic control and lowers body weight without risk of hypoglycemia in patients with type 2 diabetes. *Diabetes Care* 2007; 30:1608–1610.
105. Heymsfield SB, Greenberg AS, Fujioka K *et al*. Recombinant leptin for weight loss in obese and lean adults: a randomized, controlled, dose-escalation trial. *JAMA* 1999; 282:1568–1575.
106. Hukshorn CJ, Westerterp-Plantenga MS, Saris WH. Pegylated human recombinant leptin (PEG-OB) causes additional weight loss in severely energy-restricted, overweight men. *Am J Clin Nutr* 2003; 77:771–776.
107. Astrup A, Madsbad S, Breum L, Jensen TJ, Kroustrup JP, Larsen TM. Effect of tesofensine on body weight loss, body composition, and quality of life in obese patients: a randomised, double-blind, placebo-controlled trial. *Lancet* 2008; 372:1906–1913.
108. Hainer V, Toplak H, Mitrakou A. Treatment modalities of obesity. What fits whom? *Diabetes Care* 2008; 31:S269–S277.

6

What should be the second-line therapy after metformin in the overweight type 2 diabetic patient?

B. Gallwitz

BACKGROUND

Type 2 diabetes is a progressive disease that requires an escalation of therapeutic efforts over time as metabolic control deteriorates [1]. Metformin is considered to be the first-line drug due to its efficacy, its effect on insulin resistance, its weight neutrality, its pharmacological profile and the lack of risk for causing hypoglycaemia. In the UK Prospective Diabetes Study (UKPDS) patients treated with metformin had a very favourable outcome [2]. On the basis of these data and decades-long clinical experience with metformin, this drug was implemented in most guidelines for the treatment of type 2 diabetes as the first-line drug. In a joint recommendation for the treatment of type 2 diabetes by the American Diabetes Association (ADA) and the European Association for the Study of Diabetes (EASD) [3, 4], as well as the evidence-based treatment guidelines of the German Diabetes Association [5], metformin was proposed as the first-line drug. After this initial step of pharmacological monotherapy, the escalation of antidiabetic treatment has many options for second-line combinations. These are depicted in Figure 6.1, which shows the joint ADA/EASD guidelines for the pharmacological treatment of type 2 diabetes. Novel drugs with new mechanisms of action based on the physiological effects of incretin hormones have been introduced since then, so that it seems prudent to critically review the treatment options for obese type 2 diabetic patients with metformin monotherapy failure.

SUBSTANCES AVAILABLE FOR A SECOND-LINE THERAPY AFTER METFORMIN MONOTHERAPY

A great variety of substances are available for combination with metformin to escalate therapy after monotherapy failure on metformin (Table 6.1). Among the oral antidiabetic drugs, sulphonylureas, glinides, α-glucosidase inhibitors and glitazones have been available for at least a decade, and with dipeptidyl peptidase-4 (DPP-4) inhibitors a novel class of oral agents is available.

An option besides oral combination therapies is the possibility of combining metformin treatment with insulin as an injectable drug. Here, different forms of insulin therapy can be implemented (e.g. long-acting 'bed-time' insulin once daily, prandial insulin regimes or conventional insulin therapy).

Baptist Gallwitz, MD, PhD, Consultant Endocrinologist, Department of Medicine IV, Eberhard Karls University Tübingen, Tübingen, Germany.

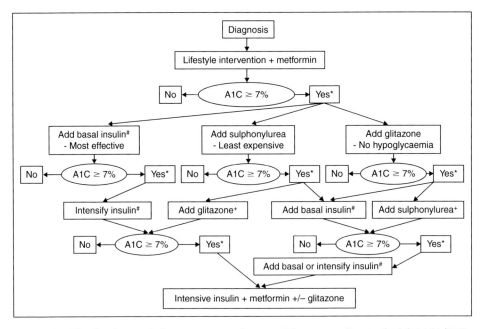

Figure 6.1 Algorithm for the metabolic management of type 2 diabetes according to the joint ADA/EASD recommendation, 2006 [3].

A novel oral/injectable agent treatment combination is available with metformin and glucagon-like peptide-1 (GLP-1) receptor agonists, either in the form of the incretin mimetic exenatide or as the human GLP-1 analogue liraglutide.

All of these treatment options will be described and discussed below.

Sulphonylureas
Sulphonylureas act by interfering with the potassium/ATP channel of the β-cell. The closure of this channel by sulphonylureas leads to a depolarization of the β-cells and a consecutive calcium influx. The rise in the intracellular calcium concentration results in insulin release independent from the actual glucose concentration [6].

The combination of metformin with sulphonylureas has been a standard combination for decades. From a theoretical point of view, it is advantageous to combine a treatment principally acting on insulin resistance with one that alters insulin secretion. Besides, a number of clinical studies have investigated cardiovascular outcomes of different cohorts of patients with type 2 diabetes being treated with this combination using different sulphonylureas. Taking these studies together, no consistent disadvantage of this combination on cardiovascular endpoints was observed.

In the UKPDS, patients receiving a combination of metformin and a sulphonylurea had a higher mortality than patients receiving sulphonylurea monotherapy [2]. This observation may be explained by the fact that patients in the sulphonylurea monotherapy group had a remarkably low incidence of mortality and cardiovascular events [2]. In a Scandinavian study, negative outcomes were also observed with the metformin–sulphonylurea combination [7]. A limitation of this study is that the patient cohort with this combination therapy had longer diabetes duration and worse metabolic control than the controls [7]. A five-year Canadian observational study showed a significantly reduced mortality risk in patients on the metformin–sulphonylurea combination (odds ratio [OR] 0.66; $n = 4684$); the overall mor-

Table 6.1 Possible therapeutic combinations after metformin failure in type 2 diabetes with advantages and disadvantages

Substance class	Advantages	Disadvantages	Remarks
Sulphonylureas	▪ Combination principle (insulin secretagogue) ▪ Long-term experience ▪ Costs ▪ Existing endpoint studies	▪ Lack of durability of control ▪ Hypoglycaemia ▪ No influence on disease progression ▪ Weight gain	▪ Promote further weight gain in obese patients
Glinides	▪ Combination principle (insulin secretagogue) ▪ Shorter duration of action compared to sulphonylureas	▪ Lack of durability of control ▪ Hypoglycaemia ▪ No influence on disease progression ▪ Weight gain ▪ Costs	▪ Promote further weight gain in obese patients
Alpha-glucosidase inhibitors	▪ Combination principle (slowing of carbohydrate resorption) ▪ Cardiovascular risk reduction shown in IGT ▪ No weight gain ▪ No hypoglycaemia with metformin combination	▪ Present lack of endpoint studies ▪ Gastrointestinal side-effects ▪ Possibly less efficacious compared to other oral antidiabetics ▪ Costs	▪ Weight loss possible with therapy, at least weight-neutral
Glitazones	▪ No increased risk of hypoglycaemia ▪ Positive pleiotropic effects (pioglitazone) ▪ Positive effects on β-cell function and survival (animal studies, in vitro data) ▪ Adipose tissue shift from visceral fat to subcutaneous fat	▪ Combination principle (also insulin resistance) ▪ Weight gain ▪ Heart failure ▪ Bone fractures ▪ Costs	▪ Promote further weight gain in obese patients

Table 6.1 Continued

Substance class	Advantages	Disadvantages	Remarks
DPP-4 inhibitors	▪ Combination principle (insulin secretagogue) ▪ No increased risk of hypoglycaemia ▪ Weight-neutral ▪ Glucose-dependent mode of action ▪ Additional effect on glucagon secretion ▪ Less need for blood glucose self-measurements	▪ Long-term effects presently unknown ▪ Lack of endpoint studies ▪ Costs	▪ May turn out to be an advantageous substitute for sulphonylureas due to glucose-dependent mode of action (no hypoglycaemia) and weight neutrality
GLP-1 receptor agonists (exenatide, liraglutide)	▪ Combination principle (insulin secretagogue) ▪ No hypoglycaemia with metformin combination ▪ Weight loss with therapy ▪ Glucose-dependent mode of action ▪ Additional effect on glucagon secretion ▪ Less need for blood glucose self-measurements	▪ Long-term effects presently unknown ▪ Lack of endpoint studies ▪ Costs ▪ Injectable therapy ▪ Transient nausea at start of therapy	▪ Significant weight loss with therapy
Insulin	▪ Combination principle (insulin substitution) ▪ Long-term experience ▪ Favourable outcomes ▪ Insulin titration allows treatment to desired target values ▪ Long-term efficacy	▪ Hypoglycaemia ▪ Weight gain ▪ Injectable therapy ▪ More need of blood glucose self-measurements ▪ Increased necessity for patient education regarding insulin titration, hypoglycaemia and metabolic control ▪ Overall costs	▪ Promotes further weight gain in obese patients

tality rate was 6.4% in this group compared to 7.0% in the metformin monotherapy group [8]. The mortality risk in the combination therapies may be dependent on the type of sulphonylurea used. An Italian observational study on more than 2000 patients showed a significantly higher 3-year mortality with a combination of metformin with glibenclamide (8.7%) than with repaglinide (3.1%; $P = 0.002$), gliclazide (2.1%; $P = 0.001$) or glimepiride (0.4%; $P < 0.0001$). Even after correcting for various confounders, the mortality risk with a metformin–glibenclamide combination was significantly higher (OR 2.09) [9]. Other retrospective studies with very large patient numbers did not reveal an increase of cardiovascular risk with a metformin–sulphonylurea combination [10].

Sulphonylureas are cheap so that a broad application in combination therapy may cause less of a financial burden to the healthcare systems provided care is taken to minimize the risk of hypoglycaemic events. This can be achieved by choosing a sulphonylurea with an action time that is not longer than necessary, and an efficacy, time course and potency that fit the patient's daily needs. Since most sulphonylureas are eliminated by the kidney, great care should be taken to adjust the dose in patients with renal impairment, if the choice falls on using a sulphonylurea [11, 12]. Some sulphonylureas are metabolized generating metabolites that are also able to lower blood glucose [13]. This fact should also be considered when choosing a sulphonylurea.

The main disadvantages of sulphonylureas are the risk of causing hypoglycaemia and weight gain [3]. The incidence of severe hypoglycaemic episodes with sulphonylurea therapy in type 2 diabetic patients was 1.4% in the UKPDS and similarly high in other studies, regardless of the sulphonylurea used [1, 14]. The weight gain observed with a sulphonylurea therapy amounted to 1.7 to 2.9 kg over the study period, also depending on the sulphonylurea used [1, 15]. Furthermore, sulphonylureas lose their efficacy over time. In the ADOPT study, the cumulative incidence of monotherapy failure at 5 years on the sulphonylurea glyburide was 34% and much higher than for metformin or rosiglitazone [16].

Glinides

Glinides have the same mode of action as sulphonylureas. Their pharmacological half-life is much shorter than that of sulphonylureas and they are mainly metabolized and eliminated by the kidneys [17, 18]. Due to their shorter action profile, they can be administered with meals and therefore allow more flexibility in dosing and action [17, 18]. To date, only two glinides are available – repaglinide and nateglinide. Weight gain and hypoglycaemia have also been described with glinide therapy. With repaglinide, the data on body weight are inconsistent – one study reported weight gain [19], another did not [20]. The present study data also do not show a significant advantage of glinides comparing hypoglycaemia risk with the sulphonylureas [19, 21, 22].

In combination therapy with metformin, both repaglinide and nateglinide lower HbA1c more effectively than metformin alone [23, 24].

Concerning cardiovascular complications of combination therapy of glinides with metformin, they have the same mode of action on β-cells as sulphonylureas. Repaglinide does not only specifically bind to the β-cell expressed sulphonylurea receptor SUR-1, but also to the cardiovascular sulphonylurea receptors SUR-2A and SUR-2B [25, 26]. In light of these preclinical findings, cardiovascular outcome studies for the glinides are needed to clarify the possible benefits and harms of a metformin–glinide combination. Presently, there are no endpoint studies available regarding cardiovascular outcomes with glinide therapy. The NAVIGATOR study, currently still running, will generate data on endpoints with nateglinide [27].

Alpha-glucosidase inhibitors

Alpha-glucosidase inhibitors are molecules with a structural similarity to tetrasaccharides. They have an affinity to intestinal disaccharidases and competitively bind to the enzyme, inhibiting disaccharide breakdown into monosaccharides. As a result, postprandial absorption of glucose is diminished, improving glycaemic control [28]. The effect of α-glucosidase inhibitors is meal-dependent, which explains their limited efficacy compared to other classes of oral antidiabetic agents. Alpha-glucosidase inhibitors do not have an intrinsic risk for causing hypoglycaemia, but in combination with sulphonylureas or insulin, hypoglycaemic events should be treated with glucose, as polysaccharides are ineffective in treating the hypoglycaemia due to the mechanism of action [29].

Alpha-glucosidase inhibitors can be combined with metformin (and any other antidiabetic treatment option). In clinical studies, an additional HbA1c reduction of 0.65–0.8% was observed in patients receiving acarbose additional to ongoing metformin therapy [30]. The results of the acarbose arm of the UKPDS showed that the additional therapy with acarbose in previously drug-treated patients with type 2 diabetes led to a 0.5% reduction in HbA1c in the group of patients receiving the drug over 3 years (39% of patients in the acarbose arm). The total acarbose cohort had an HbA1 reduction of 0.2% [31]. A multicentre observational study carried out in Germany showed an efficacy of acarbose to lower HbA1c by 1.8–2.4% in an outpatient and general practice setting [32].

High evidence class outcome studies on acarbose, miglitol or voglibose are lacking. For acarbose, there is a retrospective meta-analysis of a variety of studies showing an advantage for acarbose concerning cardiovascular endpoints with a significant relative risk reduction of 64% for myocardial infarction and 35% for all macrovascular events [33]. For subjects with impaired glucose tolerance (IGT), the use of acarbose to lower postprandial glucose has shown a 49% relative risk reduction for a combination of cardiovascular endpoints [34].

Alpha-glucosidase inhibitors do not cause weight gain [35]. In some studies a moderate weight loss was observed in patients receiving these compounds [35, 36].

Compared to sulphonylureas, the price of α-glucosidase inhibitors is higher, but it should be considered that a reduced necessity to self monitor glucose (due to the lack of intrinsic hypoglycaemia risk) may be a cost saving, as is a reduced incidence of severe hypoglycaemia necessitating emergency treatment with hospital admissions.

Glitazones

Rosiglitazone and pioglitazone are selective agonists of the peroxisomal proliferator-activated receptor gamma (PPARγ) receptor and are the only glitazones available today. They improve glucose control by lowering insulin resistance in the adipose tissue, the skeletal muscle and the liver [37]. They do not cause hypoglycaemia, but weight gain was observed in clinical studies – on average 3.3 kg with rosiglitazone and 1.5 kg with pioglitazone [38–54].

There are several studies of both substances showing an improvement of glycaemic control when either rosiglitazone or pioglitazone is added to ongoing metformin therapy [44, 45, 47]. The additional lowering of HbA1c by the glitazones was in the range between 0.33 and 1.9%, depending on the baseline HbA1c and the characteristics of the patient population [38, 40–45, 47, 55–62].

Concerning effects on lipid metabolism, pioglitazone was shown to lower low-density lipoprotein (LDL)-cholesterol by up to 4%; other studies could not confirm these changes. However, pioglitazone has beneficial effects on lipid parameters by lowering small dense LDL and raising high-density lipoprotein (HDL)-cholesterol. Rosiglitazone also has the latter two effects, but increases LDL-cholesterol [45, 63–67]. Both glitazones also lowered systolic (by 6.2 mmHg) as well as diastolic (by 4.2 mmHg) blood pressure in some clinical studies [48, 49, 51, 68].

Regarding cardiovascular outcomes, pioglitazone treatment led to a non-significant relative risk reduction of 10% in the PROActive study in the combined primary endpoint (total mortality, non-fatal myocardial infarction, acute coronary syndrome, stroke, major amputation, cardiovascular intervention [cardial or peripheral bypass operations, percutaneous angioplasties]). In this study, patients with type 2 diabetes after a macrovascular event were either treated with pioglitazone or placebo additional to their ongoing therapy. For the secondary endpoint (myocardial infarction, stroke, death) a significant risk reduction of 16% was reported. The number needed to treat was 144 per year [69]. In the pioglitazone group the need for additional insulin therapy was reduced by 46.9% compared to placebo, but a higher proportion (1.6%) of patients had to be hospitalized due to heart failure. Oedema without clinical signs of heart failure was observed in the pioglitazone group in 21.6% and in 13.0% in the placebo group [69].

A meta-analysis of glitazone therapy showed a reduction of total mortality for patients with diagnosed heart failure but a higher hospitalization rate due to a decompensation of heart failure [70]. Some recent retrospective studies and meta-analyses of rosiglitazone showed a higher incidence of myocardial infarction [71–73], whereas the RECORD study that was prematurely published after these reports, could not detect a difference in the incidence of myocardial infarction or cardiovascular death in patients treated either with a combination of metformin and a sulphonylurea or the combination of metformin and rosiglitazone [73].

Dipeptidyl peptidase-4 (DPP-4) inhibitors

Dipeptidyl peptidase-4 is a ubiquitous enzyme that is the key enzyme for degradation of the incretin hormones GLP-1 and gastric inhibitory polypeptide (GIP). These hormones are secreted from endocrine cells in the intestine postprandially and are responsible for glucose-dependent stimulation of insulin secretion. Approximately 60% of the postprandial insulin release is promoted by these two hormones [74]. Besides GLP-1 and GIP, DPP-4 has additional peptides as substrates, but the affinity of DPP-4 is higher toward GLP-1 than towards other peptides including GIP. Since DPP-4 inhibitors also inhibit the degradation of GIP, pituitary adenylate cyclase-activating polypeptide (PACAP) and other peptides involved in regulating glucose homeostasis, they could also have additional effects that are favourable in diabetes treatment. DPP-4 belongs to a whole enzyme family of endopeptidases. Therefore, DPP-4 inhibitors need to have a high selectivity to inhibit exclusively DPP-4 and not other DPPs. DPP-4 inhibitors are the first class of oral agents to have a pharmacological mechanism of action utilizing the physiology of GLP-1 [75]. The DPP-4 inhibitors, sitagliptin, saxagliptin and vildagliptin, are two compounds of the DPP-4 inhibitor class that have been approved in various countries. Further DPP-4 inhibitors are in development.

After a meal, active endogenous GLP-1 and GIP concentrations are increased two- to threefold by DPP-4 inhibitors. Across doses and multiple clinical and preclinical studies, no apparent adverse effects have been reported so far, and tolerability and safety data are good. DPP-4 inhibitors do not cause hypoglycaemia because they stimulate insulin secretion only under hyperglycaemic conditions. They also are not involved in drug–drug interactions, especially with other antihyperglycaemic oral agents [76–79].

In animal models, DPP-4 inhibitors increased the number of insulin-positive β-cells in islets, and the β- to α-cell ratio in different diabetic animals was normalized. Furthermore, islet insulin content was found to be increased and glucose-stimulated insulin secretion in isolated islets was found to be improved in comparison to glipizide-treated mice. Based on these experimental results, DPP-4 inhibitors may have the potential to delay or prevent disease progression in type 2 diabetes and to improve β-cell mass and function [76–79]. In mice deficient in DPP-4 (CD26–/–; DPP-4 knockout mice), concentrations of circulating intact GLP-1 and GIP are elevated and these animals are resistant to streptozotocin-induced β-cell destruction [80].

In monotherapy or in combination with other oral antidiabetic agents, DPP-4 inhibitors improve glycaemic control in the fasting and in the postprandial state as well as parameters of β-cell function (postprandial insulin and C-peptide responses, HOMA-B, proinsulin/ insulin ratio) in patients with type 2 diabetes. They lead to a significant reduction in HbA1c compared to placebo and to fasting plasma glucose reductions in clinical studies up to 2 years [76–79]. Treatment with DPP-4 inhibitors is weight-neutral.

As an add-on combination to ongoing metformin therapy in patients with type 2 diabetes not reaching therapeutic goals, DPP-4 inhibitors reduce HbA1c, fasting plasma glucose, and two-hour postprandial plasma glucose. A direct comparison of sitagliptin added to an ongoing treatment with metformin showed a similar efficacy to the addition of glipizide to metformin. Sitagliptin was non-inferior in this 52-week study compared to glipizide. HbA1c and fasting glucose decreased equally in both groups. The occurrence of hypoglycaemic episodes was much larger in the glipizide group than in the sitagliptin group. Body weight increased by 1.1 kg in the glipizide-treated patients, whereas the patients on sitagliptin had a weight loss of 1.5 kg [81].

In clinical studies, sitagliptin, saxagliptin and vildagliptin were well-tolerated in terms of the number of adverse events and the incidence of hypoglycaemia. The incidence of total adverse events, as well as hypoglycaemic episodes, was similar in the treatment and in the placebo groups. The addition of DPP-4 inhibitor therapy was weight-neutral [76–79].

In a study of patients with type 2 diabetes with impaired renal function, including end-stage renal disease, dose-adjusted sitagliptin (25 mg/day for patients with severely impaired renal function [creatinine clearance <30 ml/min or end-stage renal disease or 50 mg/day for moderately impaired patients]) was generally well-tolerated and appeared to be effective [76].

GLP-1 receptor agonists

Exendin-4, a peptide with a 52% amino acid sequence similarity to GLP-1, acts as a high-potency agonist at the GLP-1 receptor on β-cells [82]. Synthetic recombinant exendin-4 was named exenatide. Exenatide shares all the effects of native GLP-1, but is not enzymatically degraded by DPP-4 [83]. Subcutaneous exenatide exerts biological effects for approximately 5–7 hours in humans. Based on this prolonged *in vivo* half-life compared to GLP-1, with twice-daily subcutaneous administration, sufficient plasma concentrations can be reached to obtain the desired GLP-1-like therapeutic effects in type 2 diabetic patients [84].

In clinical trials, therapy with exenatide led to an overall improvement in glycaemic control, plus weight loss with sustained HbA1c reduction of approximately 1.0% and a decrease in body weight of approximately 5.0 kg in 2 years [83, 84]. Adverse effects were mild, mostly in the beginning of the study and generally gastrointestinal (nausea and fullness). Mild hypoglycaemia was noted only in patients receiving sulphonylureas in combination [83, 84]. In addition, exenatide treatment produced clinically significant improvements in cardiovascular risk factors in long-term treatment [85, 86]. Exenatide thus represents an efficacious supplement to failing conventional oral antihyperglycaemic agents, and the sustained effect observed in the extension studies and its continued weight-lowering effects must be considered very promising [84, 86].

In comparative studies, exenatide therapy as add-on to metformin or a sulphonylurea was compared to an insulin add-on. Both exenatide and insulin reduced HbA1c levels by approximately 1.0%. Exenatide reduced postprandial glucose excursions more than insulin, while insulin reduced fasting glucose concentrations more than exenatide. Body weight decreased 2.3 kg with exenatide and increased 1.8 kg with insulin glargine in one study. Rates of symptomatic hypoglycaemia were similar, but nocturnal hypoglycaemia occurred less frequently with exenatide [84, 86].

In animal studies, exenatide caused an increase of β-cell mass due to a stimulation of islet cell neogenesis from precursor cells on the one hand and due to an inhibition of apoptosis of β-cells on the other [87]. The improvement of β-cell function in humans receiving exenatide was demonstrated in a study showing the restoration of the first and second phases of insulin secretion after an intravenous glucose bolus [88].

Exenatide treatment leads to antibody formation. However, this is rarely associated with any reduction in efficacy and the antibodies do not cross-react with native human GLP-1. Nausea is the most common adverse reaction, but is mild, transient and most pronounced in the beginning of exenatide treatment. For this reason, a dose titration is recommended when starting therapy. Hypoglycaemia has not been reported during monotherapy, but can occur when exenatide is administered in combination with sulphonylureas [84].

Liraglutide is a long-acting DPP-4 resistant human GLP-1 analogue with two modifications in the amino acid sequence of the native GLP-1 and an attachment of a fatty acid side chain to the peptide. It is injected subcutaneously once daily [89]. The fatty acid side chain allows non-covalent binding of liraglutide to albumin after injection. This effect, as well as the protection against degradation by DPP-4, contributes to the long action profile. The biological half-life of liraglutide is approximately 13.5 hours in humans so that liraglutide is suitable for once-daily subcutaneous injection. A steady state of stable liraglutide plasma concentrations is reached after 3 days of once-daily application.

In animal studies involving diabetic rodent models, liraglutide has been shown to increase β-cell mass. Liraglutide lowers blood glucose, body weight and food intake in a broad selection of animal models [89]. In clinical studies in humans, it is efficacious and safe in the treatment of type 2 diabetes across all stages of the natural course of the disease [91–97]. More GLP-1 receptor agonists are in clinical development, some of them for once-weekly application (e.g. albiglutide, taspoglutide and others) [98].

A large and comprehensive clinical study programme called 'liraglutide effects and action in diabetes (LEAD)' has investigated the clinical efficacy and safety of liraglutide in doses of 1.2 mg and 1.8 mg once daily in monotherapy, in combinations with either metformin or a sulphonylurea or in combination with two oral antidiabetic agents. Additionally, a head-to-head study compared a liraglutide treatment with an exenatide therapy in patients with type 2 diabetes not optimally controlled under an oral therapy with metformin, a sulphonylurea, or a combination of both. In all the LEAD studies, both doses of liraglutide lowered HbA1c by up to 1.5% from a baseline of 8.0–8.4%. Other glycaemic parameters were also improved significantly, especially fasting plasma glucose, postprandial glucose and HOMA-B. In the LEAD-3 study in drug-naïve patients with type 2 diabetes receiving liraglutide as monotherapy, the glycaemic effects were sustained over a period of two years. In the LEAD-6 study comparing liraglutide to exenatide, liraglutide was non-inferior to exenatide and lead to a significantly greater reduction of fasting plasma glucose. The incidence of hypoglycaemia with liraglutide was at placebo level [91–97].

Liraglutide leads to a sustained weight loss comparable to that observed with exenatide. Weight reductions of approximately 2–3 kg were observed after 26 weeks in the LEAD studies. Furthermore, liraglutide leads to a significant reduction in blood pressure that is independent of the weight reduction. An improvement in the surrogate parameters of cardiovascular risk factors was also described with liraglutide therapy in a number of clinical studies [91–97].

Nausea and gastrointestinal side-effects (vomiting and diarrhoea) are the most common adverse events observed with liraglutide therapy. These side-effects are mostly mild-to-moderate, transient and less severe than exenatide therapy in the LEAD-6 study [91–97].

Liraglutide has been approved by the European Medicines Agency (EMEA) in 2009 and by the US Federal Drugs Administration (FDA) in 2010.

Insulin therapy

There are several studies showing favourable effects on metabolic control for the combination of insulin with metformin [99–103]. This combination has advantages in obese patients and in patients with insulin resistance. With the maintenance of metformin therapy, the amount of insulin may be lower and the effect on body weight is superior to insulin monotherapy [101, 104–106]. The incidence of hypoglycaemic events is significantly higher with insulin therapy compared to therapy with oral antidiabetic agents. In the UKPDS, the incidence of severe hypoglycaemic events with insulin therapy was 2.3 per 100 patient-years [1]. Weight gain with insulin therapy in the UKPDS amounted to a 4 kg difference in a time period of 10 years on average compared to the conventionally treated patient group [1].

When metformin is combined with a long-acting insulin given once daily as bedtime insulin, long-acting insulin analogues (insulin glargine and insulin detemir) are superior compared to NPH insulin from the point of view of incidence of hypoglycaemia, especially nocturnal hypoglycaemia [41, 107–112]. Also, insulin detemir is associated with less weight gain compared to other long-acting insulins. In a direct comparison between insulin glargine and insulin detemir, insulin glargine therapy resulted in mean weight gain of 3.5 kg compared with 2.7 kg for insulin detemir [113]. Insulin detemir was also associated with less weight gain compared to NPH insulin (1.2 kg vs. 2.8 kg, respectively) [109].

SUMMARY

Large intervention trials have demonstrated that antihyperglycaemic therapy with treatment goals aiming at normoglycaemia can reduce the risk or the progression of microvascular as well as macrovascular risk [114–119]. However, normalizing HbA1c alone is not sufficient in risk reduction. A distinct glycaemic threshold for the reduction of complications has not been found and, therefore, the goal of antidiabetic treatment should be to achieve near-normoglycaemia as safely as possible regarding HbA1c, fasting plasma glucose and postprandial glucose concentrations. Since normal HbA1c levels cannot be reached by treating fasting plasma glucose alone, postprandial glucose must also be considered in therapeutic strategies. At lower HbA1c concentrations, the proportional contribution of postprandial glucose to HbA1c is greater than at higher HbA1c values [120]. In addition, a prospective intervention study in a cohort with IGT demonstrated that by reducing post-meal glucose with pharmacological intervention using an α-glucosidase inhibitor, macrovascular events could be significantly reduced [34].

All of the drugs discussed above have shown their efficacy in combination with metformin.

Sulphonylureas, glinides and insulin therapy are associated with an increased risk of hypoglycaemia and are also associated with weight gain. Therefore, these agents should not be considered first-line for combination therapy in overweight patients with type 2 diabetes and metformin monotherapy failure. Sulphonylureas and glinides are insulin secretagogues that, from a theoretical angle, may be a good combination with a drug like metformin acting on insulin resistance, but their glucose-independent mode of action is definitely a disadvantage compared to the novel incretin-based therapies that are safe regarding hypoglycaemia and that are weight-neutral (DPP-4 inhibitors) or even allow weight loss (GLP-1 receptor agonists). The only advantage of the sulphonylureas may be their low cost, but this has to be weighed against the costs of more frequent blood glucose testing and the financial and personal costs of severe hypoglycaemic events.

Insulin has the advantage that it can be dosed in a manner to lower glycaemic parameters to any desired goal, but also has the limitations of weight gain and hypoglycaemia. The latter problem may be reduced by using insulin analogues, but weight gain remains a problem that is only less severe when insulin detemir is used as a long-acting insulin [121]. Here, incretin-based therapies, especially injectable GLP-1 receptor agonists, may be an alternative leading to an improvement of overall glycaemia while allowing weight loss [92, 93, 122].

Acarbose specifically acts on post-meal hyperglycaemia, is weight-neutral and has lowered cardiovascular events in a prospective, randomized double-blind clinical trial in subjects with IGT. In type 2 diabetic patients, a meta-analysis also showed a reduction of cardiovascular events in patients treated with acarbose. Gastrointestinal side-effects and costs, however, are a barrier to broad use of this compound [33, 34].

Glitazones may not appear to be ideal candidates for combination with metformin as the next escalation step, since they act on insulin resistance like metformin and are also associated with weight gain, although they do not cause hypoglycaemia [16]. In a prospective trial on cardiovascular outcomes, pioglitazone failed to show a significant improvement of cardiovascular events defined in the primary endpoint of the study (although the principal secondary endpoint of cardiovascular death, myocardial infarction and stroke was reached) [67].

Presently, many epidemiological studies show an association of post-meal- or post-challenge hyperglycaemia and cardiovascular risk. However, data on the beneficial effects of a pharmacological intervention on cardiovascular endpoints is scarce and still missing for the recently released compounds (DPP-4 inhibitors, GLP-1 receptor agonists).

In recent long-term trials addressing glycaemic goals for the treatment of type 2 diabetes, a lowering of HbA1c to levels not below 6.5% led to a significant reduction in microvascular endpoints, but macrovascular endpoints were not reduced significantly. A very vigorous reduction of the HbA1c to levels below 6.5% lowered non-fatal cardiovascular events but increased mortality for reasons that are most likely associated with hypoglycaemia and unfavourable multiple combinations of oral antidiabetic agents with insulin. In this intensively treated group of patients, the majority of participants with a baseline HbA1c >8.0% received a antidiabetic combination therapy of more than two drugs and gained significantly more weight than the patient group having a higher HbA1c goal [123, 124]. In this respect, a safe antihyperglycaemic treatment not leading to hypoglycaemia and weight gain may be favourable, especially in patients with HbA1c values below 7.5%, where postprandial hyperglycaemia contributes to a high degree to the HbA1c reduction. Here, the incretin-based therapies may become attractive and effective treatment options, especially for overweight patients with type 2 diabetes. DPP-4 inhibitors have been shown to be weight-neutral, and if weight loss is an additional therapeutic goal in obese patients, GLP-1 receptor agonists would appear to be ideal in combination with metformin. Furthermore, DPP-4 inhibitors demonstrated a sustained durability of efficacy in combination with metformin over 2 years [125, 126]. Exenatide also showed a durable HbA1c reduction in a small cohort of patients treated in an open study for 3 years with a baseline oral therapy of metformin or sulphonylureas or a combination of both [85].

In general, however, we need long-term intervention studies to investigate the durability of the effect of these drugs and their effect on vascular outcomes and hard endpoints. These studies will have to be very large and will need to have a long duration to clarify the open questions that still remain.

REFERENCES

1. Intensive blood-glucose control with sulphonylureas or insulin compared with conventional treatment and risk of complications in patients with type 2 diabetes (UKPDS 33). UK Prospective Diabetes Study (UKPDS) Group. *Lancet* 1998; 352:837–853.
2. Effect of intensive blood-glucose control with metformin on complications in overweight patients with type 2 diabetes (UKPDS 34). UK Prospective Diabetes Study (UKPDS) Group. *Lancet* 1998; 352:854–865.
3. Nathan DM, Buse JB, Davidson MB *et al.* Management of hyperglycaemia in type 2 diabetes: a consensus algorithm for the initiation and adjustment of therapy. A consensus statement from the American Diabetes Association and the European Association for the Study of Diabetes. *Diabetologia* 2006; 49:1711–1721.
4. Nathan DM, Buse JB, Davidson MB *et al*, American Diabetes Association; European Association for the Study of Diabetes. Medical management of hyperglycemia in type 2 diabetes: a consensus algorithm for the initiation and adjustment of therapy: a consensus statement of the American Diabetes Association and the European Association for the Study of Diabetes. *Diabetes Care* 2009; 32:193–203.

5. German Diabetes Association, Matthaei S, Bierwirth R et al. Medical antihyperglycaemic treatment of type 2 diabetes mellitus: update of the evidence-based guideline of the German Diabetes Association. *Exp Clin Endocrinol Diabetes* 2009; 117:522–557.

6. Bryan J, Crane A, Vila-Carriles WH, Babenko AP, Aguilar-Bryan L. Insulin secretagogues, sulfonylurea receptors and K(ATP) channels. *Curr Pharm Des* 2005; 11:2699–2716.

7. Olsson J, Lindberg G, Gottsäter M et al. Increased mortality in Type II diabetic patients using sulphonylurea and metformin in combination: a population-based observational study. *Diabetologia* 2000; 43:558–560.

8. Johnson JL, Wolf SL, Kabadi UM. Efficacy of insulin and sulfonylurea combination therapy in type II diabetes. A meta-analysis of the randomized placebo-controlled trials. *Arch Intern Med* 1996; 156:259–264.

9. Monami M, Luzzi C, Lamanna C et al. Three-year mortality in diabetic patients treated with different combinations of insulin secretagogues and metformin. *Diabetes Metab Res Rev* 2006; 22:477–482.

10. Gulliford M, Latinovic R. Mortality in type 2 diabetic subjects prescribed metformin and sulphonylurea drugs in combination: cohort study. *Diabetes Metab Res Rev* 2004; 20:239–245.

11. Graal MB, Wolffenbuttel BH. The use of sulphonylureas in the elderly. *Drugs Aging* 1999; 15:471–481.

12. Krentz AJ. Comparative safety of newer oral antidiabetic drugs. *Expert Opin Drug Saf* 2006; 5:827–834.

13. Rosenkranz B. Pharmacokinetic basis for the safety of glimepiride in risk groups of NIDDM patients. *Horm Metab Res* 1996; 28:434–439.

14. Draeger KE, Wernicke-Panten K, Lomp HJ, Schüler E, Rosskamp R. Long-term treatment of type 2 diabetic patients with the new oral antidiabetic agent glimepiride (Amaryl): a double-blind comparison with glibenclamide. *Horm Metab Res* 1996; 28:419–425.

15. Hermansen K, Mortensen LS. Bodyweight changes associated with antihyperglycaemic agents in type 2 diabetes mellitus. *Drug Saf* 2007; 30:1127–1142.

16. Kahn SE, Haffner SM, Heise MA et al, ADOPT Study Group. Glycemic durability of rosiglitazone, metformin, or glyburide monotherapy. *N Engl J Med* 2006; 355:2427–2443.

17. Derosa G, Sibilla S. Optimizing combination treatment in the management of type 2 diabetes. *Vasc Health Risk Manag* 2007; 3:665–671.

18. Blickle JF. Meglitinide analogues: a review of clinical data focused on recent trials. *Diabetes Metab* 2006; 32:113–120.

19. Marbury T, Huang WC, Strange P, Lebovitz H. Repaglinide versus glyburide: a one-year comparison trial. *Diabetes Res Clin Pract* 1999; 43:155–166.

20. Moses RG, Gomis R, Frandsen KB, Schlienger JL, Dedov I. Flexible meal-related dosing with repaglinide facilitates glycemic control in therapy-naïve type 2 diabetes. *Diabetes Care* 2001; 24:11–15.

21. Landgraf R, Bilo HJ, Muller PG. A comparison of repaglinide and glibenclamide in the treatment of type 2 diabetic patients previously treated with sulphonylureas. *Eur J Clin Pharmacol* 1999; 55:165–171.

22. Hanefeld M, Bouter KP, Dickinson S, Guitard C. Rapid and short-acting mealtime insulin secretion with nateglinide controls both prandial and mean glycemia. *Diabetes Care* 2000; 23:202–207.

23. Moses R, Slobodniuk R, Boyages S et al. Effect of repaglinide addition to metformin monotherapy on glycemic control in patients with type 2 diabetes. *Diabetes Care* 1999; 22:119–124.

24. Horton ES, Clinkingbeard C, Gatlin M, Foley J, Mallows S, Shen S. Nateglinide alone and in combination with metformin improves glycemic control by reducing mealtime glucose levels in type 2 diabetes. *Diabetes Care* 2000; 23:1660–1665.

25. Meyer M, Chudziak F, Schwanstecher C, Schwanstecher M, Panten U. Structural requirements of sulphonylureas and analogues for interaction with sulphonylurea receptor subtypes. *Br J Pharmacol* 1999; 128:27–34.

26. Dabrowski M, Wahl P, Holmes WE, Ashcroft FM. Effect of repaglinide on cloned beta cell, cardiac and smooth muscle types of ATP-sensitive potassium channels. *Diabetologia* 2001; 44:747–756.

27. Califf RM, Boolell M, Haffner SM et al. Prevention of diabetes and cardiovascular disease in patients with impaired glucose tolerance: rationale and design of the Nateglinide And Valsartan in Impaired Glucose Tolerance Outcomes Research (NAVIGATOR) Trial. *Am Heart J* 2008; 156:623–632.

28. Hanefeld M, Schaper F. Acarbose: oral anti-diabetes drug with additional cardiovascular benefits. *Expert Rev Cardiovasc Ther* 2008; 6:153–163.

29. Holstein A, Egberts EH. Risk of hypoglycaemia with oral antidiabetic agents in patients with Type 2 diabetes. *Exp Clin Endocrinol Diabetes* 2003; 111:405–414.

30. Lebovitz HE. Postprandial hyperglycaemic state: importance and consequences. *Diabetes Res Clin Pract* 1998; 40:S27–S28.

31. Holman RR, Cull CA, Turner RC. A randomized double-blind trial of acarbose in type 2 diabetes shows improved glycemic control over 3 years (U.K. Prospective Diabetes Study 44). *Diabetes Care* 1999; 22:960–964.

32. Mertes G. Safety and efficacy of acarbose in the treatment of Type 2 diabetes: data from a 5-year surveillance study. *Diabetes Res Clin Pract* 2001; 52:193–204.

33. Hanefeld M, Cagatay M, Petrowitsch T, Neuser D, Petzinna D, Rupp M. Acarbose reduces the risk for myocardial infarction in type 2 diabetic patients: meta-analysis of seven long-term studies. *Eur Heart J* 2004; 25:10–16.

34. Chiasson JL , Josse RG, Gomis R, Hanefeld M, Karasik A, Laakso M, STOP-NIDDM Trial Research Group. Acarbose treatment and the risk of cardiovascular disease and hypertension in patients with impaired glucose tolerance: the STOP-NIDDM trial. *JAMA* 2003; 290:486–494.

35. Scheen AJ. Clinical efficacy of acarbose in diabetes mellitus: a critical review of controlled trials. *Diabetes Metab* 1998; 24:311–320.

36. Krentz AJ, Bailey CJ. Oral antidiabetic agents: current role in type 2 diabetes mellitus. *Drugs* 2005; 65:385–411.

37. Kintscher U, Law RE. PPARgamma-mediated insulin sensitization: the importance of fat versus muscle. *Am J Physiol Endocrinol Metab* 2005; 288:E287–E291.

38. Hanefeld M , Brunetti P, Schernthaner GH, Matthews DR, Charbonnel BH, QUARTET Study Group. One-year glycemic control with a sulfonylurea plus pioglitazone versus a sulfonylurea plus metformin in patients with type 2 diabetes. *Diabetes Care* 2004; 27:141–147.

39. Umpierrez G, Issa M, Vlajnic A. Glimepiride versus pioglitazone combination therapy in subjects with type 2 diabetes inadequately controlled on metformin monotherapy: results of a randomized clinical trial. *Curr Med Res Opin* 2006; 22:751–759.

40. Nagasaka S, Aiso Y, Yoshizawa K, Ishibashi S. Comparison of pioglitazone and metformin efficacy using homeostasis model assessment. *Diabet Med* 2004; 21:136–141.

41. Rosenstock J, Dailey G, Massi-Benedetti M, Fritsche A, Lin Z, Salzman A. Reduced hypoglycemia risk with insulin glargine: a meta-analysis comparing insulin glargine with human NPH insulin in type 2 diabetes. *Diabetes Care* 2005; 28:950–955.

42. Zhu XX, Pan CY, Li GW et al. Addition of rosiglitazone to existing sulfonylurea treatment in chinese patients with type 2 diabetes and exposure to hepatitis B or C. *Diabetes Technol Ther* 2003; 5:33–42.

43. Kerenyi Z , Samer H, James R, Yan Y, Stewart M. Combination therapy with rosiglitazone and glibenclamide compared with upward titration of glibenclamide alone in patients with type 2 diabetes mellitus. *Diabetes Res Clin Pract* 2004; 63:213–223.

44. Matthews DR , Charbonnel BH, Hanefeld M, Brunetti P, Schernthaner G. Long-term therapy with addition of pioglitazone to metformin compared with the addition of gliclazide to metformin in patients with type 2 diabetes: a randomized, comparative study. *Diabetes Metab Res Rev* 2005; 21: 167–174.

45. Bailey CJ, Bagdonas A, Rubes J et al. Rosiglitazone/metformin fixed-dose combination compared with uptitrated metformin alone in type 2 diabetes mellitus: a 24-week, multicenter, randomized, double-blind, parallel-group study. *Clin Ther* 2005; 27:1548–1561.

46. Charbonnel BH , Matthews DR, Schernthaner G, Hanefeld M, Brunetti P, QUARTET Study Group. A long-term comparison of pioglitazone and gliclazide in patients with type 2 diabetes mellitus: a randomized, double-blind, parallel-group comparison trial. *Diabet Med* 2005; 22:399–405.

47. Jung HS, Youn BS, Cho YM et al. The effects of rosiglitazone and metformin on the plasma concentrations of resistin in patients with type 2 diabetes mellitus. *Metabolism* 2005; 54:314–320.

48. Natali A, Baldeweg S, Toschi E et al. Vascular effects of improving metabolic control with metformin or rosiglitazone in type 2 diabetes. *Diabetes Care* 2004; 27:1349–1357.

49. Pavo I, Jermendy G, Varkonyi TT et al. Effect of pioglitazone compared with metformin on glycemic control and indicators of insulin sensitivity in recently diagnosed patients with type 2 diabetes. *J Clin Endocrinol Metab* 2003; 88:1637–1645.

50. Schernthaner G, Matthews DR, Charbonnel B, Hanefeld M, Brunetti P, Quartet [corrected] Study Group. Efficacy and safety of pioglitazone versus metformin in patients with type 2 diabetes mellitus: a double-blind, randomized trial. *J Clin Endocrinol Metab* 2004; 89:6068–6076.

51. St John Sutton M, Rendell M, Dandona P et al. A comparison of the effects of rosiglitazone and glyburide on cardiovascular function and glycemic control in patients with type 2 diabetes. *Diabetes Care* 2002; 25:2058–2064.

52. Tan M, Johns D, González Gálvez G *et al*, GLAD Study Group. Effects of pioglitazone and glimepiride on glycemic control and insulin sensitivity in Mexican patients with type 2 diabetes mellitus: A multicenter, randomized, double-blind, parallel-group trial. *Clin Ther* 2004; 26:680–693.

53. Tan MH, Johns D, Strand J *et al*, GLAC Study Group. Sustained effects of pioglitazone vs. glibenclamide on insulin sensitivity, glycaemic control, and lipid profiles in patients with Type 2 diabetes. *Diabet Med* 2004; 21:859–866.

54. Tan MH, Baksi A, Krahulec B *et al*, GLAL Study Group. Comparison of pioglitazone and gliclazide in sustaining glycemic control over 2 years in patients with type 2 diabetes. *Diabetes Care* 2005; 28:544–550.

55. Hanefeld M, Pfützner A, Forst T, Lübben G. Glycemic control and treatment failure with pioglitazone versus glibenclamide in type 2 diabetes mellitus: a 42-month, open-label, observational, primary care study. *Curr Med Res Opin* 2006; 22:1211–1215.

56. Derosa G, Cicero AF, Gaddi AV *et al*. Long-term effects of glimepiride or rosiglitazone in combination with metformin on blood pressure control in type 2 diabetic patients affected by the metabolic syndrome: a 12-month, double-blind, randomized clinical trial. *Clin Ther* 2005; 27:1383–1391.

57. Garber A, Klein E, Bruce S, Sankoh S, Mohideen P. Metformin-glibenclamide versus metformin plus rosiglitazone in patients with type 2 diabetes inadequately controlled on metformin monotherapy. *Diabetes Obes Metab* 2006; 8:156–163.

58. Pfutzner A, Forst T. Pioglitazone: an antidiabetic drug with the potency to reduce cardiovascular mortality. *Expert Opin Pharmacother* 2006; 7:463–476.

59. Fonseca V, Grunberger G, Gupta S, Shen S, Foley JE. Addition of nateglinide to rosiglitazone monotherapy suppresses mealtime hyperglycemia and improves overall glycemic control. *Diabetes Care* 2003; 26:1685–1690.

60. Raskin P, McGill J, Saad MF *et al*, Repaglinide/Rosiglitazone Study Group. Combination therapy for type 2 diabetes: repaglinide plus rosiglitazone. *Diabet Med* 2004; 21:329–335.

61. Dailey GE 3rd, Noor MA, Park JS, Bruce S, Fiedorek FT. Glycemic control with glyburide/metformin tablets in combination with rosiglitazone in patients with type 2 diabetes: a randomized, double-blind trial. *Am J Med* 2004; 116:223–229.

62. Orbay E, Sargin M, Sargin H, Gözü H, Bayramiçli OU, Yayla A. Addition of rosiglitazone to glimepirid and metformin combination therapy in type 2 diabetes. *Endocr J* 2004; 51:521–527.

63. Wagstaff AJ, Goa KL. Rosiglitazone: a review of its use in the management of type 2 diabetes mellitus. *Drugs* 2002; 62:1805–1837.

64. Goldberg RB, Kendall DM, Deeg MA *et al*, GLAI Study Investigators. A comparison of lipid and glycemic effects of pioglitazone and rosiglitazone in patients with type 2 diabetes and dyslipidemia. *Diabetes Care* 2005; 28:1547–1554.

65. Freed MI, Ratner R, Marcovina SM *et al*, Rosiglitazone Study 108 investigators. Effects of rosiglitazone alone and in combination with atorvastatin on the metabolic abnormalities in type 2 diabetes mellitus. *Am J Cardiol* 2002; 90:947–952.

66. King AB, Armstrong DU. Lipid response to pioglitazone in diabetic patients: clinical observations from a retrospective chart review. *Diabetes Technol Ther* 2002; 4:145–151.

67. van Wijk JP, de Koning EJ, Castro Cabezas M, Rabelink TJ. Rosiglitazone improves postprandial triglyceride and free fatty acid metabolism in type 2 diabetes. *Diabetes Care* 2005; 28:844–849.

68. Yosefy C, Magen E, Kiselevich A *et al*. Rosiglitazone improves, while Glibenclamide worsens blood pressure control in treated hypertensive diabetic and dyslipidemic subjects via modulation of insulin resistance and sympathetic activity. *J Cardiovasc Pharmacol* 2004; 44:215–222.

69. Dormandy JA, Charbonnel B, Eckland DJ *et al*, PROactive investigators. Secondary prevention of macrovascular events in patients with type 2 diabetes in the PROactive Study (PROspective pioglitAzone Clinical Trial In macroVascular Events): a randomised controlled trial. *Lancet* 2005; 366:1279–1289.

70. Eurich DT, McAlister FA, Blackburn DF *et al*. Benefits and harms of antidiabetic agents in patients with diabetes and heart failure: systematic review. *BMJ* 2007; 335:497.

71. Singh S, Loke YK, Furberg CD. Long-term risk of cardiovascular events with rosiglitazone: a meta-analysis. *JAMA* 2007; 298:1189–1195.

72. Lago RM, Singh PP, Nesto RW. Congestive heart failure and cardiovascular death in patients with prediabetes and type 2 diabetes given thiazolidinediones: a meta-analysis of randomised clinical trials. *Lancet* 2007; 370:1129–1136.

73. Home PD, Pocock SJ, Beck-Nielsen H *et al*. Rosiglitazone evaluated for cardiovascular outcomes in oral agent combination therapy for type 2 diabetes (RECORD): a multicentre, randomised, open-label trial. *Lancet* 2009; 373:2125–2135.

74. Creutzfeldt W. Entero-insular axis and diabetes mellitus. *Horm Metab Res Suppl* 1992; 26:13–18.
75. Drucker DJ, Nauck MA. The incretin system: glucagon-like peptide-1 receptor agonists and dipeptidyl peptidase-4 inhibitors in type 2 diabetes. *Lancet* 2006; 368:1696–1705.
76. Karasik A, Aschner P, Katzeff H *et al*. Sitagliptin, a DPP-4 inhibitor for the treatment of patients with type 2 diabetes: a review of recent clinical trials. *Curr Med Res Opin* 2008; 24:489–496.
77. Ahrén B. Clinical results of treating type 2 diabetic patients with sitagliptin, vildagliptin or saxagliptin– diabetes control and potential adverse events. *Best Pract Res Clin Endocrinol Metab* 2009; 23:487–498.
78. Shubrook JH, Colucci RA, Schwartz FL. Exploration of the DPP-4 inhibitors with a focus on saxagliptin. *Expert Opin Pharmacother* 2009; 10:2927–2934.
79. Banerjee M, Younis N, Soran H. Vildagliptin in clinical practice: a review of literature. *Expert Opin Pharmacother* 2009; 10:2745–2757.
80. Conarello SL, Li Z, Ronan J *et al*. Mice lacking dipeptidyl peptidase IV are protected against obesity and insulin resistance. *Proc Natl Acad Sci USA* 2003; 100:6825–6830.
81. Nauck MA, Meininger G, Sheng D, Terranella L, Stein PP, Sitagliptin Study 024 Group. Efficacy and safety of the dipeptidyl peptidase-4 inhibitor, sitagliptin, compared with the sulfonylurea, glipizide, in patients with type 2 diabetes inadequately controlled on metformin alone: a randomized, double-blind, non-inferiority trial. *Diabetes Obes Metab* 2007; 9:194–205.
82. Göke R, Fehmann HC, Linn T *et al*. Exendin-4 is a high potency agonist and truncated exendin-(9–39)-amide an antagonist at the glucagon-like peptide 1-(7–36)-amide receptor of insulin-secreting beta-cells. *J Biol Chem* 1993; 268:19650–19655.
83. Gallwitz B. Exenatide in type 2 diabetes: treatment effects in clinical studies and animal study data. *Int J Clin Pract* 2006; 60:1654–1661.
84. Gallwitz B. Benefit-risk assessment of exenatide in the therapy of type 2 diabetes mellitus. *Drug Saf* 2010; 33:87–100. doi: 10.2165/11319130-000000000-00000.
85. Klonoff DC, Buse JB, Nielsen LL *et al*. Exenatide effects on diabetes, obesity, cardiovascular risk factors and hepatic biomarkers in patients with type 2 diabetes treated for at least 3 years. *Curr Med Res Opin* 2008; 24:275–286.
86. Blonde L, Klein EJ, Han J *et al*. Interim analysis of the effects of exenatide treatment on A1C, weight and cardiovascular risk factors over 82 weeks in 314 overweight patients with type 2 diabetes. *Diabetes Obes Metab* 2006; 8:436–447.
87. Brubaker PL, Drucker DJ. Minireview: Glucagon-like peptides regulate cell proliferation and apoptosis in the pancreas, gut, and central nervous system. *Endocrinology* 2004; 145:2653–2659.
88. Fehse F, Trautmann M, Holst JJ *et al*. Exenatide augments first- and second-phase insulin secretion in response to intravenous glucose in subjects with type 2 diabetes. *J Clin Endocrinol Metab* 2005; 90: 5991–5997.
89. Agersø H, Jensen LB, Elbrønd B, Rolan P, Zdravkovic M. The pharmacokinetics, pharmacodynamics, safety and tolerability of NN2211, a new long-acting GLP-1 derivative, in healthy men. *Diabetologia* 2002; 45:195–202.
90. Sturis J, Gotfredsen CF, Rømer J *et al*. GLP-1 derivative liraglutide in rats with beta-cell deficiencies: influence of metabolic state on beta-cell mass dynamics. *Br J Pharmacol* 2003; 140:123–132.
91. Garber AJ, Spann SJ. An overview of incretin clinical trials. *J Fam Pract* 2008; 57:S10–S18.
92. Garber A, Henry R, Ratner R *et al*. Liraglutide versus glimepiride monotherapy for type 2 diabetes (LEAD-3 Mono): a randomised, 52-week, phase III, double-blind, parallel-treatment trial. *Lancet* 2009; 373:473–481.
93. Nauck M, Frid A, Hermansen K *et al*, LEAD-2 Study Group. Efficacy and safety comparison of liraglutide, glimepiride, and placebo, all in combination with metformin, in type 2 diabetes: the LEAD (liraglutide effect and action in diabetes)-2 study. *Diabetes Care* 2009; 32:84–90.
94. Marre M, Shaw J, Brändle M *et al*. Liraglutide, a once-daily human GLP-1 analogue, added to a sulphonylurea over 26 weeks produces greater improvements in glycaemic and weight control compared with adding rosiglitazone or placebo in subjects with Type 2 diabetes (LEAD-1 SU). *Diabet Med* 2009; 26:268–278.
95. Zinman B, Gerich J, Buse JB *et al*. Efficacy and safety of the human glucagon-like peptide-1 analog liraglutide in combination with metformin and thiazolidinedione in patients with type 2 diabetes (LEAD-4 Met+TZD). *Diabetes Care* 2009; 32:1224–1230.
96. Russell-Jones D, Vaag A, Schmitz O *et al*. Liraglutide vs insulin glargine and placebo in combination with metformin and sulfonylurea therapy in type 2 diabetes mellitus (LEAD-5 met+SU): a randomised controlled trial. *Diabetologia* 2009; 52:2046–2055.

97. Buse JB, Rosenstock J, Sesti G *et al.* Liraglutide once a day versus exenatide twice a day for type 2 diabetes: a 26-week randomised, parallel-group, multinational, open-label trial (LEAD-6). *Lancet* 2009; 374:39–47.

98. Kapitza C, Heise T, Birman P *et al.* Pharmacokinetic and pharmacodynamic properties of taspoglutide, a once-weekly, human GLP-1 analogue, after single-dose administration in patients with Type 2 diabetes. *Diabet Med* 2009; 26:1156–1164.

99. Yki-Jarvinen H, Kauppila M, Kujansuu E *et al.* Comparison of insulin regimens in patients with non-insulin-dependent diabetes mellitus. *N Engl J Med* 1992; 327:1426–1433.

100. Yki-Jarvinen H, Ryysy L, Nikkilä K, Tulokas T, Vanamo R, Heikkilä M. Comparison of bedtime insulin regimens in patients with type 2 diabetes mellitus. A randomized, controlled trial. *Ann Intern Med* 1999; 130:389–396.

101. Yki-Jarvinen H. Combination therapies with insulin in type 2 diabetes. *Diabetes Care* 2001; 24:758–767.

102. Aviles-Santa L, Sinding J, Raskin P. Effects of metformin in patients with poorly controlled, insulin-treated type 2 diabetes mellitus. A randomized, double-blind, placebo-controlled trial. *Ann Intern Med* 1999; 131:182–188.

103. Makimattila S, Nikkila K, Yki-Jarvinen H. Causes of weight gain during insulin therapy with and without metformin in patients with Type II diabetes mellitus. *Diabetologia* 1999; 42:406–412.

104. Ponssen HH, Elte JW, Lehert P, Schouten JP, Bets D. Combined metformin and insulin therapy for patients with type 2 diabetes mellitus. *Clin Ther* 2000; 22:709–718.

105. Fritsche A, Schmülling RM, Häring HU, Stumvoll M. Intensive insulin therapy combined with metformin in obese type 2 diabetic patients. *Acta Diabetol* 2000; 37:13–18.

106. Goudswaard AN, Furlong NJ, Rutten GE, Stolk RP, Valk GD. Insulin monotherapy versus combinations of insulin with oral hypoglycaemic agents in patients with type 2 diabetes mellitus. *Cochrane Database Syst Rev* 2004: CD003418.

107. Yki-Jarvinen H, Dressler A, Ziemen M. Less nocturnal hypoglycemia and better post-dinner glucose control with bedtime insulin glargine compared with bedtime NPH insulin during insulin combination therapy in type 2 diabetes. HOE 901/3002 Study Group. *Diabetes Care* 2000; 23:1130–1136.

108. Riddle MC, Rosenstock J, Gerich J. The treat-to-target trial: randomized addition of glargine or human NPH insulin to oral therapy of type 2 diabetic patients. *Diabetes Care* 2003; 26:3080–3086.

109. Hermansen K, Davies M, Derezinski T, Martinez Ravn G, Clauson P, Home P. A 26-week, randomized, parallel, treat-to-target trial comparing insulin detemir with NPH insulin as add-on therapy to oral glucose-lowering drugs in insulin-naïve people with type 2 diabetes. *Diabetes Care* 2006; 29:1269–1274.

110. Fritsche A, Schweitzer MA, Haring HU. Glimepiride combined with morning insulin glargine, bedtime neutral protamine hagedorn insulin, or bedtime insulin glargine in patients with type 2 diabetes. A randomized, controlled trial. *Ann Intern Med* 2003; 138:952–959.

111. Tschritter O *et al.* Langwirkende Insulinanaloga in der Therapie des Diabetes mellitus Typ 1 und Typ 2. *Diabetes Stoffw* 2005; 6:375–382.

112. Mullins P, Sharplin P, Yki-Jarvinen H, Riddle MC, Haring HU. Negative binomial meta-regression analysis of combined glycosylated hemoglobin and hypoglycemia outcomes across eleven Phase III and IV studies of insulin glargine compared with neutral protamine Hagedorn insulin in type 1 and type 2 diabetes mellitus. *Clin Ther* 2007; 29:1607–1619.

113. Rosenstock J, Davies M, Home PD, Larsen J, Koenen C, Schernthaner G. A randomised, 52-week, treat-to-target trial comparing insulin detemir with insulin glargine when administered as add-on to glucose-lowering drugs in insulin-naïve people with type 2 diabetes. *Diabetologia* 2008; 51:408–416.

114. Nathan DM, Cleary PA, Backlund JY *et al*, Diabetes Control and Complications Trial/Epidemiology of Diabetes Interventions and Complications (DCCT/EDIC) Study Research Group. Intensive diabetes treatment and cardiovascular disease in patients with type 1 diabetes. *N Engl J Med* 2005; 353:2643–2653.

115. The absence of a glycemic threshold for the development of long-term complications: the perspective of the Diabetes Control and Complications Trial. *Diabetes* 1996; 45:1289–1298.

116. Stratton IM, Adler AI, Neil HA *et al.* Association of glycaemia with macrovascular and microvascular complications of type 2 diabetes (UKPDS 35): prospective observational study. *BMJ* 2000; 321:405–412.

117. Khaw KT, Wareham N, Luben R *et al.* Glycated haemoglobin, diabetes, and mortality in men in Norfolk cohort of european prospective investigation of cancer and nutrition (EPIC-Norfolk). *BMJ* 2001; 322:15–18.

118. DECODE Study Group, the European Diabetes Epidemiology Group. Glucose tolerance and cardiovascular mortality: comparison of fasting and 2-hour diagnostic criteria. *Arch Intern Med* 2001; 161:397–405.

119. Nakagami T, Qiao Q, Tuomilehto J et al. Screen-detected diabetes, hypertension and hypercholesterolemia as predictors of cardiovascular mortality in five populations of Asian origin: the DECODA study. *Eur J Cardiovasc Prev Rehabil* 2006; 13:555–561.
120. Monnier L, Lapinski H, Colette C. Contributions of fasting and postprandial plasma glucose increments to the overall diurnal hyperglycemia of type 2 diabetic patients: variations with increasing levels of HbA(1c). *Diabetes Care* 2003; 26:881–885.
121. Fakhoury W, Lockhart I, Kotchie RW, Aagren M, LeReun C. Indirect comparison of once daily insulin detemir and glargine in reducing weight gain and hypoglycaemic episodes when administered in addition to conventional oral anti-diabetic therapy in patients with type-2 diabetes. *Pharmacology* 2008; 82:156–163.
122. Heine RJ, Van Gaal LF, Johns D et al. Exenatide versus insulin glargine in patients with suboptimally controlled type 2 diabetes: a randomized trial. *Ann Intern Med* 2005; 143:559–569.
123. Action to Control Cardiovascular Risk in Diabetes Study Group, Gerstein HC, Miller ME, Byington RP et al. Effects of intensive glucose lowering in type 2 diabetes. *N Engl J Med* 2008; 358:2545–2559.
124. ADVANCE Collaborative Group, Patel A, MacMahon S, Chalmers J et al. Intensive blood glucose control and vascular outcomes in patients with type 2 diabetes. *N Engl J Med* 2008; 358:2560–2572.
125. Williams-Herman D, Johnson J, Teng R et al. Efficacy and safety of initial combination therapy with sitagliptin and metformin in patients with type 2 diabetes: a 54-week study. *Curr Med Res Opin* 2009; 25:569–583.
126. Gallwitz B, Häring HU. Future perspectives for insulinotropic agents in the treatment of type 2 diabetes-DPP-4 inhibitors and sulphonylureas. *Diabetes Obes Metab* 2010; 12:1–11.

7

The place of incretin-based therapies in patients with type 2 diabetes

M. Evans, R. Peter

SUMMARY

The management of blood glucose in patients with type 2 diabetes remains a considerable therapeutic challenge, with less than 50% of patients achieving the desired HbA1c target of 7%. This may be related to the progressive nature of the condition along with inherent limitations of currently available therapies, in particular hypoglycaemia and weight gain.

Pharmacotherapies that augment the incretin pathway have recently become available, which include incretin mimetics in the form of glucagon like peptide-1 (GLP-1) analogues (exenatide) and incretin enhancers (vildagliptin and sitagliptin) that inhibit the breakdown of endogenous GLP-1 by blocking the peptidase involved in its degradation, dipeptidyl peptidase-4 (DPP-4). Their role in the management of type 2 diabetes is not clearly defined yet. In this chapter we review the rationale, mechanism of action, efficacy and safety profiles of this class of agents with a view to defining their role in the treatment paradigm of type 2 diabetes.

The results of the randomized, multicentre United Kingdom Prospective Diabetes Study (UKPDS) confirmed the importance of long-term glycaemic control in limiting the complications associated with type 2 diabetes [1]. Such data drive current clinical practice in which treatment is directed towards the attainment of near normal glycaemia (HbA1c concentrations <7%). While such targets may be difficult to attain for many patients, there is clear consensus that chronic hyperglycaemia should be optimally managed, weighing safety and quality of life considerations on an individual basis.

Insulin resistance along with defective insulin secretion are the cardinal metabolic features of type 2 diabetes, with subtle abnormalities of both being evident even at the earliest stages of glucose intolerance. Whilst insulin resistance is highly prevalent, linked to obesity and physical inactivity, near normal glucose tolerance can be maintained as long as β-cell insulin secretion is maintained. The development of glucose intolerance and type 2 diabetes is thus dependent on progressive β-cell dysfunction. The initial management of a person newly diagnosed with type 2 diabetes involves advice and education relating to the potential benefits of dietary modification and lifestyle change, the objectives of these being to improve metabolic control through reductions in body weight that may help

Marc Evans, MD, MRCP, Consultant Diabetologist, Department of Diabetes, University Hospital Llandough, Cardiff, UK.

Raj Peter, MD, MRCP, Consultant Diabetologist, Department of Diabetes, Neath Port Talbot Hospital, Port Talbot, UK.

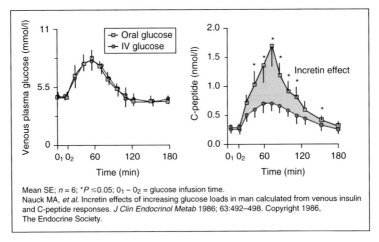

Mean SE; $n = 6$; $^*P \leq 0.05$; $0_1 - 0_2$ = glucose infusion time.
Nauck MA, *et al.* Incretin effects of increasing glucose loads in man calculated from venous insulin and C-peptide responses. *J Clin Endocrinol Metab* 1986; 63:492–498. Copyright 1986, The Endocrine Society.

Figure 7.1 The incretin effect results in increased insulin release in response to an oral glucose stimulus.

improve insulin sensitivity. The majority of patients will, however, require pharmacological therapy in the medium- to long-term. In the UKPDS, only 25% of patients maintained an HbA1c level <7% after 9 years without either oral agents or exogenous insulin [2]. Indeed, in routine clinical practice, fewer than half of patients with type 2 diabetes achieve an HbA1c target of <7% [3]. Ineffective implementation of existing pharmacotherapies may be a significant factor contributing to suboptimal glucose control; however, efficacy of available therapies, even when used appropriately, diminishes as the disease progresses because of a steady, relentless decline in pancreatic β-cell function [2]. The limitations of traditional blood glucose-lowering therapies were illustrated in the ADOPT study, in which only 21.9%, 21% and 16.5%, respectively, of patients treated with either rosiglitazone, metformin or glyburide monotherapy demonstrated sustained blood glucose control after 4 years of treatment [4].

Furthermore, current therapies for type 2 diabetes are often limited by adverse effects such as weight gain, oedema, or hypoglycaemia, and most do not target postprandial hyperglycaemias effectively. Therefore, therapies that improve glucose control, while reducing both postprandial and fasting plasma glucose, without causing weight gain and with minimal adverse effects are desirable. In this chapter we assess the potential role of new therapies targeting the incretin pathway in the treatment strategy of type 2 diabetes.

THE INCRETINS AS A THERAPY IN TYPE 2 DIABETES

Recently, improved understanding of the incretin effect on the pathophysiology of type 2 diabetes has led to the development of a variety of new hypoglycaemic agents. The incretin effect is the augmentation of glucose-stimulated insulin secretion by intestinally derived peptides, which are released in the presence of glucose or nutrients in the gut [5]. The theory evolved from the observation that an oral glucose load was more effective at releasing insulin compared with the same amount of glucose given intravenously [6] (Figure 7.1). GLP-1 and glucose-dependent insulinotropic polypeptide, also called gastric inhibitory polypeptide (GIP), are the two main physiological incretins synthesized in the intestinal tract. Research has focused on GLP-1 as a candidate antidiabetic agent for several reasons. First, it is estimated that GLP-1 accounts for at least 50% of the total incretin activity [7]. Second, on a molar basis, the effect of exogenous GLP-1 on insulin secretion in healthy

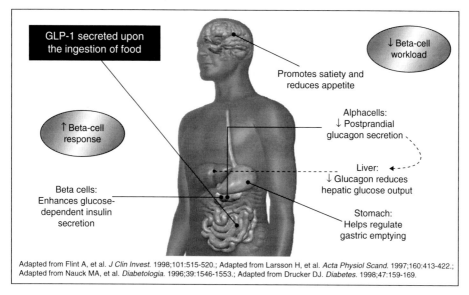

GLP-1 secreted upon the ingestion of food

↓ Beta-cell workload

Promotes satiety and reduces appetite

↑ Beta-cell response

Alphacells:
↓ Postprandial glucagon secretion

Beta cells:
Enhances glucose-dependent insulin secretion

Liver:
↓ Glucagon reduces hepatic glucose output

Stomach:
Helps regulate gastric emptying

Adapted from Flint A, et al. *J Clin Invest.* 1998;101:515-520.; Adapted from Larsson H, et al. *Acta Physiol Scand.* 1997;160:413-422.; Adapted from Nauck MA, et al. *Diabetologia.* 1996;39:1546-1553.; Adapted from Drucker DJ. *Diabetes.* 1998;47:159-169.

Figure 7.2 Multiple physiological actions of GLP-1.

subjects is substantially greater than that of GIP [7]. Third, in addition to its insulinotropic action, GLP-1, but not GIP, inhibits glucagon release, delays gastric emptying, and may promote early satiety [7] (Figure 7.2). Fourth, in patients with type 2 diabetes, GLP-1 administered in physiological [7] and supraphysiological [8] doses proved a potent insulin secretagogue, whereas GIP given in approximate equimolar doses had minimal [8, 9], or no effect on insulin secretion. Finally, the response of native GLP-1 to meals in type 2 diabetes is decreased or absent [7, 10], a defect that may exacerbate postprandial hyperglycaemia. These factors coupled with the fact that the insulinotropic actions of incretins are glucose-dependent, with their function ceasing when serum glucose levels are below 3.0525 mmol/l (55 mg/dl) [7], has made the incretin pathway an appealing therapeutic target. Despite the beneficial actions of GLP-1 and GIP on glucose control, their use as anti-diabetic agents was impractical due to their short half-lives as a result of their rapid inactivation by a protease called dipeptidyl peptidase type 4 [7], with the half-life of GLP-1 being around 2 min [11]. Thus, two approaches have been undertaken to overcome this problem. The first consists in the development of GLP-1 analogues, also called incretin mimetics, that bind to GLP-1 receptors with the same affinity as GLP-1 but resist degradation by DPP-4. The second is to design drugs that inhibit the action of DPP-4, which prolong the effects of native GLP-1 and GIP, and increase their serum levels approximately two-fold.

In April 2005, the US Food and Drug Administration approved the first incretin mimetic, exenatide, an exendin-based GLP-1 receptor mimetic, as adjunctive therapy for patients with type 2 diabetes at initial doses of 5 µg b.i.d. for 4 weeks increasing to 10 µg b.i.d. Liraglutide is an injectable GLP-1 analogue rendered resistant to DPP-4-mediated degradation due to enhanced albumin binding which is in late stage clinical development with a dose range 0.6 to 1.8 mg daily, while a long-acting version of exenatide (LAR) is also undergoing clinical evaluation. Two DPP-4 inhibitors sitagliptin and vildagliptin are currently available in the UK and Europe for use in combination with other oral hyperglycaemic agents, while a variety of other such agents, including saxagliptin and alogliptin, are in late-stage clinical development.

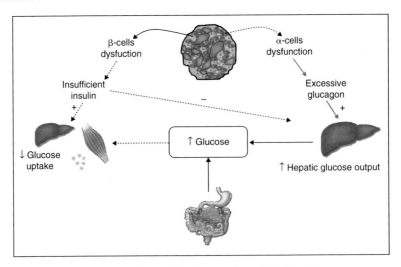

Figure 7.3 Pathophysiology of type 2 diabetes includes β- and α-cell dysfunction.

LIMITATIONS OF CURRENT THERAPIES

Prior to considering the role of these newer agents, it is reasonable to evaluate the utility and limitations of established agents and strategies. Islet cell dysfunction, including defective β-cell insulin secretion and inappropriate α-cell glucagon secretion resulting in suboptimal suppression of hepatic gluconeogenesis, are key elements in the pathophysiology of type 2 diabetes (Figure 7.3). While metformin improves hepatic insulin sensitivity, thiazolidine-diones (TZDs) improve both hepatic and peripheral insulin sensitivity and sulphonylureas stimulate β-cell insulin secretion, none of the currently available therapies address both β- and α-cell dysfunction.

The results of the UKPDS and ADOPT studies [2, 4] have demonstrated the limitations of current therapies with respect to the maintenance of long-term blood glucose control. Exogenous insulin is accepted as the most efficacious means of reducing blood glucose in patients with type 2 diabetes. Insulin initiation is, however, often a late event in the natural history of type 2 diabetes, with mean HbA1c on commencement of insulin of over 9% [12], resulting in often disappointing effects of insulin therapy on glycaemic control in patients with type 2 diabetes. This delay in insulin initiation is largely related to the inherent limitations associated with exogenous insulin therapy, in particular fear of injection and concerns around weight gain and hypoglycaemia.

The effectiveness of oral therapies in patients with type 2 diabetes may also be limited by their tolerability and adverse event profile. Metformin is widely accepted as the first-line oral blood glucose-lowering therapy for the majority of patients with type 2 diabetes. Its use is contraindicated in patients with impaired renal function (serum creatinine >150 μmol/l; GFR <60 ml/min), along with conditions pre-disposing to tissue hypoxia, includ-ing severe liver disease, alcohol abuse and previous history of metabolic acidosis. Gastrointestinal side-effects are the commonest adverse event associated with metformin, occurring at a frequency of up to 50% [13]. Furthermore, metformin may also reduce gas-trointestinal absorption of vitamin B_{12}; while anaemia is very rare, an annual haemoglobin measurement and B_{12} assessment is prudent. Sulphonylureas are commonly used second-line agents stimulating glucose-independent β-cell insulin secretion. Consequent weight gain of up to 3 kg [13], and in particular hypoglycaemia, are the commonest sulphonylurea side-effects, with the reported incidence of sulphonylurea-related hypoglycaemia ranging from 10–40% [13].

Thiazolidinediones improve glucose control by improving insulin sensitivity and are widely used as either monotherapy or in combination therapy. TZDs are associated with multiple adverse effects including weight gain of up to 5 kg [4], oedema at a frequency of 5–15% and fluid retention-related congestive heart failure [13]. TZD therapy may also be associated with an increase in bone fracture risk [14], while there is persisting debate relating to the cardiovascular safety of rosiglitazone [15].

HYPOGLYCAEMIA

Hypoglycaemia is a major consideration in the management of blood glucose. Severe hypoglycaemia is associated with increased mortality rates [16] and it has been speculated that the excess mortality reported in the ACCORD study [17] may have been precipitated by hypoglycaemia. Furthermore, hypoglycaemia and the fear of hypoglycaemia are recognized barriers to the achievement of glucose control and have a markedly negative impact on quality of life [16].

There are also a number of specific patient groups in whom hypoglycaemia is of particular concern:

- Vocational drivers and those in jobs where hypoglycaemia may be particularly detrimental (e.g. heavy machine operators).
- Those living alone.
- Those where cultural or lifestyle factors may increase the risk of hypoglycaemia.
- Those with a previous history of hypoglycaemic episodes.

WEIGHT GAIN

The majority of people with type 2 diabetes have excess body weight or are obese [18]. While much attention has focused on the adverse health consequences of excess body weight, little consideration has been given to the effects of weight gain in people with type 2 diabetes. Weight gain in this group has a detrimental effect on the physiological capacity of these people to achieve glycaemic targets but also has significant adverse effects on psychological health, quality of life and adherence to therapy [19]. Thus, while weight gain is undesirable for any patient with type 2 diabetes, it is of particular concern in specific patient groups:

- Those whose body weight is already high.
- Those from certain ethnic groups in whom definitions of obesity and excess weight are reflective of an increased cardiometabolic risk.
- Those where further weight gain may exacerbate or complicate comorbid conditions (e.g. obstructive sleep apnoea, polycystic ovarian syndrome).

Based on the foregoing discussion, blood glucose-lowering therapies with positive effects on body weight and minimal hypoglycaemia risk may have an important role in the treatment paradigm of type 2 diabetes.

EXENATIDE

Exenatide is available in a pre-loaded pen (5 µg and 10 µg) and is currently indicated for use as add-on therapy for type 2 diabetes subjects inadequately controlled with metformin and/or sulphonylureas. Exenatide rapidly and significantly reduces both fasting and postprandial glucose levels and, in principle, should be associated with a low rate of hypoglycaemia since its therapeutic effects are glucose-dependent. Exenatide demonstrates an 11-fold longer half-life and 14-fold plasma clearance rate compared with human GLP-1. It is exclusively eliminated by the kidneys primarily via glomerular filtration followed by proteolytic inactivation in the renal tubules. It has a half-life of 2.4 h and drug concentrations are detectable for up to 10 h following a single injection. Exenatide pharmacokinetics are unaffected by age, sex, race or obesity. Exenatide clearance is significantly reduced in subjects with end-stage renal disease precluding its use in these subjects. A number of potential drug interactions may occur primarily due to the delay in gastric emptying. Although dose adjustment is not necessary, careful monitoring is advised for agents with a narrow therapeutic window (e.g. digoxin).

Exenatide does not appear to have any impact on the pharmacokinetic properties of metformin and sulphonylureas. The effect on gastric emptying is influenced by the timing of administration, with a significant delay in gastric emptying occurring within 1 hour of exenatide administration. Thus, any oral therapies which may be affected by a delay in gastric emptying should be taken >1 hour prior to exenatide administration.

CLINICAL EFFICACY

Exenatide has been assessed as adjunctive therapy in three trials of similar design, including >1400 obese patients with type 2 diabetes uncontrolled with metformin [20], sulphonylurea (SU) [21], or both [22]. After 30 weeks, average reductions in HbA1c levels with a high dose of exenatide (10 µg b.i.d.) were approximately 0.8% and 1.0% compared with baseline and placebo, respectively. Similar reductions in HbA1c values were reported in a smaller trial ($n =$ 232) of shorter duration (16 weeks), in which exenatide was evaluated as add-on therapy in patients with type 2 diabetes suboptimally controlled on a TZD and metformin [23]. At the end of the previous five trials, the average proportions of subjects who achieved HbA1c value of $\leq 7.0\%$, were 45% and 10% in the exenatide and placebo groups, respectively, an observation which relates both to drug efficacy and baseline HbA1c. In subgroup analysis of subjects with baseline HbA1c >9% compared with <9%, greater reductions were seen with exenatide (5 µg dose, -0.8% vs. -0.4%, respectively; and 10 µg, -1.5% vs. -0.6%).

Exenatide was compared with insulin glargine in 549 patients with type 2 diabetes (baseline HbA1c 8.3%) on a background therapy of SU plus metformin [24]. After 26 weeks, HbA1c was reduced by 1.1% in both groups. In another trial, exenatide was compared with biphasic insulin aspart (formed of 30% short-acting insulin aspart and 70% intermediate-acting insulin) as adjunctive therapy in patients with type 2 diabetes ($n = 501$) inadequately controlled on metformin plus SU (mean baseline HbA1c 8.6%) [25]. After 52 weeks, no significant differences in HbA1c reductions were found between the exenatide and biphasic insulin aspart groups: 1% and 0.9%, respectively. At 52 weeks, significantly more subjects achieved an HbA1c <7 % in the exenatide group (32%) vs. the biphasic aspart group (24%). In both studies, better postprandial control was achieved with exenatide (difference -0.7 to -1.7 mmol/l).

In the previous two studies, the mean daily doses of insulin glargine and biphasic insulin aspart at the study ends were 26 and 24 units, respectively, suggesting that exenatide efficacy (10 µg b.i.d.) may be equivalent to mean daily insulin doses close to that range. However, more studies are needed to examine the benefits and risks of switching from insulin to exenatide therapy. Until these studies become available, such a strategy is not recommended, particularly in patients whose diabetes is not controlled on relatively high doses of insulin. For instance, in an exploratory study of 49 subjects with type 2 diabetes having mean baseline HbA1c values of approximately 8.1% while receiving insulin doses >40 units/day, the substitution of exenatide for insulin resulted in further deterioration of glycaemic control in 40% of patients, and lack of improvement in the remaining 60% of patients [26]. Open-label long-term extension data have demonstrated a sustained reduction in HbA1c and progres-

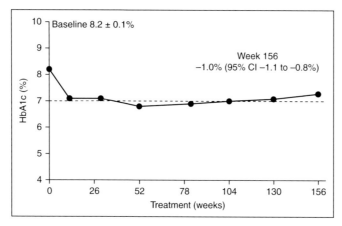

Figure 7.4 Long-term glucose-lowering effects of exenatide: completer analysis.

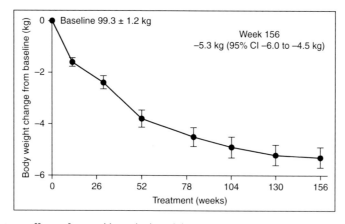

Figure 7.5 Long-term effects of exenatide on body weight.

sive weight loss (Figures 7.4 and 7.5), with reductions in HbA1c of 1.1% achieved after 12 weeks being maintained after 3 years [27].

In clinical studies, exenatide was associated with progressive and dose-dependent weight loss. After 30 weeks, subjects receiving 10 μg b.i.d. exenatide had lost more weight than those receiving placebo (mean 1.6 kg or 2.8 kg) compared with 0.3 kg and 0.9 kg for placebo [22]. There was no correlation between reported nausea and weight loss. Weight loss was progressive throughout the study period and persisted through the 104-week open-label completer analysis. In this study there was progressive reduction in body weight of 1.6, 2.4 and 4.7 kg at weeks 12, 30 and 104, respectively [27]. A similar pattern of weight loss was seen in an 82-week open-label completer analysis study (2.9 kg at 30 weeks, 5.3 kg at 82 weeks) [28]. At week 156, patients completing 3 years of exenatide treatment ($n = 217$) continued to lose body weight (-5.3 ± 0.4 kg; 95% confidence interval [CI] -6.0 to -4.5 kg; $P < 0.0001$) [27]. In both insulin comparator trials, weight change favoured exenatide after only 2 weeks [24, 25] (Figures 7.6 and 7.7).

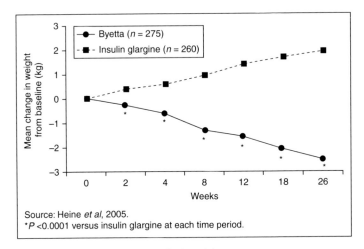

Source: Heine *et al*, 2005.
*P <0.0001 versus insulin glargine at each time period.

Figure 7.6 Effect of exenatide vs. basal insulin on body weight.

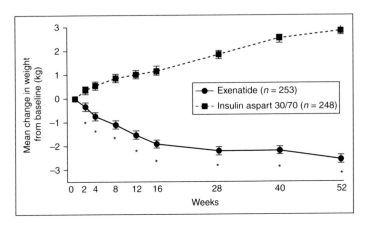

Figure 7.7 Effect of exenatide vs. biphasic insulin aspart on body weight.

Significant reductions in apolipoprotein B (apoB) (−5.2 mg/dl) and triglycerides (−73 mg/dl), and increases in high-density lipoprotein cholesterol (HDL-C) (+4.5 mg/dl) have been seen compared to placebo [28]. Total and low-density lipoprotein cholesterol (LDL-C) were also reduced (−7.3 mg/dl and −4.4 mg/dl), while LDL-C/HDL-C and TC/HDL-C ratios both fell (−0.37 and −0.73, respectively). Systolic and diastolic blood pressures were also reduced using exenatide for 82 weeks by 6.3 mmHg and 4.1 mmHg, respectively. These effects appear to have been maintained after up to 3.5 years of therapy (Table 7.1)

SAFETY AND TOLERABILITY

The main reported adverse events are gastrointestinal, occurring in a dose-dependent manner in 39% and 48% of subjects receiving 5 µg or 10 µg exenatide, respectively. Symptoms peaked after 8 weeks and declined thereafter, resulting in study withdrawal in only 2% (5 µg) and 4% (10 µg) of subjects, respectively. The aetiology of nausea is not fully clear, but may be related to the delay in gastric emptying. Nausea did not seem to be the predominant

Table 7.1 Effects of exenatide on cardiovascular risk factors

Cardiovascular risk factor	Baseline (mean ± SEM)	Change from baseline (mean ± SEM)	Mean % change	95% CI	P-value
Triglycerides (mg/dl)	225.1 ± 11.6	−44.4 ± 12.1	−12	−68.3 to −20.5	0.0003
Total cholesterol (mg/dl)	184.4 ± 3.0	−10.8 ± 3.1	−5	−17.0 to −4.6	0.0007
HDL-C (mg/dl)	38.6 ± 0.8	8.5 ± 0.6	+24	7.2 to 9.7	<0.0001
LDL-C (mg/dl)	113.7 ± 2.7	−11.8 ± 2.9	−6	−17.5 to −6.1	<0.0001
Systolic blood pressure (mmHg)	129.3 ± 1.0	−3.5 ± 1.2	−2	−5.9 to −1.0	0.0063
Diastolic blood pressure (mmHg)	79.2 ± 0.6	−3.3 ± 0.8	−4	−4.9 to −1.7	<0.0001

factor in the weight loss induced by exenatide, as there was no significant correlation between change in body weight and the duration of nausea [20, 22].

Consistent with the glucose-dependent insulinotropic effect of exenatide, hypoglycaemia caused by the drug is generally uncommon and mild-to-moderate in severity. Studies in healthy volunteers suggest that glucagon and other hormonal counter-regulatory responses to hypoglycaemia are preserved with short-term administration of exenatide [29]. In clinical trials using metformin alone as background treatment, the frequency of hypoglycaemia in the exenatide and placebo groups was similar [20]. However, hypoglycaemia was more frequent with exenatide compared with placebo in trials that included a SU as background therapy [22]. The incidence and severity of hypoglycaemia with exenatide treatment were similar when compared with insulin glargine [24] and biphasic insulin aspart [25], which may be due in part to the moderate insulin doses used in these studies. Nocturnal hypoglycaemia was however lower with exenatide compared with either glargine or biphasic insulin (−1.6 and −0.9 events per patient-year) [24, 25].

Anti-exenatide antibodies were present in 41% to 49% of subjects receiving exenatide, although the clinical significance is unclear [30]. The antibodies were generally in low titre and were not predictive of glycaemic control or adverse events.

In the post-marketing period, 30 cases of pancreatitis possibly caused by exenatide were reported from the date of the drug's approval through to 31 December 2006 [31], although the frequency of pancreatitis did not appear to be significantly greater than that observed in the background population of patients with type 2 diabetes.

LIRAGLUTIDE

Liraglutide is another GLP-1 analog with a long duration of action (half-life of around 12 hours) owing to its stability against DPP-4, albumin-binding acylated side chain and self-association, resulting in slow absorption from subcutaneous tissue [32]. It is given by a single daily subcutaneous injection [33], and has recently been licensed for use in Europe for use in combination therapy with metformin, metformin and a TZD or metformin and a sulphonylurea. In the US, liraglutide also has a license indication for use as monotherapy in patients with suboptimal glycaemic control following appropriate lifestyle modifications.

The clinical profile of liraglutide has been extensively studied in the Liraglutide Effect and Action in Diabetes (LEAD) study programme. In the largest of these studies, LEAD-3 [33], 746 patients with early type 2 diabetes were randomly assigned to once daily liraglutide (1.2 mg [n = 251] or 1.8 mg [n = 247]) or glimepiride 8 mg (n = 248) for 52 weeks, with the primary outcome being change in HbA1c. At 52 weeks, HbA1c decreased by 0.51% with glimepiride, compared with 0.84% with liraglutide 1.2 mg (difference –0.33%; 95% CI –0.53 to –0.13, P = 0.0014) and 1.14% with liraglutide 1.8 mg (–0.62; –0.83 to –0.42, P <0.0001). Five patients in the liraglutide 1.2 mg, and one in the 1.8 mg group discontinued treatment because of vomiting, whereas none in the glimepiride group did so, while subjects receiving liraglutide 1.8 mg od had a reduction in body weight of 3.5 kg as opposed to 0.8 kg weight gain in the glimeparide group.

The effectiveness of liraglutide compared with exenatide has also been evaluated as part of the LEAD programme. In the LEAD-6 study [34] adults with inadequately controlled type 2 diabetes on maximally tolerated doses of metformin, sulphonylurea, or both, were stratified by previous oral antidiabetic therapy and randomly assigned to receive additional liraglutide 1.8 mg once a day (n = 233) or exenatide 10 µg twice a day (n = 231) in a 26-week open-label, parallel-group, multinational study with an intention to treat efficacy analysis. Mean baseline HbA1c for the study population was 8.2%. Liraglutide reduced mean HbA1c significantly more than did exenatide (–1.12% [SE 0.08] vs –0.79% [0.08]; estimated treatment difference –0.33; 95% CI –0.47 to –0.18; P <0.0001) and more patients achieved an HbA1c value of less than 7% (54% vs. 43%, respectively; odds ratio 2.02; 95% CI 1.31 to 3.11; P = 0.0015). Liraglutide reduced mean fasting plasma glucose more than did exenatide (–1.61 mmol/l [SE 0.20] vs. –0.60 mmol/l [0.20]; estimated treatment difference –1.01 mmol/l; 95% CI –1.37 to –0.65; P <0.0001) but postprandial glucose control was less effective after breakfast and dinner. Both drugs promoted similar weight losses (liraglutide –3.24 kg vs. exenatide –2.87 kg). Both drugs were well tolerated, but nausea was less persistent (estimated treatment rate ratio 0.448, P <0.0001) and minor hypoglycaemia less frequent with liraglutide than with exenatide (1.93 vs. 2.60 events per patient per year; rate ratio 0.55; 95% CI 0.34 to 0.88; P = 0.0131; 25.5% vs. 33.6% had minor hypoglycaemia). Liraglutide in this study thus appeared to both provide significantly greater improvements in glycaemic control and be better tolerated compared with twice daily exenatide.

The results of the LEAD clinical trial program suggest that liraglutide may be a particularly useful treatment option for people with type 2 diabetes, particularly when hypoglycaemia and weight gain are major considerations. Indeed analysis of the LEAD study program demonstrates that a greater number of patients achieve a composite endpoint of an HbA1c target of <7% with no hypoglycaemia and no weight gain with liraglutide at doses of 1.2 and 1.8 mg daily than with active comparators (Figure 7.8).

GLP-1: ANALOGUES UNDER DEVELOPMENT

A variety of long acting GLP-1 analogue preparations are under late stage clinical evaluation. Taspoglutide is a new antidiabetic drug from Hoffmann-La Roche. The compound is to be administered as a subcutaneous injection once weekly and is also effective given bi-weekly. It is a long acting 10% formulation of (Aib 8-35) human glucagon-like polypeptide-1 (7-36 amides) with 93% homology with the native polypeptide. In clinical studies taspoglutide reduces blood glucose and has favourable effects on body weight and significantly reduces three of five diagnostic criteria for metabolic syndrome, namely glucose, waist circumference and fasting triglyceride [35].

The effects of a long-acting release (LAR) formulation were assessed in a 15-week placebo-controlled study [36] in which exenatide LAR was given once weekly at doses of 0.8 mg and 2.0 mg to patients suboptimally controlled with metformin and/or diet and exercise with mean duration of diabetes of around 5 years and mean baseline HbA1c 8.5%. From baseline to week 15, exenatide LAR reduced mean HbA1c by –1.4 +/– 0.3% (0.8 mg) and –1.7 +/– 0.3% (2.0 mg), compared with +0.4 +/– 0.3% with placebo LAR (P <0.0001 for both). HbA1c of ≤7% was achieved by 36% and 86% of subjects receiving 0.8 mg and 2.0 mg

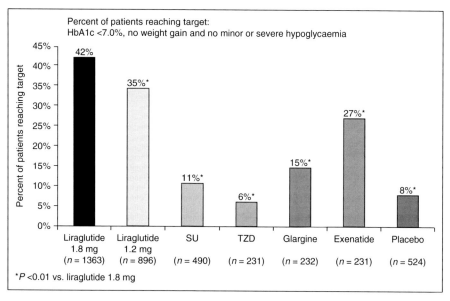

Figure 7.8 Composite endpoint of HbA1c target achievement with no hypoglycaemia and no weight gain for liraglutide versus active comparators in the LEAD study program.

exenatide LAR, respectively, compared with 0% of subjects receiving placebo LAR. Fasting plasma glucose was reduced by $-2.4 +/- 0.9$ mmol/l (0.8 mg) and $-2.2 +/- 0.5$ mmol/l (2.0 mg) compared with $+1.0 +/- 0.7$ mmol/l with placebo LAR ($P <0.001$ for both). Exenatide LAR reduced self-monitored postprandial hyperglycaemia. Subjects receiving 2.0 mg exenatide LAR had body weight reductions ($-3.8 +/- 1.4$ kg) ($P <0.05$), whereas body weight was unchanged with both placebo LAR and the 0.8 mg dose. Mild nausea was the most frequent adverse event, with no subjects withdrawing from the study. Thus, based on these early results, both liraglutide and exenatide LAR appear to be promising therapeutic entities.

DPP-4 INHIBITORS

Dipeptidyl peptidase-4 inhibitors lowered HbA1c compared with placebo (weighted mean difference, -0.74%; 95% CI, -0.85% to -0.62%) with similar efficacy as monotherapy or add-on therapy. The two available DPP-4 inhibitors have not been compared directly, but both appeared to lower HbA1c similarly compared with placebo (-0.74% vs. -0.73% for sitagliptin and vildagliptin, respectively). Tables 7.2 and 7.3 list the comparative mechanisms of action and clinical effects of exenatide/GLP-1 analogues and DPP-4 inhibitors.

In a study formed of six groups of patients, sitagliptin was evaluated as monotherapy as well as part of initial combination therapy with metformin. At 24 weeks, the mean decreases in HbA1c values from a mean baseline of 8.8% were 0.7, 0.8, 1.1, 1.4, 1.9, and a slight increase of 0.2% in the groups randomized to sitagliptin 100 mg od, metformin 500 mg b.i.d., metformin 1000 mg b.i.d., sitagliptin 50 mg b.i.d. + metformin 500 mg b.i.d., sitagliptin 50 mg b.i.d. + metformin 1000 mg b.i.d. and placebo, respectively [37]. The effects of metformin and sitagliptin on HbA1c reduction were additive, with metformin increasing GLP-1 levels [38], possibly by acting as a weak DPP-4 inhibitor [39]. Vildagliptin when added to metformin produced similar effects on glucose control [40].

Table 7.2 Summary of differences in mechanisms of action between GLP-1 analogues and DPP-4 inhibitors

	Exenatide/GLP-1 analogues	DPP-4 inhibitors
Overall mechanism of action	Exogenous supply of GLP-1 analogue that exerts its effects via the GLP-1 receptor	Inhibition of DPP-4 enzyme, resulting in increased levels of endogenous incretion hormones, GLP-1 and GIP
Level of GLP-1/GLP-1 analogue	Supraphysiological, concentration relating to meals about 5 times that of DPP-4 inhibitors	Near physiological
Improves β-cell mass and function	Yes	Yes
Glucose-dependent increase in insulin release	Yes	Yes
Glucose-dependent lowering of glucagon endocrine secretion	Yes	Yes
Reduced production and release of glucose from liver	Yes	Yes
Delayed stomach emptying	Yes	No
Decreased appetite and increased feeling of satiety (resulting in less food intake and giving the body smaller amounts of nutrients to deal with)	Yes	No

Table 7.3 Comparative summary of clinical effects of exenatide and DPP-4 inhibitors

Proven effects	Exenatide	DPP-4 inhibitors
Average lowering of HbA1c	0.6% to 1.43%	0.48% to 0.74%
Effect on postprandial glucose rise	Substantial lowering	Moderate lowering
Effect on fasting glucose	Yes	Yes
Improved proinsulin/insulin ratio	Yes	Yes
Long-term effect	Stable HbA1c lowering proven for up to three years [17]	Only studied for one year
Hypoglycaemic risk inherent in treatment	No, but increased risk in combination with, for example, sulphonylurea	No, but increased risk in combination with, for example, sulphonylurea
Weight decrease	Yes, average about 2 kg after 6 months, about 5 kg after 2 years	No, weight-neutral
Lowering of triglycerides	Yes	Little or no effect
Lowering of LDL-cholesterol	Yes	Little or no effect
Increase in HDL-cholesterol	Yes	Little or no effect
Lowering of liver values (ALT and AST)	Yes, in subjects with raised values	No
Lowering of blood pressure	Yes, moderate effect (6/4 mmHg)	No
Feeling unwell	Yes, slight to moderate and usually passing with continued treatment [16, 18, 19, 31]	No

Hermansen and colleagues [41] evaluated the additional effect of sitagliptin versus placebo in 441 patients with uncontrolled type 2 diabetes (baseline HbA1c 8.3%) on glimepiride alone or on glimepiride plus metformin. After 24 weeks, the addition of sitagliptin to glimepiride resulted in mean HbA1c reductions of 0.3% and 0.6% compared with baseline and placebo, respectively. In the subgroup of patients randomized to triple therapy formed of metformin, glimepiride and sitagliptin, the corresponding reductions in HbA1c values were 0.6% and 0.9%. Likewise, in patients with type 2 diabetes uncontrolled on glimepiride (baseline HbA1c 8.5%), the addition of vildagliptin 50 mg once daily ($n = 170$) and 50 mg twice daily ($n = 169$) resulted in reductions in HbA1c values of around 0.6% after 24 weeks, compared with the addition of placebo ($n = 176$) [42]. The results of the previous two trials suggest that DPP-4 inhibitors may have some value in improving glycaemic control when used in conjunction with metformin or sulphonylurea, despite the fact that both sulphonylureas and DDP-4 inhibitors stimulate insulin secretion. This improvement may result from the glucagon-suppressive effect of DPP-4 inhibitors, and perhaps by boosting the action of sulphonylureas on postprandial insulin secretion.

The addition of sitagliptin (100 mg od) to ongoing pioglitazone therapy (30 mg or 45 mg od) for 24 weeks was associated with a mean reduction in HbA1c values of 0.8% and 0.7% compared with baseline (8.0%) and placebo, respectively [43]. Similar results were obtained with the addition of vildagliptin to patients with inadequately controlled type 2 diabetes (average baseline HbA1c 8.7%) on maximal pioglitazone doses (45 mg/day). The mean reductions in HbA1c values with vildagliptin 50 mg b.i.d. were 1.0% and 0.7% compared with baseline and placebo, respectively [44]. In a third trial, 607 drug-naïve patients with uncontrolled type 2 diabetes (mean baseline HbA1c 8.7%) were randomized to four groups to receive pioglitazone 30 mg od, vildagliptin 50 mg od + pioglitazone 15 mg od., vildagliptin 100 mg od plus pioglitazone 30 mg od, and vildagliptin 100 mg od. [45]. After 24 weeks, mean reductions in HbA1c from baseline were 1.4, 1.7, 1.9, and 1.1% in the pioglitazone monotherapy, 50/15 mg combination, 100/30 mg combination and the vildagliptin monotherapy groups, respectively. Thus, contrary to the potential synergistic effect of metformin/DPP-4 inhibitor therapy, the efficacy of thiazolidinedione/DPP-4 combination appears to be less than additive. In one trial, the addition of vildagliptin (50 mg b.i.d.) to ongoing insulin therapy in patients with advanced type 2 diabetes modestly reduced HbA1c values by 0.5% and 0.3% after 24 weeks compared with baseline and placebo, respectively [46]. However, for unclear reasons, this reduction in HbA1c values was limited to the subgroup of patients aged >65 years.

There were no consistent changes in lipid profile with either sitagliptin or vildagliptin compared with placebo, but there were some improvements in triglycerides and LDL- and HDL-cholesterol. Relative to rosiglitazone, vildagliptin decreased total cholesterol, triglycerides, and LDL-cholesterol but produced a smaller increase in HDL-cholesterol. Relative to pioglitazone, vildagliptin decreased total and LDL-cholesterol. Vildagliptin also had a favourable change in triglycerides compared with metformin [37].

DPP-4 INHIBITORS IN COMPARISON WITH EXISTING THERAPY

Sulphonylureas

In a non-inferiority trial, sitagliptin was compared with glipizide as add-on therapy in >1000 patients with inadequate glycaemic control on metformin [47]. After 52 weeks, both groups had similar reductions in HbA1c values of approximately 0.7% versus baseline. However, the mean daily dose of glipizide was submaximal (around 10 mg), and withdrawal rates due to lack of efficacy were higher with sitagliptin compared with glipizide: 86 of 588 patients (15%) versus 58 of 584 (10%) patients [47]. On the other hand, sitagliptin was associated with lower rates of hypoglycaemia (5% vs. 32% of patients), and weight loss of 1.5 kg compared with 1.1 kg of weight gain with glipizide [47].

Metformin

In a non-inferiority trial, vildagliptin (50 mg b.i.d.) was compared with metformin (1000 mg b.i.d.) in 780 drug-naïve patients. After 52 weeks, the average reductions in HbA1c values from baseline were significantly greater with metformin compared with vildagliptin: 1.4% and 1.0%, respectively [48]. In another trial of 24-weeks duration, the placebo-subtracted reductions in HbA1c values with sitagliptin (100 mg od), metformin (500 mg b.i.d.) and metformin (1000 mg b.i.d.) were 0.8%, 1.0%, and 1.3%, respectively [39]. However, levels of statistical significance were not reported. In these studies there was no significant difference in hypoglycaemia or weight between metformin and DPP-4 inhibitor-treated groups, however, gastrointestinal side-effects were significantly greater with metformin.

Thiazolidinediones

In drug-naïve patients with type 2 diabetes, vildagliptin (50 mg b.i.d.) and rosiglitazone (8 mg od) decreased HbA1c values by 1.1% and 1.3%, respectively, after 24 weeks, meeting the statistical criterion of non-inferiority of vildagliptin relative to rosiglitazone. Patients on rosiglitazone had an average weight gain of 1.6 kg, while vildagliptin had no effect on weight [49]. In another trial including patients with type 2 diabetes inadequately controlled on metformin (mean HbA1c 8.4%), additional treatment with vildagliptin (50 mg b.i.d.) was compared with pioglitazone given in submaximal doses (30 mg/day) [50]. After 24 weeks, the reductions in mean HbA1c values were similar in the vildagliptin and pioglitazone groups: 0.9% and 1.0%, respectively. Mean weight gain was significantly greater in the pioglitazone group compared with the vildagliptin group: 1.9 kg and 0.3 kg, respectively.

SAFETY OF DPP-4 INHIBITORS

Both sitagliptin and vildagliptin appear to be well-tolerated [37], withdrawal rates in patients randomized to either agent being similar to placebo. A recent meta-analysis suggested that the commonest adverse effects reported in slightly higher proportions of patients receiving sitagliptin or vildagliptin were nasopharyngitis (6.4 vs. 6.1% vs. comparator, risk ratio 1.2), urinary tract infection (3.2 vs. 2.4% with placebo, risk ratio 1.5) and headache (5.1 vs. 3.9% with placebo, risk ratio 1.4) [23]. Available data suggest that DPP-4 inhibitors may be better tolerated than metformin, glipizide, and acarbose [37]. There was no difference in reported mild-to-moderate hypoglycaemia between DPP-4 inhibitors and a comparator group (1.6% vs. 1.4%, respectively; risk ratio 1.0). Hypoglycaemia did become more evident when DPP-4 inhibitors were used in conjunction with SU, with the proportions of patients reporting hypoglycaemia being 12% (27 of 222) and 1.8% (4 of 219) in patients receiving sitagliptin plus glimepiride versus patients receiving glimepiride plus placebo, respectively [41].

The efficacy and safety of saxagliptin has also been studied in patients with type 2 diabetes inadequately controlled by treatment with metformin, a TZD, or an SU alone [51]. At week 24, once-daily saxagliptin (2.5–10 mg) as an add-on treatment to stable metformin provided significant ($P <0.0001$) reductions in HbA1c (0.71–0.83%) compared with placebo [52]. In the TZD study, 565 patients with inadequate glycaemic control (HbA1c, 7–10.5%) were randomized to receive add-on therapy with saxagliptin (2.5 or 5 mg) or placebo once daily, in addition to either pioglitazone (30 mg or 45 mg) or rosiglitazone (4 mg or 8 mg) for 24 weeks [53]. At week 24, saxagliptin (2.5 mg and 5 mg) add-on treatment provided significant adjusted-mean reductions in HbA1c from baseline (–0.66% and –0.94%, respectively) compared with placebo (–0.30%; both $P <0.001$). In the SU study, 768 patients with T2DM inadequately controlled (HbA1c 7.5–10%) with glyburide 7.5 mg alone were randomized to receive saxagliptin 2.5 mg or 5 mg, or glyburide 2.5 mg in addition to open-label glyburide for 24 weeks. Blinded up-titration of glyburide to a maximum of 15 mg daily was permitted in the glyburide treatment arm only. At week 24, saxagliptin 2.5 mg and 5 mg add-on treatment provided significant (P <0.0001) adjusted mean reductions in HbA1c (–0.54% and –0.64%, respectively), compared with an increase for up-titrated glyburide (0.08%). In all of these studies, saxagliptin resulted in more patients achieving an HbA1c target of <7%, along with significant reductions in both fasting and postprandial plasma glucose levels.

Initial combination therapy with saxagliptin plus metformin has also been investigated in drug-naïve patients with inadequate blood glucose control (HbA1c, 8–12%; n = 1306). Patients were treated with saxagliptin (5 mg or 10 mg) plus metformin 500 mg, or placebo, in addition to either saxagliptin 10 mg alone or metformin 500 mg alone, for 24 weeks. Saxagliptin (5 mg and 10 mg) initial combination therapy with metformin provided significant (P <0.001) reductions in HbA1c (–2.53% and –2.49%, respectively), FPG (–59.8 and–62.2 mg/dl, respectively), PPG at 120 minutes during an OGTT (–137.9 and –137.3 mg/dl, respectively), and improved beta-cell function (HOMA–2β; 33% and 38%, respectively), compared with saxagliptin 10 mg alone (HbA1c –1.69%; FPG –30.9 mg/dl; PPG –106.3 mg/dl; HOMA–2β 18.2%) or metformin 500 mg alone (HbA1c –1.99%; FPG –47.3 mg/dl; PPG –96.8 mg/dl; HOMA–2β 22.6%).

ROLE OF INCRETIN THERAPIES IN CLINICAL PRACTICE

There is no doubt that incretin-based drugs represent a useful addition to the existing armamentarium of antidiabetic drugs. These agents have several advantages. First, because of their distinct mechanism of action, they generally exert a beneficial effect on glycaemic control, irrespective of the type of background oral agents. Second, by targeting postprandial hyperglycaemia more than fasting or pre-meal hyperglycaemia, they complement the action of metformin, TZD, and long-acting SU, which act mainly by lowering fasting plasma glucose. A third advantage is the progressive weight loss caused by exenatide, and the weight-neutral effect of the DPP-4 inhibitors. Fourth, the use of incretin-related agents is uncommonly associated with severe hypoglycaemia. Moreover, the use of DPP-4 inhibitors is simple, with once- or twice-daily oral dosing irrespective of meal intake.

Meanwhile, exenatide and current DPP-4 inhibitors have important limitations. First, it should be emphasized that 50% of patients in clinical trials failed to achieve HbA1c levels <7.0%. Second, exenatide has to be injected twice daily, and is associated with high rates of nausea, although tolerance to nausea appears to develop over time and a dose escalation protocol for exenatide appears to minimize the gastrointestinal adverse effects. Third, while the short-term (≤1 year) safety profile of two DPP-4 inhibitors – sitagliptin and vildagliptin – is reassuring, there are still some unresolved issues related to their safety. For instance, the enzyme DPP-4 plays an important role in the immune system, being a T-cell co-stimulator [54]; this raises concern about possible immune suppression as a result of DPP-4 inhibition. In addition to GLP-1 and GIP, DPP-4 inhibits the degradation of other peptides *in vitro,* such as substance P [54]. Thus, there is a possibility that serum levels of such peptides may rise with the use of DPP-4 inhibitors leading to potential undesired effects. There are also two other enzymes, DPP-8 and DPP-9, structurally related to DPP-4 but with largely unknown functions [54]. Although *in-vitro* data suggest that DPP-4 inhibitors display high selectivity for DPP-4, no *in-vivo* data are available.

In individual studies, DPP-4 inhibitors showed no characteristic pattern of adverse effects. However, a recent meta-analysis showed an increased risk of infections, such as urinary tract infection and nasopharyngitis. Although the observed relative risk was small, its implications in clinical practice are unclear and longer-term evaluation is required. Potential skin toxicity also remains a consideration with DPP-4 inhibitors with a few serious cases of hypersensitivity reactions being reported possibly related to sitagliptin, including anaphylaxis, angioedema, and Stevens-Johnson syndrome [55].

On balance, incretin-based therapies, with modest glucose-lowering effects, favourable weight profile, low hypoglycaemia risk and potentially positive effects on cardiovascular risk factors for exenatide, represent a useful alternative to, and may offer an advantage over, currently available hypoglycaemic agents. Hypoglycaemia may still be an issue, especially if incretin therapy is combined with an insulin secretagogue; therefore, when incretin therapy is co-administered with such agents, the dose of the latter should be adjusted to minimize hypoglycaemia.

Metformin will remain the drug of choice for initial treatment of type 2 diabetes due to its long-term safety, efficacy, and low cost [56]. Meanwhile, based on the available data, and while longer-term efficacy, safety and cost-effectiveness evaluation is awaited, incretin-based therapies may be of particular benefit in specific situations.

EXENATIDE/GLP-ANALOGUE THERAPY

The most recent blood glucose-lowering guidelines from the National Institute of Clinical Excellence (NICE) in the UK [57] suggest that such agents may be considered for use in patients with suboptimal glycaemic control with ongoing metformin/sulphonylurea combination therapy if a person is:

- Obese (a body mass index [BMI] ≥35 kg/m^2) in those of European descent, with appropriate adjustment for other ethnic groups and other specific psychological or medical problems associated with high body weight.
- Overweight (BMI <35 kg/m^2) and for whom initiation of insulin therapy would have significant occupational implications, or where weight loss would benefit other significant comorbidities such as sleep apnoea.
- Therapy should be only be continued following an appropriate assessment of efficacy and safety (e.g. 1% reduction in HbA1c at 6 months and 5% weight loss after 1 year).

The above approach to the use of these agents, while providing some useful guidance, may be considered as somewhat over-prescriptive in nature. Given their high cost and subcutaneous method of administration, it is unlikely that they would gain widespread support for second-line use following metformin monotherapy failure. However, such agents would make a sensible second-line therapy choice for people in whom weight loss is a crucial therapeutic priority (e.g. obstructive sleep apnoea and non-alcoholic steatohepatitis).

When considering stipulations around discontinuation of therapy, this is an area where the effects of therapy on both weight and glycaemic control should be assessed on an individual patient basis with the decision to continue treatment or otherwise based on the overall clinical picture, including an evaluation of the potential limitations of alternative therapy options.

The most recent ADA/EASD consensus algorithm for the management of blood glucose in type 2 diabetes [58], suggests that exenatide should only be considered when weight loss is a major consideration and the HbA1c level close to target (<8%). This suggested approach is based on reductions in HbA1c of 0.5–1% seen in clinical trials with exenatide [26, 27]. It is, however, noteworthy that greater reductions in HbA1c have been noted (1–1.5%) in patients with higher baseline HbA1c levels [28] and that these reductions may be maintained for up to 82 weeks of therapy. Thus, to define the clinical indication for such agents based on the minimal reported glucose-lowering effects set in the context of a population-based glycaemic target approach as opposed to a more individualized approach may lead to significant numbers of patients, who would otherwise gain benefit either in terms of weight and glucose reduction, being denied treatment.

When deciding between the use of GLP-analogue therapy and insulin, the progression of type 2 diabetes along with the expected improvement in HbA1c as compared with the individualized patient glycaemic are important considerations. In particular, if hyperglycaemia is sufficiently pronounced that the addition of GLP-analogue therapy is unlikely to

Table 7.4 Range of circumstances where a DPP-4-inhibitor would be preferable to a sulphonylurea

People where further weight gain would be disadvantageous
- People with already elevated BMI
- Sleep apnoea
- Multiple cardiovascular risk factors
- Established cardiovascular / peripheral vascular disease
- Poor mobility due to musculoskeletal problems

People at risk of hypoglycaemia
- People living alone
- Vocational drivers
- People working at heights or with machinery
- People with irregular eating habits (e.g. fasting during Ramadan)

achieve the desired HbA1c target, then insulin would be a more appropriate therapy choice.

DPP-4 INHIBITORS

Their relatively high cost, limited long-term safety data and modest glucose-lowering efficacy suggest that DPP-4 inhibitors should not generally replace a sulphonylurea as second-line therapy at this time. These agents may, however, be considered as an alternative to a sulphonylurea in a range of circumstances (Table 7.4). These include people for whom hypoglycaemia and/or weight gain are of particular concern, although there are insufficient data currently available to define a threshold BMI above which the use of a DPP-4 inhibitor would be particularly appropriate. Instead, the potential weight/hypoglycaemia benefits of these agents should be evaluated on an individual patient basis. When considering the use of second-line oral agents in patients with suboptimal glycaemic control on metformin monotherapy, a DPP-4 inhibitor may be more appropriate than a TZD in patients where fracture risk or congestive cardiac failure is a concern, or in whom further weight gain would exacerbate psychological or medical problems associated with a high body weight. A DPP-4 inhibitor may be considered as add-on therapy for patients with suboptimal glucose control receiving sulphonylurea monotherapy, where the person does not tolerate metformin or it is contraindicated.

If metformin in combination with a sulphonylurea does not adequately control blood glucose (HbA1c $\leq 7.5\%$), and injection-based therapies such as insulin or GLP-1 analogues are inappropriate, then a DPP-4 inhibitor is an appropriate third-line therapy alternative to a TZD based on the considerations outlined above.

The most recent ADA/EASD consensus guidance on the management of blood glucose in type 2 diabetes [58] does not include DPP-4 inhibitors due to their limited clinical data and relative expense. While the absence of long-term data currently precludes the widespread adoption of this class as a preferred second-line therapy, it is important to remember that these agents have been studied in a wide variety of clinical scenarios over periods of up to 1 year. Furthermore, in an era of ever tighter glycaemic targets, there is not only considerable patient morbidity but also cost implications associated with managing hypoglycaemia, weight gain and congestive heart failure risk associated with achieving HbA1c targets of <7% with the more established therapies such as sulphonylureas and TZDs.

The decision to continue DPP-4 inhibitor therapy should be based on individual patient assessment and not simply guided by the achievement of a prespecified HbA1c reduction, taking into consideration the individualized HbA1c target, comorbid conditions and the limitations of alternative therapy options.

REFERENCES

1. UK Prospective Diabetes Study group. Intensive blood glucose control with sulphonylureas or insulin compared with conventional treatment and risk of complications in patients with type 2 diabetes (UKPDS 33). *Lancet* 1998; 352:837–853.
2. Turner RC, Cull CA, Frighi V, Holman RR, UK Prospective Diabetes Study Group. Glycaemic control with diet, sulphonylureas, metformin or insulin in patients with type 2 diabetes: progressive requirements for multiple therapies. *JAMA* 1999; 281:2005–2012.
3. Resnick HE, Foster GL, Bardsley J, Ratner RE. Achievement of American Diabetes Association clinical practice recommendations among US adults with diabetes, 1999–2002: the National Health and Nutrition Examination Survey. *Diabetes Care* 2006; 29:531–537.
4. Khan SE, Haffner SM, Heise MA *et al*, ADOPT Study Group. Glycaemic durability of rosiglitazone, metformin, or glyburide monotherapy. *N Engl J Med* 2006; 355:2427–2443.
5. Habener JF. Insulinotropic glucagon-like peptides. In: LeRoith D, Taylor SI, Olefsky JM (eds). *Diabetes Mellitus: A Fundamental and Clinical Text*, 3rd edition. Lippincott Williams and Wilkins, Philadelphia, 2003.
6. Elrick H, Stimmler L, Hlad CJ Jr, Arai Y. Plasma insulin response to oral and intravenous glucose administration. *J Clin Endocrinol Metab* 1964; 24:1076–1082.
7. Drucker DJ, Nauck MA. The incretin system: glucagon-like peptide-1 receptor agonists and dipeptidyl peptidase-4 inhibitors in type 2 diabetes. *Lancet* 2006; 368:1696–1705.
8. Nauck MA, Heimesaat MM, Orskov C *et al*. Preserved incretin activity of GLP-1 (7–36 amide) but not of synthetic human GIP in patients with type 2 diabetes mellitus. *J Clin Invest* 1993; 91:301–307.
9. Nathan DM, Schreiber E, Fogel H *et al*. Insulinotropic action of glucagon-like peptide-I-(7–37) in diabetic and nondiabetic subjects. *Diabetes Care* 1992; 15:270–276.
10. Lugari R, Dei Cas A, Ugolotti D *et al*. Evidence for early impairment of glucagon like peptide 1-induced insulin secretion in human type 2 (non-insulin dependent diabetes. *Horm Metab Res* 2002; 34:150–154.
11. Vilsbøll T, Agersø H, Krarup T, Holst JJ. Similar elimination rates of glucagon-like peptide-1 in obese type 2 diabetic patients and healthy subjects. *J Clin Endocrinol Metab* 2003; 88:220–224.
12. McEwan P, Evans M. 44th Annual Meeting of the EASD European Association for the Study of Diabetes (EASD): Rome, Italy, 2008.
13. Krentz AJ, Bailey CJ. Oral antidiabetic agents – Current role in type 2 diabetes. *Drugs* 2006; 65:385–411.
14. Khan Se, Zinman Lachin JM. Rosiglitazone associated fractures in type 2 diabetes in an analysis from the ADOPT study. *Diabetes Care* 2008; 31:845–851.
15. Nissen SE, Wolski K. Effect of rosiglitazone on the risk of myocardial infarction and death from cardiovascular causes. *N Engl J Med* 2007; 356:2457–2471.
16. Amiel SA, Dixon T, Mann R, Jameson K. Hypoglycaemia in type 2 diabetes. *Diabet Med* 2008; 25: 245–254.
17. Dluhy RG, McMahon GT. Intensive glycaemic control in the ACCORD and ADVANCE trials. *N Engl J Med* 2008; 358:2360–2363.
18. Lusignan S, Sismanidis C, Carey IM *et al*. Trends in the prevalence and management of diagnosed type 2 diabetes in England and Wales. *BMC Family Practice* 2005; 6:13.
19. Barnett A, Allswort J, Jameson K, Mann R. A review of the effects of antihyperglycaemic agents on body weight: The potential effect of incretin based therapies. *Curr Med Res Opin* 2007; 23:1493–1507.
20. DeFronzo RA, Ratner RE, Han J *et al*. Effects of exenatide (exendin-4) on glycemic control and weight over 30 weeks in metformin-treated patients with type 2 diabetes. *Diabetes Care* 2005; 28:1092–1100.
21. Buse JB, Henry RR, Han J *et al*. Effects of exenatide (exendin-4) on glycemic control over 30 weeks in sulfonylurea-treated patients with type 2 diabetes. *Diabetes Care* 2004; 27:2628–2635.
22. Kendall DM, Riddle MC, Rosenstock J *et al*. Effects of exenatide (exendin-4) on glycemic control over 30 weeks in patients with type 2 diabetes treated with metformin and a sulfonylurea. *Diabetes Care* 2005; 28:1083–1091.
23. Zinman B, Hoogwerf BJ, Garcia SD *et al*, The effect of adding exenatide or a thiazolidinedione in suboptimally controlled type 2 diabetes. *Ann Intern Med* 2007; 146:477–485.

24. Heine RJ, Van Gaal LF, Johns D et al, GWAA Study Group. Exenatide versus insulin glargine in patients with suboptimally controlled type 2 diabetes. A randomized trial. Ann Intern Med 2005; 143:559–569.

25. Nauck MA, Duran S, Kim D et al. A comparison of twice-daily exenatide and biphasic insulin aspart in patients with type 2 diabetes who were suboptimally controlled with sulfonylurea and metformin: a non-inferiority trial. Diabetologia 2007; 50:259–267.

26. Davis SN, Johns D, Maggs D et al. Exploring the substitution of exenatide for insulin in patients with type 2 diabetes treated with insulin in combination with oral antidiabetes agents. Diabetes Care 2007; 30:2767–2772.

27. Klonoff DC, Buse JB, Nielsen LL et al. Exenatide effects on diabetes, obesity, cardiovascular risk factors and hepatic biomarkers in patients with type 2 diabetes treated for at least 3 years. Curr Med Res Opin 2008; 24:275–286.

28. Ratner RE, Maggs D, Nielsen LL et al. Long-term effects of exenatide therapy over 82 weeks on glycaemic control and weight in over-weight metformin-treated patients with type 2 diabetes mellitus. Diabetes Obes Metab 2006; 8:419–428.

29. Degn KB, Brock B, Juhl CB et al. Effect of intravenous infusion of exenatide (synthetic exendin-4) on glucose-dependent insulin secretion and counterregulation during hypoglycemia. Diabetes 2004; 53:2397–2403.

30. Cvetković RS, Plosker GL. Exenatide: a review of its use in patients with type 2 diabetes mellitus (as an adjunct to metformin and/or a sulfonylurea). Drugs 2007; 67:935–954.

31. Ahmad SR, Swann J. Exenatide and rare adverse events [letter]. N Engl J Med 2008; 358:1970–1972.

32. Harder H, Nielsen L, Tu DT, Astrup A. The effect of liraglutide, a long-acting glucagon-like peptide 1 derivative, on glycemic control, body composition, and 24-h energy expenditure in patients with type 2 diabetes. Diabetes Care 2004; 27:1915–1921.

33. Garber A, Henry R, Ratner R et al. Liraglutide versus glimepiride monotherapy for type 2 diabetes (LEAD-3 Mono): a randomised, 52-week, phase III, double-blind, parallel-treatment trial. Lancet 2009; 373:473–481.

34. Buse JB, Rosenstock J, Sesti G et al. Liraglutide once a day versus exenatide twice a day for type 2 diabetes: a 26-week randomised, parallel-group, multinational, open-label trial (LEAD-6). Lancet 2009; 374:39–44.

35. Retterstøl K. Taspoglutide: a long acting human glucagon-like polypeptide-1 analogue. Expert Opin Investig Drugs 2009; 18:1405–1411.

36. Kim D, McConnell L, Zhunag D et al. Effects of once-weekly dosing of a long-acting release formulation of exenatide on glucose control and body weight in subjects with type 2 diabetes. Diabetes Care 2007; 30:1487–1493.

37. Goldstein BJ, Feinglos MN, Lunceford JK et al, Sitagliptin 036 Study Group. Effect of initial combination therapy with sitagliptin, a dipeptidyl peptidase-4 inhibitor, and metformin on glycemic control in patients with type 2 diabetes. Diabetes Care 2007; 30:1979–1987.

38. Mannuci E, Ognibene A, Cremasco F et al. Effect of metformin on glucagon-like peptide (GLP-1) and leptin levels in obese nondiabetic subjects. Diabetes Care 2001; 24:489–494.

39. Amori RE, Lau J, Pittas AG. Efficacy and safety of incretin therapy in type 2 diabetes. JAMA 2007; 298:194–206.

40. Green BD, Irwin N, Duffy NA et al. Inhibition of dipeptidyl peptidase-IV activity by meformin enhances the antidiabetic effects of glucagon-like peptide-1. Eur J Pharmacol 2006; 547:192–199.

41. Hermansen K, Kipnes M, Luo E et al, Sitagliptin Study 035 Group. Efficacy and safety of the dipeptidyl peptidase-4-inhibitor, sitagliptin, in patients with type 2 diabetes inadequately controlled on glimepiride and metformin. Diabetes Obes Metab 2007; 9:733–745.

42. Garber AJ, Foley JE, Banerji MA et al. Effects of vildagliptin on glucose control in patients with type 2 diabetes inadequately controlled with a sulphonylurea. Diabetes Obes Metab 2008; 10:1047–1056.

43. Rosenstock J, Brazg R, Andryuk PJ et al, Sitagliptin Study 019 Group. Efficacy and safety of the dipeptidyl peptidase-4 inhibitor sitagliptin added to ongoing pioglitazone therapy in patients with type 2 diabetes: a 24-week, multicenter, randomized, double-blind, placebo-controlled, parallel-group study. Clin Ther 2006; 28:1556–1568.

44. Garber AJ, Schweizer A, Baron A et al. Vildagliptin in combination with pioglitazone improves glycaemic control in patients with type 2 diabetes failing thiazolidinedione monotherapy: a randomized, placebo-controlled study. Diabetes Obes Metab 2007; 9:166–174.

45. Rosenstock J, Baron MA, Camisasca RP *et al.* Effi cacy and tolerability of initial combination therapy with vildagliptin and pioglitazone compared with component monotherapy in patients with type 2 diabetes. *Diabetes Obes Metab* 2007; 9:175–185.
46. Fonesca V, Schweizer A, Albrecht D, Baron MA, Chang I, Dejager S. Addition of vildagliptin to insulin improves glycaemic control in type 2 diabetes. *Diabetologia* 2007; 50:1148–1155.
47. Nauck MA, Meininger G, Sheng D *et al*, Sitagliptin Study 024 Group. Efficacy and safety of the dipeptidyl peptidase-4 inhibitor, sitagliptin, compared with the sulfonylurea, glipizide, in patients with type 2 diabetes inadequately controlled on metformin alone: a randomized, double-blind, non-inferiority trial. *Diabetes Obes Metab* 2007; 9:194–205.
48. Schweizer A, Couturier A, Foley JE, Dejager S. Comparison between vildagliptin and metformin to sustain reductions in HbA(1c) over 1 year in drug-naïve patients with type 2 diabetes. *Diabet Med* 2007; 24:955–961.
49. Rosenstock J, Baron MA, Dejager S *et al.* Comparison of vildagliptin and rosiglitazone monotherapy in patients with type 2 diabetes. *Diabetes Care* 2007; 30:217–223.
50. Bolli G, Dotta F, Rochette E, Cohen SE. Efficacy and tolerability of vildagliptin vs. pioglitazone when added to metformin: a 24-week, randomized, double-blind study. *Diabetes Obes Metab* 2008; 10:82–90.
51. Gallwitz B. Saxagliptin, a dipeptidyl peptidase IV inhibitor for the treatment of type 2 diabetes. *Drugs* 2008; 11:906–917.
52. Defronzo RA, Hissa M, Blauwet MB *et al.* Saxagliptin added to metformin improves glycemic control in patients with type 2 diabetes. Presented at the 67th Scientific Sessions of the American Diabetes Association; June 22–26, 2007; Chicago, IL. 2007.
53. Allen E, Hollander P, Li L *et al.* Saxagliptin added to a thiazolidinedione improves glycemic control in patients with inadequately controlled type 2 diabetes. Presented at the 44th annual meeting of the European Society for the Study of Diabetes; September 7–11, 2008; Rome, Italy (abstract).
54. Barnett A. DPP-4 inhibitors and their potential role in the management of type 2 diabetes. *Int J Clin Pract* 2006; 60:1454–1470.
55. Januvia (sitagliptin phosphate). Product insert. Merk & Co., Station, NJ, USA, 2007.
56. Bolen S, Feldman L, Vassy J *et al.* Systemic review: comparative effectiveness and safety of oral medications for type 2 diabetes mellitus. *Ann Intern Med* 2007; 147:386–399.
57. NICE blood glucose lowering guidelines, May 2008.
58. Nathan D, Buse JB, Davidson MB *et al.* Medical management of hyperglycaemia in type 2 diabetes: A consensus algorithm for the initiation and adjustment of therapy. *Diabetes Care* 2008; 31:1–11.

8

How should we manage a diabetic patient who has recently had a myocardial infarction?

M. Fisher

BACKGROUND

The excessive cardiovascular risk of diabetes mellitus is well established. Epidemiological studies from many geographical areas have confirmed an increase in morbidity and mortality from cardiovascular disease (CVD), particularly myocardial infarction (MI), in people with diabetes compared to people without diabetes. It remains controversial, however, whether a person with diabetes and no clinically evident CVD really has the same risk of myocardial infarction and death as a non-diabetic patient who has already survived one MI, as suggested following analysis of a population-based cohort study from Finland [1]. A recent meta-analysis [2] has confirmed that the cardiovascular risk of people with diabetes is greatly increased compared to non-diabetic subjects, but this falls short of being a true coronary heart disease (CHD) equivalent. Analysis of 13 studies involving 45 108 patients showed that patients with diabetes without prior MI had a 43% lower risk of developing CHD events compared with patients without diabetes with previous myocardial infarction [2].

All are agreed, however, that an even greater risk of further MI and death is seen in patients with diabetes who have already sustained a MI [1].

The newer classification of acute coronary syndromes (ACS) based on clinical presentation, electrocardiogram (ECG) changes and increases in troponin concentrations, coupled with newer imaging techniques, has led to a greater understanding of the pathophysiology underlying acute MI [3].

Most ACS do not occur as a result of stable narrowing of coronary arteries but as a consequence of spontaneous rupture or erosion of an atheromatous coronary plaque. Exposure of plaque contents leads to platelet aggregation and thrombosis, which occludes the vessel causing damage to cardiac myocytes and release of troponin. Detailed examination of plaque numbers and morphology in people with diabetes has shown a greater number of plaques with a more distal location in the coronary arteries and a larger necrotic core, which is more prone to rupture [4]. Plaques from people with diabetes have increased vascular inflammation, with a greater infiltration of lymphocytes, increased production of inflammatory cytokines, and higher levels of matrix metalloproteinases making the plaque unstable and liable to rupture. At the same time, abnormalities of platelet function, coagulation and fibrinolysis

Miles Fisher, MD, FRCP (Glas), FRCP (Ed), MB ChB, Consultant Physician, Department of Medicine, Glasgow Royal Infirmary, Glasgow, UK.

result in increased thrombosis upon a ruptured plaque, increasing the risk of vessel occlusion or of distal embolization [4].

Diabetes is becoming increasingly common in patients presenting with ACS as heart disease is reduced in the non-diabetic population. Data from individual coronary care units and registries indicate that one-quarter to one-third of patients with an ACS will have diabetes, many previously undiagnosed, and if formal glucose tolerance testing is performed another one-quarter to one-third will have impaired glucose tolerance [5].

Many modifiable and non-modifiable risk factors for MI have been identified in people with diabetes. In the United Kingdom Prospective Diabetes Study (UKPDS), baseline diastolic blood pressure, raised low-density lipoprotein (LDL) cholesterol and HbA1c were independent predictors of future fatal MI and, in addition, smoking and low high-density lipoprotein (HDL) cholesterol were predictors of fatal or non-fatal MI [6]. In a separate analysis of the UKPDS dataset, patients with a fatal myocardial infarction had a higher HbA1c in the first years of diagnosis compared to patients with a non-fatal infarction, and increased age, blood pressure and urine albumin level were also risk factors for a fatal infarction [7].

The prognosis following ACS and MI is much worse in people with diabetes and most studies show almost a doubling of short-term and long-term mortality with acute MI in people with diabetes. An explanation for this excessive mortality following MI remains elusive. Undoubtedly, people with diabetes have more extensive and diffuse coronary artery disease at the time of MI, and concomitant diabetic autonomic neuropathy and a diabetic cardiomyopathy may increase the risk of sudden death, arrhythmias and heart failure. Other complications of infarction that are also increased include left ventricular systolic dysfunction without clinical heart failure, recurrent myocardial ischaemia and re-infarction, cardiogenic shock, renal failure and stroke [4].

IMMEDIATE CARDIOVASCULAR MANAGEMENT

Diabetic patients are more likely to have atypical symptoms of MI so the first management priority in a diabetic patient with a suspected MI is to confirm the suspected diagnosis with a careful history, cardiovascular examination, electrocardiography and measurement of cardiac markers. The immediate management of a diabetic patient with an ACS is cardiological and depends on the changes that are seen in the presenting ECG, and in particular whether ST segment elevation is present or not.

Antiplatelet therapy

All diabetic patients with suspected ACS should be treated immediately with aspirin 300 mg, and in the presence of ischaemic changes or elevation of cardiac markers, should also receive clopidogrel 300 mg. This was first proven for patients with non-ST elevation MI in the CURE trial where the combination of aspirin and clopidogrel was more effective than aspirin alone and produced a 20% reduction in numbers of patients achieving the first primary endpoint (composite of cardiovascular death, MI and stroke) after 12 months of follow-up [8]. Of the 12 562 patients in CURE, 2840 had diabetes. The diabetic subgroup had a higher event rate than their non-diabetic counterparts and the event rate was reduced by a similar amount to non-diabetic subjects.

In the subsequent CLARITY-TIMI 28 [9] and COMMIT trials [10], similar increased benefits were seen when comparing the combination of aspirin and clopidogrel with aspirin alone in patients with ST-elevation MI. CLARITY-TIMI 28 randomized 3491 patients to aspirin or combination therapy, and a 36% reduction in the composite of death, recurrent MI or occluded artery on angiography was observed with combination therapy. Sixteen per cent of subjects in CLARITY had diabetes but subgroup data were not provided. Rather surprisingly, no information is given on diabetes status or effects in diabetic patients in the COMMIT study, which included 45 852 patients from China and showed similar further reductions in the primary endpoint of death, re-infarction or stroke.

Prasugrel is a newer oral antiplatelet agent that is similar in action to clopidogrel. In the TRITON-TIMI 38 trial, aspirin plus prasugrel was compared to aspirin plus clopidogrel in 13 608 patients with ACS who were scheduled for percutaneous coronary intervention (PCI) [11]. There was a significant reduction in the primary endpoint of cardiovascular death, non-fatal MI and non-fatal stroke, but at the expense of an increase in major and life-threatening bleeding. A total of 3146 subjects had pre-existing diabetes and diabetic patients tended to have a greater reduction in ischaemic events with prasugrel compared with clopidogrel, without an observed increase in major bleeding [12]. MI was reduced with prasugrel by 18% in subjects without diabetes and by 40% in subjects with diabetes. The full clinical role for prasugrel is yet to be established, but in people with diabetes there appears to be an acceptable balance of increased efficacy versus side-effects.

ST-elevation myocardial infarction

Once combination antiplatelet therapy has been started the optimal reperfusion therapy for diabetic patients with ST-elevation acute MI is a primary PCI as the typical pathology is a ruptured plaque causing total occlusion. Systematic reviews and meta-analyses of randomized controlled trial (RCT) data has shown that primary PCI is superior to thrombolysis, and further reduces short- and long-term mortality, re-infarction, strokes and the need for coronary artery bypass grafting (CABG) [13]. A recent meta-analysis compared the data for individual subjects with diabetes in 19 trials comparing primary PCI and thrombolysis [14]. The 30-day mortality was greater in patients with diabetes, but similar reductions in relative risk were seen for most outcomes comparing diabetic and non-diabetic subjects, including death, recurrent MI and stroke.

Diabetic patients undergoing primary PCI should also be treated with glycoprotein IIb/IIIa receptor antagonists, and intracoronary stenting rather than balloon angioplasty should be used. There have been several meta-analyses comparing drug-eluting stents with bare-metal stents in diabetic patients undergoing PCI. The majority of studies were in subjects undergoing an arranged PCI rather than an emergency PCI for MI. Nevertheless, drug-eluting stents appear to offer considerable benefits in diabetic patients as restenosis following PCI is particularly common in diabetic patients. There is now evidence of late stent thrombosis once combination antiplatelet therapy is discontinued, and combination antiplatelet therapy may need to be continued long-term in patients who have received drug-eluting stents.

Thrombolysis has been shown in meta-analysis to reduce mortality and complications following MI in patients with diabetes [15], but is inferior to primary angioplasty so is now reserved for patients with ST-elevation MI who do not have access to the expertise to perform this intervention, or where this cannot be delivered within the desired time frame. The presence of diabetic retinopathy is not a contraindication to potentially life-saving thrombolytic treatment as retinal haemorrhage is rare, and can be treated surgically if it occurs.

Non-ST-elevation myocardial infarction

Patients with non-ST-elevation MI usually have a plaque rupture that has caused a non-occlusive thrombus and neither immediate primary PCI nor thrombolysis improve outcomes. Diabetic patients require maximum therapy to dissipate the thrombosis, including combination antiplatelet therapy with aspirin and clopidogrel, possible use of glycoprotein IIb/IIIa receptor antagonists, antithrombotic therapy with low molecular weight heparin or unfractionated heparin, and anti-ischaemic therapy with β-blockers. In a meta-analysis of glycoprotein IIb/IIIa receptor antagonists for non-ST-elevation MI, treatment with an antagonist reduced mortality and a composite of death or MI in diabetic subjects whereas there was no mortality benefit in non-diabetic subjects [16]. Patients with diabetes are at high risk so should be considered for coronary angiography and revascularization with CABG for left main stem disease or triple vessel disease, or PCI where the coronary anatomy is appropriate.

IMMEDIATE GLYCAEMIA MANAGEMENT

Once appropriate cardiological management has been started, the next management consideration is the emergency control of glycaemia. Obtaining evidence for the best cardiological treatments for MI in people with diabetes has been relatively straightforward as it has relied on subgroup analysis of single interventions, many of which can be gathered together into systematic reviews and meta-analyses. The management of glycaemia following MI is much more complex, as there are multiple variables including the use of intravenous or subcutaneous insulin therapy, the use of individual antidiabetic drugs, the rate and intensity of insulin administration, accompanying fluid volumes and constituents, and potassium supplementation. Unfortunately, many of the studies in this area have yielded negative results.

These studies can broadly be grouped into two categories [17]:

1. 'Insulin focus' where insulin is given for its potential metabolic effects on suppressing free fatty acid concentrations, stimulating potassium re-uptake and enhancing glycolysis in ischaemic myocardium. Examples of this are the use of a combined solution of glucose, insulin and potassium (GIK).
2. 'Glycaemia focus' where insulin is given for the control of hyperglycaemia. Studies which have adopted the latter approach include the DIGAMI studies, the HI-5 study and the HEART2D study.

DIGAMI studies

The first DIGAMI study used a combination of intensive intravenous insulin in glucose followed by four times daily multidose insulin for at least three months compared to conventional insulin treatment in 620 patients with diabetes who were admitted to Swedish coronary care units between 1990 and 1993. There was no statistically significant benefit at three month follow-up but by one year there was a statistically significant reduction in total mortality [18] that persisted for the mean follow-up of 3.4 years [19].

A second DIGAMI study was set up in an attempt to try and replicate the results of the first study, and also to try and identify which components of the strategy were required for mortality benefit [20]. This study randomized 1253 patients between 1998 and 2003 to one of three possible treatment strategies:

1. Intensive intravenous insulin and glucose infusion followed by multidose subcutaneous insulin similar to the intensive treatment group in the first DIGAMI study.
2. Immediate insulin glucose infusion followed by conventional therapy.
3. Conventional therapy throughout.

A major deficiency of the study was that recruitment was exceedingly slow and eventually the study was halted when less than half of the desired subjects had been recruited and it was clear that the planned number of study entrants would not be reached in a reasonable timescale. Secondly, only minor differences were obtained in HbA1c concentrations on follow-up, which is probably explained by the frequent use of twice-daily insulin and the infrequent use of multidose insulin in the group of patients that were supposed to be receiving intensive subcutaneous insulin.

Table 8.1 Results from the DIGAMI 2 trial

Principal result
- ▦ DIGAMI 2 did not support the fact that acutely introduced long-term insulin improves survival in patients with type 2 diabetes following MI.

Other results from *post hoc* analysis:
- ▦ Controlling for confounders there was no difference in mortality between patients treated with sulphonylureas, metformin and insulin following discharge. Metformin reduced the risk of non-fatal MI and stroke and the risks were significantly increased by insulin treatment.
- ▦ Initiation of insulin treatment after MI was associated with a significant increase in weight and incidence of re-infarction. The increase in weight, however, did not explain the increased rate of re-infarction.
- ▦ Hypoglycaemia during the initial hospitalization was not an independent risk factor for morbidity or mortality on follow-up.
- ▦ High levels of insulin-like growth factor-binding protein 1 (IGFBP-1) at admission were associated with an increased risk for cardiovascular mortality and cardiovascular events (CV death, re-infarction or stroke).

The study was therefore statistically underpowered to demonstrate benefit in either intervention group. In fact, survival was non-significantly reduced in the control group that received conventional treatment throughout, but this can be explained by baseline inequalities with significantly less prior vascular disease in that group. Overall, there was a high use of aspirin and β-blockers in the study, whereas use of angiotensin-converting enzyme (ACE) inhibitors and cholesterol-lowering therapies was less than might be expected. Epidemiological observations from the whole cohort showed a significant adverse effect of raised admission blood glucose and HbA1c, and benefit from β-blockers and statins [20]. There have been several recent *post hoc* analyses of data from DIGAMI 2 that have given useful information on MI in diabetes [21–24] (Table 8.1).

HI-5 study

The Hyperglycemia: Intensive Insulin Infusion In Infarction (HI-5) study examined the effects of an insulin/dextrose infusion given for at least 24 h versus conventional therapy in 240 patients with an acute MI and a random blood glucose concentration of >7.8 mmol/l [25]. Half of the participants had known diabetes. The insulin/dextrose infusion had no significant effect on mortality, but there was a lower incidence of cardiac failure and re-infarction within three months in the insulin/dextrose infusion patients [25]. A subsequent *post hoc* analysis showed that mortality was lower in subjects who attained an average blood glucose below 8 mmol/l in the first 24 h compared to subjects with a mean blood glucose above 8 mmol/l [26]. The authors suggested that tight glycaemic control with a blood glucose target <8 mmol/l improves outcomes, but an alternative explanation is that glycaemia is more difficult to manage in patients with worse outcomes.

In HI-5 ECGs were performed at admission and 24 h. In the conventional treatment group there was prolongation of the QT interval after 24 h, but this did not occur in the insulin infusion group. In the patients with a mean blood glucose above 8 mmol/l in the first 24 h, new ECG conduction abnormalities were significantly more common than in those with a mean glucose <8 mmol/l [27].

HEART2D study

The Hyperglycaemia and its Effects after Acute Myocardial Infarction on Cardiovascular Outcomes in Patients with Type 2 Diabetes Mellitus (HEART2D) study examined two subcutaneous insulin strategies following MI in patients with type 2 diabetes [28]. A total of

Table 8.2 Protocol used by coronary care unit nurses for insulin–glucose infusions in the DIGAMI study

Infusion: 500 ml 5% glucose with 80 IU of soluble insulin (~1 IU/6 ml).
Start with 30 ml/h. Check blood glucose after 1 h. Adjust infusion rate according to the protocol and aim for a blood glucose level of 7 to 10 mmol/l. Blood glucose should be checked after 1 h if infusion rate has been changed, otherwise every 2 h. If the initial decrease in blood glucose exceeds 30%, the infusion rate should be left unchanged if blood glucose is >11 mmol/l and reduced by 6 ml/h if blood glucose is within the targeted range of 7 to 10.9 mmol/l. If blood glucose is stable and <10.9 mmol/l after 10pm, reduce infusion rate by 50% during night.

Blood glucose >15 mmol/l:	Give 8 IU of insulin as an intravenous bolus injection and increase infusion rate by 6 ml/h.
11 to 14.9 mmol/l:	Increase infusion rate by 3 ml/h.
7 to 10.9 mmol/l:	Leave infusion rate unchanged.
4 to 6.9 mmol/l:	Decrease infusion rate by 6 ml/h.
<4 mmol/l:	Stop infusion for 15 min. Then test blood glucose and continue testing every 15 min until blood glucose is >7 mmol/l. In the presence of symptoms of hypoglycaemia, administer 20 ml of 30% glucose intravenously. The infusion is restarted with an infusion rate decreased by 6 ml/h when blood glucose is >7 mmol/l.

1115 patients were randomized within 21 days of an acute MI to either a prandial insulin strategy, which comprised three premeal doses of insulin lispro with a target postprandial glucose of less than 7.5 mmol/l, or to a basal strategy of twice-daily isophane insulin or once-daily glargine, with a target fasting and premeal glucose of less than 6.7 mmol/l. Most subjects were recruited from Central and Eastern Europe, and only a small number of patients were recruited from Western Europe and Canada. Similar to the DIGAMI 2 study, the study was halted because of a lack of effect on the primary endpoint which included cardiovascular death, non-fatal MI, stroke, ACS and revascularizations, and a less than expected separation in blood glucose concentrations between the two groups. In the prandial group, the mean postprandial blood glucose of 7.8 mmol/l was significantly less than 8.6 mmol/l in the basal group, but well above the targets. In the basal group, the mean fasting blood glucose of 7.0 was also significantly lower than the 8.1 mmol/l in the prandial group, but again was above target. There were no differences in HbA1c comparing the two groups.

A detailed description of the DIGAMI regimen is shown in Table 8.2.

In the absence of definitive answers from RCTs, data from cohort studies have provided some support for benefit of glucose normalization following MI. One large cohort study identified 7820 hyperglycaemic patients with MI admitted to 40 US hospitals. Around half had known diabetes [29]. After multivariable adjustment, lower mean post-admission glucose levels were associated with better survival. Mortality rates were similar between insulin-treated and non-insulin-treated patients. The results were similar for people with and without diabetes. In a separate publication from the same cohort, hypoglycaemia was associated with an increased mortality, but not in those treated with insulin; patients with hypoglycaemia were older and had more comorbidity [30].

SECONDARY PREVENTION OF MYOCARDIAL INFARCTION IN DIABETIC PATIENTS

There is clear evidence that patients with diabetes benefit from the use of secondary preventive therapies following MI. Meta-analysis has demonstrated that people with diabetes benefit from the early and continued use of β-blockers which reduce mortality and sudden death in people with diabetes [31], but data from individual centres and registries shows that these therapies are often less used than in non-diabetic subjects, especially patients treated with insulin [32]. This is probably because of misunderstanding of the effects of β-blockers on the symptoms and recovery from hypoglycaemia. Beta-blockers have only a minor effect on the symptom profile produced by hypoglycaemia, and as sweating is a sympathetic cholinergic response, it is unaffected. Similarly, modern cardioselective β-blockers that been proven to reduce mortality have no significant effect on the metabolic recovery from hypoglycaemia.

Registry data shows a much greater use of ACE inhibitors following MI in patients with diabetes, probably because of the perception that these will reduce future cardiovascular and renal events [32]. Angiotensin receptor blockers (ARBs) are better tolerated than ACE inhibitors, but studies comparing ACE inhibitors and ARBs for the treatment of heart failure or left ventricular systolic dysfunction following MI have yielded conflicting results, so ARBs should be used if patients are intolerant of ACE inhibitors.

Eplerenone is a selective mineralocorticoid receptor antagonist. In the EPHESUS study eplerenone was compared to placebo in 6632 patients with heart failure following MI [33]. Non-diabetic subjects had a low ejection fraction and clinical evidence of heart failure, whereas the one-third of the subjects with diabetes was recruited on the basis of a reduced ejection fraction following MI without necessarily having clinical evidence of heart failure. The results overall showed that eplerenone reduced total mortality following MI. This reduction was not significant in the diabetic subjects, probably because of a lack of statistical power, but there was a significant reduction in a composite endpoint of cardiovascular death and hospitalization due to cardiovascular events.

Statin treatment is one of the longest established evidence-based therapies to reduce mortality following MI. The original 4S (Scandinavian Simvastatin Survival Study) study compared simvastatin 20 mg with placebo in patients with a raised cholesterol and previous MI or angina, increasing to 40 mg if target cholesterol was not achieved [34]. Total mortality was reduced, as were the major coronary events of CHD-related death and non-fatal MI. In two diabetes subgroup analyses, simvastatin reduced major coronary events but not total mortality in diabetic subjects [35, 36].

More recent studies have compared low-dose versus high-dose statins following MI. The Pravastatin or Atorvastatin Evaluation and Infection Therapy–Thrombolysis in Myocardial Infarction 22 (PROVE-IT TIMI 22) trial compared 40 mg of pravastatin versus 80 mg of atorvastatin in patients with recent ACS [37]. At the start of the study they had modestly elevated total and LDL-cholesterol levels of 4.7 and 2.7 mmol/l, respectively. After a mean follow-up period of 24 months, the atorvastatin group achieved a 32% reduction in LDL-cholesterol (2.7 to 1.6 mmol/l) compared to minor reductions seen with pravastatin (2.7 to 2.4 mmol/l). There was a 16% reduction in the primary endpoint of time to first major cardiovascular event, including death from any cause, MI, unstable angina, stroke and revascularization procedures. There were 978 subjects with diabetes in the study (23%). There was a non-significant reduction in the time to first major cardiovascular event within this subgroup, probably reflecting the relatively small number of patients with diabetes [38]. Acute coronary events were significantly reduced by 25%.

In the TNT (Treating to New Targets) study atorvastatin 80 mg/day was compared with atorvastatin 10 mg/day in patients with previous MI, objective evidence of CHD or previous coronary revascularization procedures [39]. In people with diabetes, the use of atorvastatin 80 mg was associated with a significant reduction in major cardiovascular events (CHD death, MI, cardiac arrest or stroke). A marked reduction in cardiovascular events was particularly demonstrated in diabetic patients with chronic kidney disease (CKD). In both PROVE-IT and TNT the main side-effect of high-dose atorvastatin was an increase in abnormalities of liver function tests.

LONGER-TERM GLYCAEMIA MANAGEMENT

The conflicting results of the studies examining the immediate and short-term management of glycaemia following MI are described above. There is also uncertainty about the optimal strategy for the longer-term management of glycaemia in these patients. In the DIGAMI studies, four times daily insulin was to be continued for at least three months [16], but in the second DIGAMI study, many patients in the intensive treatment group were treated with twice-daily insulin [18].

PROactive

The PROactive trial examined the use of pioglitazone 45 mg in 5238 diabetic patients with evidence of macrovascular disease [40]. Inclusion criteria included MI at least 6 months prior to entry in the study, and approximately half of the subjects (2445; 46%) had evidence of previous MI. In the overall trial there was a statistically insignificant reduction of 10% in the primary endpoint comprising disease endpoints (death, MI, ACS and stroke) and procedural endpoints (coronary revascularization, leg revascularization, leg amputation). Before the study was completed and unblinded, the investigators defined a main or principal secondary endpoint comprising death, MI and stroke and this was significantly reduced by 16% comparing pioglitazone with placebo [40]. Detailed subgroup analysis of patients with a previous MI showed a 28% relative risk reduction in fatal and non-fatal MI, and a 37% relative risk reduction in ACS [41]. A 19% relative risk reduction was seen in a composite endpoint of non-fatal MI, coronary revascularization, ACS, and cardiac death. The main side-effect was an increase in non-fatal heart failure. Pioglitazone should therefore be considered for glycaemic management following MI in patients without heart failure, as glitazones are contraindicated in heart failure. A detailed description of the controversy surrounding rosiglitazone and a possible increase in MIs is beyond the scope of this chapter; suffice to indicate that there is no evidence that rosiglitazone reduces MIs either when used following previous MI or as primary prevention.

Studies of intensive insulin therapy

More recently three studies of intensive insulin therapy in diabetic patients with established vascular disease or high vascular risk have cast doubt on the desirability of intensively treating hyperglycaemia in these subjects. The ACCORD study examined the effects of intensive and rapid glucose lowering in 10 251 patients with type 2 diabetes [42]. One-third had baseline CVD but the number with previous MI was not published. The study was stopped early after 3.5 years because of an increase in total mortality in the intensive treatment group compared to the standard treatment group. In particular, there was an increase in unexpected or presumed CVD, which may have been a fatal consequence of hypoglycaemia. At the time the study was stopped the primary outcome of non-fatal MI, non-fatal stroke and cardiovascular death was not significantly reduced, but a significant reduction in non-fatal MIs was observed, which occurred in 3.6% of the intensive therapy group and 4.6% of the standard therapy group ($P = 0.004$).

The ADVANCE study examined the effects of less rapid intensive blood glucose control in 10 251 patients with type 2 diabetes, and again one-third had established CVD [43]. No major harmful effects of intensive glucose control were observed in the ADVANCE study, and there was a significant reduction in the primary endpoint of major macrovascular and microvascular events in the intensive treatment group. Further analysis showed that the significant reduction was in microvascular events, and there was no significant effect on macrovascular events, non-fatal MI or cardiovascular death.

The smaller VADT trial of 1791 military veterans recruited patients with poorly controlled diabetes and around half of the subjects had previous cardiovascular events [44]. Intensive glucose control had no significant effect on the rates of major cardiovascular

Table 8.3 Management of the diabetic patient with no known vascular disease, stable cardiovascular disease, and following a recent myocardial infarction

	No known vascular disease	Stable CHD and stroke	ACS and myocardial infarction
Glycaemia	Intensive treatment with metformin, sulphonylurea or pioglitazone	Intensive treatment with pioglitazone	Intensive treatment with multi-dose insulin, pioglitazone
Cholesterol	Simvastatin 40 mg or atorvastatin 10 mg	Consider atorvastatin 80 mg	Atorvastatin 80 mg
Blood pressure	ACE inhibitor, calcium channel blocker or diuretic	Beta-blocker or calcium channel for symptom control	Beta-blocker for prognosis
RAS inhibition (ACE inhibitor, ARB)	For blood pressure or microalbuminuria	ACE inhibitor for prognosis	ACE inhibitor for prognosis
Antiplatelet therapy	None	Aspirin (or clopidogrel)	Aspirin plus clopidogrel

events, death or microvascular complications, and there were 78 infarctions in the standard treatment group and 64 infarctions in the intensive therapy group (not statistically significant).

A recent meta-analysis included data from UKPDS, PROactive, ADVANCE, VADT and ACCORD [45]. A 17% reduction in non-fatal MI was observed comparing intensive treatment with standard treatment (95% confidence interval 0.75–0.93), and there was a 15% reduction in CHD events. Taken together, the results of these studies suggest that there may be benefit in intensive control of glucose in reducing MIs in patients with previous CVD or high cardiovascular risk, but that this should not be done rapidly, and should avoid hypoglycaemia and excessive weight gain.

PRIMARY PREVENTION OF MYOCARDIAL INFARCTION IN DIABETES

As described in the introduction, it is now clear that not all patients with diabetes have the same immediate and long-term cardiovascular risk, and patients can now be staged according to the presence and type of CVD (Table 8.3). Patients with recent MI were excluded from the UKPDS and most subjects had no vascular disease at baseline. The results from the UKPDS [46, 47] and the recently published post-trial monitoring (UKPDS-PTM) [48] indicate that early intensive treatment based on monotherapy with metformin will reduce MIs, diabetes-related deaths and all-cause mortality, and that the benefit is not directly related to control of blood glucose. In the main UKPDS group, intensive treatment based on monotherapy with sulphonylureas or insulin did not reduce MIs during the course of the study [47], but during post-trial monitoring a significant reduction in MIs leading to a significant reduction in all-cause mortality was observed [48]. HbA1c concentrations were similar to conventional control during post-trial monitoring and this late benefit was described as a legacy effect of early intensive glycaemic control. As similar reductions were seen with sulphonylureas and insulin that were consistent with epidemiological observations, this can be considered to be a benefit of controlling hyperglycaemia separate from the effect of any specific drug. The results of UKPDS post-trial monitoring are also consistent with the results of DCCT/EDIC in patients with type 1 diabetes, where intensive insulin therapy reduced the risk of any cardiovascular event by 42% and the risk of non-fatal MI, stroke or death from CVD by 57% [49]. In DCCT/EDIC, the investigators described the prolonged benefits of previous intensive treatment as a 'metabolic memory'.

In diabetic patients with hypertension, aggressive treatment of blood pressure has been particularly useful in reducing stoke events, but reductions in MIs have also been observed [50, 51]. Statin treatment with atorvastatin or simvastatin in diabetic patients with no known vascular disease significantly reduced MIs in the CARDS study [52] and HPS [53]. The possible benefits of antiplatelet drugs are less clear in diabetic patients without known vascular disease. The only study showing benefit was the HOT study [54] where aspirin reduced non-fatal MI but had no effect on cardiovascular or total mortality, and meta-analysis of primary prevention trials of antiplatelet therapy in people with diabetes has been negative [55]. At this point in time, aspirin is not recommended for the prevention of CVD in diabetic patients without established vascular disease. The differing management approaches to diabetes patients without CVD, with stable CVD, and following MI are summarized in Table 8.3.

SUMMARY

Myocardial infarction is a common medical emergency in people with diabetes, carries a high mortality compared to people without diabetes, and is a common cause of death. Diabetic patients with a suspected MI should receive early treatment with a combination of aspirin and clopidogrel. Diabetic patients with ST-elevation MI should undergo primary angioplasty and stenting, complemented by the use of glycoprotein IIb/IIIa antagonists. Thrombolysis should now be reserved for patients with ST-elevation MI where timely primary angioplasty cannot be performed, and there are no specific contraindications to thrombolysis in diabetic patients. Patients with non-ST-elevation MI and unstable angina should be treated with combination antiplatelet therapy and low molecular weight heparin. Diabetes increases the level of risk, and high-risk patients should receive early coronary angiography with a view to further intervention or surgical revascularization. The optimal short- and medium-term glycaemic management strategies remain uncertain. In the first DIGAMI study, a strategy of intensive intravenous insulin followed by intensive multidose subcutaneous insulin reduced total mortality in patients with diabetes following MI, but the follow-up DIGAMI 2 study and other studies using different glycaemic management regimens failed to show any benefit. Secondary preventive therapies including the appropriate use of β-blockers, ACE inhibitors, eplerenone and high-dose statins all have an important role following MI in diabetic patients, and cardiac rehabilitation is of benefit. There remains a high residual risk even when employing all of these evidence-based therapies, and to reduce the mortality from MI in people with diabetes will also require early attention to proven primary preventive therapies.

To optimally manage the diabetic patient who has recently had a MI requires attention to cardiovascular and metabolic factors, including the appropriate use of cardiovascular interventions and drugs, intensive treatment with statins, and the management of glycaemia.

REFERENCES

1. Haffner SM, Lehto S, Ronnemaa T, Pyorala K, Laakso M. Mortality from coronary heart disease in subjects with type 2 diabetes and in nondiabetic subjects with and without prior myocardial infarction. *N Engl J Med* 1998; 339:229–234.
2. Bulugahapitiya U, Siyambalapitiya S, Sithole J, Idris I. Is diabetes a coronary risk equivalent? Systematic review and meta-analysis. *Diabet Med* 2009; 26:142–148.
3. White HD, Chew DP. Acute myocardial infarction. *Lancet* 2008; 372:570–584.
4. Kahn M, Wheatcroft S. Acute coronary syndromes in diabetes. In: Fisher M (ed.). *Heart Disease and Diabetes*. Oxford University Press, Oxford, 2008.
5. Norhammer A, Tenerz A, Nilsson G *et al*. Glucose metabolism in patients with acute myocardial infarction and no previous diagnosis of diabetes mellitus: a prospective study. *Lancet* 2002; 359:2140–2144.

6. Turner RC, Millns H, Neil HAW *et al*, for the United Kingdom Prospective Diabetes Study Group. Risk factors for coronary artery disease in non-insulin dependent diabetes mellitus: United Kingdom Prospective Diabetes Study (UKPDS: 23). *BMJ* 1998; 316:823–828.

7. Stevens RJ, Coleman RL, Adler AI *et al*. Risk factors for myocardial infarction case fatality and stroke case fatality in type 2 diabetes. *Diabetes Care* 2004; 27:201–207.

8. The Clopidogrel in Unstable Angina to Prevent Recurrent Events Trial Investigators. Effects of clopidogrel in addition to aspirin in patients with acute coronary syndromes without ST-segment elevation. *N Engl J Med* 2001; 345:494–502.

9. Sabatine MS, Cannon CP, Gibson CM *et al*, for the CLARITY-TIMI 28 Investigators. Addition of clopidogrel to aspirin and fibrinolytic therapy for myocardial infarction with ST-segment elevation. *N Engl J Med* 2005; 352:1179–1189.

10. COMMIT (ClOpidogrel and Metoprolol in Myocardial Infarction Trial) collaborative group. Addition of clopidogrel to aspirin in 45,852 patients with acute myocardial infarction: randomised placebo-controlled trial. *Lancet* 2005; 366:1607–1621.

11. Wiviott SD, Braunwald E, McCabe CH *et al*, for the TRITON-TIMI 38 Investigators. Prasugrel versus clopidogrel in patients with acute coronary syndromes. *N Engl J Med* 2007; 357:2001–2015.

12. Wiviott SD, Braunwald E, Angiolillo DJ *et al*, for the TRITON-TIMI 38 Investigators. Greater clinical benefit of more intensive oral antiplatelet therapy with prasugrel in patients with diabetes mellitus in the trial to assess improvement in therapeutic outcomes by optimizing platelet inhibition with prasugrel-thrombolysis in Myocardial Infarction 38. *Circ* 2008; 118:1626–1636.

13. Keeley EC, Boura JA, Grines CL. Primary angioplasty versus intravenous thrombolytic therapy for acute myocardial infarction: a quantitative review of 23 randomised trials. *Lancet* 2003; 361:13–20.

14. Timmer JR, Ottervanger JP, de Boer MJ *et al*. Primary percutaneous coronary intervention compared with fibrinolysis for myocardial infarction in diabetes mellitus: results from the Primary Coronary Angioplasty vs Thrombolysis-2 trial. *Arch Intern Med* 2007; 167:1353–1359.

15. Fibrinolytic Therapy Trialists' (FTT) Collaborative Group. Indications for fibrinolytic therapy in suspected acute myocardial infarction: collaborative overview of early mortality and major morbidity from randomised trials of more than 1000 patients. *Lancet* 1994; 343:311–322.

16. Roffi M, Chew DP, Mukherjee D *et al*. Platelet glycoprotein IIb/IIIa inhibitors reduce mortality in diabetic patients with non-ST-segment-elevation acute coronary syndromes. *Circ* 2001; 104:2767–2771.

17. Cheung NW. Glucose control during myocardial infarction. *Intern Med J* 2008; 38:345–348.

18. Malmberg K, Ryden L, Efendic S *et al*. Randomized trial of insulin-glucose infusion followed by subcutaneous insulin treatment in diabetic patients with acute myocardial infarction (DIGAMI study): effects on mortality at 1 year. *J Am Coll Cardiol* 1995; 26:57–65.

19. Malmberg K for the DIGAMI (Diabetes Mellitus, Insulin Glucose Infusion in Acute Myocardial Infarction) Study Group. Prospective randomised study of intensive insulin treatment on long term survival after acute myocardial infarction in patients with diabetes mellitus. *BMJ* 1997; 314:1512–1515.

20. Malmberg K, Ryden L, Wedel H *et al*. Intense metabolic control by means of insulin in patients with diabetes mellitus and acute myocardial infarction (DIGAMI 2): effects on mortality and morbidity. *Eur Heart J* 2005; 26:650–661.

21. Melbin LG, Malmberg K, Norhammer *et al*, for the DIGAMI 2 Investigators. The impact of glucose lowering treatment on long-term prognosis in patients with type 2 diabetes and myocardial infarction: a report from the DIGAMI 2 trial. *Eur Heart J* 2008; 29:166–176.

22. Melbin LG, Malmberg K, Waldenstrom A *et al*, for the DIGAMI 2 Investigators. Prognostic implications of hypoglycaemic episodes during hospitalisation for myocardial infarction in patients with type 2 diabetes: a report from the DIGAMI 2 trial. *Heart* 2009; 95:721–727.

23. Aas A-M, Ohrvik J, Malmberg K *et al*, for the DIGAMI 2 Investigators. Insulin-induced weight gain and cardiovascular events in patients with type 2 diabetes. A report from the DIGAMI 2 study. *Diabetes Obes Metab* 2009; 11:323–329.

24. Wallander M, Norhammer A, Malmberg K *et al*. IGF binding protein 1 predicts cardiovascular morbidity and mortality in patients with acute myocardial infarction and type 2 diabetes. *Diabetes Care* 2007; 30:2343–2348.

25. Cheung NW, Wong VW, McLean M. The Hyperglycemia: Intensive Insulin Infusion In Infarction (HI-5) Study. A randomized controlled trial of insulin infusion therapy for myocardial infarction. *Diabetes Care* 2006; 29:765–770.

26. Cheung NW, Wong VW, McLean M. What glucose target should we aim for in myocardial infarction? *Diabetes Res Clin Pract* 2008; 80:411–415.

27. Gan RM, Wong V, Cheung NW, McLean M. Effect of insulin infusion on electrocardiographic findings following acute myocardial infarction: importance of glycaemic control. *Diabet Med* 2009; 26:174–176.

28. Raz I, Wilson PWF, Strojek K *et al*. Effects of prandial versus fasting glycemia on cardiovascular outcomes in type 2 diabetes: the HEART2D trial. *Diabetes Care* 2009; 32:381–386.

29. Kosiborod M, Inzucchi SE, Krumholz HM *et al*. Glucose normalization and outcomes in patients with acute myocardial infarction. *Arch Intern Med* 2009; 169:438–446.

30. Kosiborod M, Inzucchi SE, Goyal *et al*. Relationship between spontaneous and iatrogenic hypoglycaemia and mortality in patients hospitalized with acute myocardial infarction. *JAMA* 2009; 301:1556–1564.

31. Zuanetti G, Latini R. Impact of pharmacological treatment on mortality after myocardial infarction in diabetic patients. *J Diabetes Complications* 1997; 11:131–136.

32. Brogan GX, Peterson ED, Mulgund J *et al*. Treatment disparities in the care of patients with and without diabetes presenting with non-ST-segment elevation acute coronary syndromes. *Diabetes Care* 2006; 29:9–14.

33. Pitt B, Remme W, Zannad F *et al*. Eplerenone, a selective aldosterone blocker, in patients with left ventricular dysfunction after myocardial infarction. *N Engl J Med* 2003; 348:1309–1321.

34. Scandinavian Simvastatin Survival Study Group. Randomised trial of cholesterol lowering in 4444 patients with coronary heart disease: the Scandinavian Simvastatin Survival Study (4S). *Lancet* 1994; 344:1383–1389.

35. Pyorala K, Pedersen TR, Kjekshus J, Faergeman O, Olsson AG, Thorgeirsson G, for the Scandinavian Simvastatin Survival Study (4S) Group. Cholesterol lowering with simvastatin improves prognosis of diabetic patients with coronary heart disease. A subgroup analysis of the Scandinavian Simvastatin Survival Study (4S). *Diabetes Care* 1997; 20:614–620.

36. Haffner SM, Alexander CM, Cook TJ *et al*, for the Scandinavian Simvastatin Survival Study Group. Reduced coronary events in simvastatin-treated patients with coronary heart disease and diabetes or impaired fasting glucose levels. Subgroup analyses in the Scandinavian Simvastatin Survival Study. *Arch Intern Med* 1999; 159:2661–2667.

37. Cannon CP, Braunwald E, McCabe CH *et al*, for the Pravastatin or Atorvastatin Evaluation and Infection Therapy–Thrombolysis in Myocardial Infarction 22 Investigators. Intensive versus moderate lipid lowering with statins after acute coronary syndromes. *N Engl J Med* 2004; 350:1495–1504.

38. Ahmed S, Cannon CP, Murphy SA, Braunwald E. Acute coronary syndromes and diabetes: is intensive lipid lowering beneficial? Results of the PROVE IT-TIMI 22 trial. *Eur Heart J* 2006; 27:2323–2329.

39. Shepherd J, Barter P, Carmena R *et al*, for the Treating to New Targets Investigators. Effect of lowering LDL cholesterol substantially below currently recommended levels in patients with coronary heart disease and diabetes: the Treating to New Targets (TNT) study. *Diabetes Care* 2006; 29:1220–1226.

40. Dormandy JA, Charbonnel B, Eckland DJ *et al*. Secondary prevention of macrovascular events in patients with type 2 diabetes in the PROactive study (PROspective pioglitAzone Clinical Trial in MacroVascular events): a randomised controlled trial. *Lancet* 2005; 366:1279–1289.

41. Erdmann E, Dormandy JA, Charbonnel B *et al*. The effect of pioglitazone on recurrent myocardial infarction in 2,445 patients with type 2 diabetes and previous myocardial infarction: results from the PROactive (PROactive 5) Study. *J Am Coll Cardiol* 2007; 49:1772–1780.

42. The Action to Control Cardiovascular Risk in Diabetes Study Group. Effects of intensive glucose lowering in type 2 diabetes. *N Engl J Med* 2008; 358:2545–2559.

43. The ADVANCE Collaborative Group. Intensive blood glucose control and vascular outcomes in patients with type 2 diabetes. *N Engl J Med* 2008; 358:2560–2572.

44. Duckworth W, Abraira C, Moritz T *et al*, for the VADT Investigators. Glucose control and vascular complications in veterans with type 2 diabetes. *N Engl J Med* 2009; 360:129–139.

45. Ray KK, Seshasai SRK, Wijesuriya S *et al*. Effect of intensive control of glucose on cardiovascular outcomes and death in patients with diabetes mellitus: a meta-analysis of randomised controlled trials. *Lancet* 2009; 373:1765–1772.

46. UK Prospective Diabetes Study (UKPDS) Group. Effect of intensive blood-glucose control with metformin on complications in overweight patients with type 2 diabetes (UKPDS 34). *Lancet* 1998; 352:854–865.

47. UK Prospective Diabetes Study (UKPDS) Group. Intensive blood-glucose control with sulphonylureas or insulin compared with conventional treatment and risk of complications in patients with type 2 diabetes (UKPDS 33). *Lancet* 1998; 352:837–853.

48. Holman RR, Paul SK, Bethel A, Matthews DR, Neil HAW. 10-year follow-up of intensive glucose control in type 2 diabetes. *N Engl J Med* 2008; 359:1577–1589.

49. The Diabetes Controls and Complications Trial/Epidemiology of Diabetes Interventions and Complications (DCCT/EDIC) Study Research Group. Intensive diabetes treatment and cardiovascular disease in patients with type 1 diabetes. *N Engl J Med* 2005; 353:2643–2653.

50. Dahlof B, Sever PS, Poulter NR *et al.* Prevention of cardiovascular events with an antihypertensive regimen of amlodipine adding perindopril as required versus atenolol adding bendroflumethiazide as required, in the Anglo-Scandinavian Cardiac Outcomes Trial-Blood Pressure Lowering Arm (ASCOT-BPLA): a multicentre randomised controlled trial. *Lancet* 2005; 366:895–906.

51. ADVANCE Collaborative Group. Effects of a fixed dose combination of perindopril and indapamide on macrovascular and microvascular outcomes in patients with type 2 diabetes mellitus (the ADVANCE trial): a randomised controlled trial. *Lancet* 2007; 370:829–840.

52. Colhoun HM, Betteridge DJ, Durrington PN *et al.* Primary prevention of cardiovascular disease with atorvastatin in type 2 diabetes in the Collaborative Atorvastatin Diabetes Study (CARDS): multicentre randomised placebo-controlled trial. *Lancet* 2004; 364:685–696.

53. Heart Protection Study Collaborative Group. MRC / BHF Heart Protection Study of cholesterol-lowering with simvastatin in 5963 people with diabetes: a randomised placebo-controlled trial. *Lancet* 2003; 361:2005–2016.

54. Hansson L, Lennart Zanchetti A, Alberto Carruthers SG *et al.* Effects of intensive blood-pressure lowering and low-dose aspirin in patients with hypertension: prinicipal results of the Hypertension Optimal Treatment (HOT) randomised trial. *Lancet* 1998; 351:1755–1762.

55. De Berardis G, Sacco M, Strippoli GFM *et al.* Aspirin for primary prevention of cardiovascular events in people with diabetes: meta-analysis of randomised controlled trials. *BMJ* 2009; 339:64531.

9

Can we prevent problems in the at-risk diabetic foot?

M. J. Stevens, R. Pop-Busui, C. M. Holmes

INTRODUCTION

Diabetes is a contributing factor in up to 70% of lower limb amputations [1, 2]. In the majority of diabetic subjects, the underlying factor contributing to eventual amputation is diabetic foot disease and diabetic foot ulcer [3]. Amongst persons with diabetes, the lifetime risk of developing a foot ulcer is estimated to be 5–15% [4, 5]. Based on recent studies, the annual population-based incidence of foot ulcers ranges from 1.0% to 4.1% and the prevalence ranges from 4% to 10% [6]. The burden of diabetic foot disease and ulceration is set to further increase due to the coexistence of contributory comorbidities including peripheral arterial disease and peripheral neuropathy. Lower extremity amputation is twice as common in subjects with diabetes compared with non-diabetic persons, affecting 30% of subjects with diabetes 40 years and older [7].

Foot ulcers cause substantial emotional, physical, productivity and financial losses [8, 9]. The most costly and feared consequence of a foot ulcer is limb amputation, which occurs 10 to 30 times more often in diabetes than in the general population [10, 11]. In diabetes, 85% of non-traumatic amputations follow a foot ulcer [4]. Furthermore, a diabetes-related amputation markedly worsens quality of life and increases the risk of further amputations [12]. Most ominously, the mortality rate after amputation is about 40% at 1 year and 80% at 5 years – worse than for most malignancies [6, 13].

MECHANISMS INVOLVED IN THE ONSET AND PROGRESSION OF DIABETIC FOOT DISEASE

Peripheral somatic neuropathy can be identified in over 80% of subjects with diabetic foot ulcers [14–16]. High mechanical pressure [17, 18] resulting from structural deformities in the insensate foot, is a fundamental contributing factor to foot ulceration in these patients. Inadequate arterial perfusion associated with peripheral arterial disease is a contributing factor in approximately 60% of diabetic subjects with non-healing foot ulcers and 46% of those who have a major amputation [14]. In addition to macrovascular disease, microvessel disease also contributes to the chronicity of the diabetic foot ulcer [19]. Although multiple

Martin J. Stevens, MD, FRCP, Professor of Medicine, Honorary Consultant Physician, School of Clinical and Experimental Medicine, University of Birmingham and Heart of England NHS Foundation Trust, Birmingham, UK.

Rodica Pop-Busui, MD, PhD, Assistant Professor of Internal Medicine, Division of Metabolism, Endocrinology and Diabetes, Department of Internal Medicine, University of Michigan, Ann Arbor, Michigan, USA.

Crystal M. Holmes, DPM, CWS, Clinical Instructor, Podiatry, University of Michigan, Department of Internal Medicine, Division of Metabolism, Endocrinology and Diabetes, Ann Arbor, Michigan, USA.

factors contribute to the formation of foot ulcers in diabetes, oxidative/nitrosative stress, altered inflammatory responses and impairment of the skin microcirculation have also emerged as critical intermediates [20–23]. In the diabetic foot ulcer, infection is usually polymicrobial, and may not present with systemic manifestations despite extensive, limb-threatening sepsis [24].

Dermal atrophy: occurrence in diabetic skin and a common intermediate in chronic wound formation

Progressive atrophy of dermal connective tissue is a critical intermediate in the formation of a foot ulcer [25–27]. Proliferation of skin fibroblasts is reduced in diabetic patients [25–27]. Chronic, non-healing skin wounds of multiple aetiologies demonstrate similar connective tissue abnormalities, including reduced fibroblast numbers and proliferative capacity, reduced procollagen synthesis and increased levels of connective tissue-degrading matrix metalloproteinases (MMPs) [28, 29].

Less well understood is the role of epidermal changes in diabetes as contributors to the formation of non-healing wounds. Reduced keratinocyte proliferation may contribute directly to the atrophic changes occurring in the epidermis of diabetic subjects [30, 31]. Keratinocyte motility is also impaired in diabetes [32]. Since epidermal motility and proliferation contribute to wound closure [30], it is easy to envisage how alterations in these responses directly contribute to slowed repair of wounds in diabetic skin.

Structural and functional skin deficits in diabetes

Recent studies have shown that in diabetes dermal atrophy of the hip and ankle skin is associated with increased elaboration of MMP-1 (interstitial collagenase) and MMP-9 (gelatinase B) compared to age-matched healthy control skin [27]. Increased MMP elaboration precedes overt changes in skin structure and can be considered an 'early event' in skin degeneration. Sustained reduction in collagen synthesis occurs subsequently and concomitantly with evidence of widespread collagen destruction [28, 33, 34].

Oxidative stress and nitric oxide

Oxidative stress is implicated in the development of diabetic complications [35, 36] including neuropathy [35] and foot ulceration [37, 38]. Hyperglycaemia results in the increased production of vascular superoxide (O^{2-}), thereby inactivating nitric oxide (NO) and contributing to vascular dysfunction [39]. Additionally, NO plays an important role in wound repair [40] by promoting angiogenesis [41], migration and proliferation of fibroblasts [42], epithelial [43] and endothelial cells [41] and keratinocytes [40]. In diabetic mice, impaired wound healing is associated with decreased wound NO synthase expression and NO levels, and L-arginine improves wound healing [44]. Skin biopsies from the dorsum of the foot in diabetic subjects demonstrate a decrease in endothelial NO synthase expression [42]. However, the precise mechanisms whereby NO deficiency impairs wound healing are unclear.

The role of advanced glycosylation end-products (AGEs)

Accumulation of AGEs have also been implicated in the pathogenesis of diabetic complications [45], including impaired wound healing [46]. Increased skin AGEs have been identified in diabetic subjects with neuropathic foot ulceration compared to healthy diabetic subjects [47]. AGEs accumulate in diabetic wounds, and after interaction with the receptor for AGEs (RAGE) lead to expression of proinflammatory molecules including endothelin-1, tumour necrosis factor alpha (TNF-α) and MMPs [46–48]. TNF-α decreases the formation and tensile strength of granulation tissue potentially by enhancing the generation of activated MMPs, an effect involving interleukin (IL)-1 [23]. RAGE can be upregulated in cells important in the inflammatory response, including fibroblasts, vascular endothelial cells and mononuclear phagocytes [46]. The result is reduced angiogenesis, decreased collagen deposition and reduced quality and quantity of granulation tissue, ultimately resulting in poor wound healing and neovascularization in diabetic wounds [46, 49, 50]. The AGE precursor methylglyoxal impairs wound healing in rats by impairing the granulative tissue response [51]. Blockage of RAGE suppresses levels of inflammatory cytokines, TNF-α, IL-6 and MMPs [21] and promotes wound healing [46].

Oxidative stress and skin perfusion

Oxidative stress in the diabetic vasculature [52, 53] may increase diacylglycerol and protein kinase C (PKC) [54] thereby contributing to vascular dysfunction, skin small vessel disease and impaired skin perfusion [35]. Increased lipid hydroperoxides may increase cyclooxygenase activity and thromboxane synthesis [55, 56] but decrease prostacyclin synthase activity [56, 57] with resultant vasoconstriction [56, 57]. Skin vasodilatation in diabetes is reduced in response to occlusive ischaemia [58], local heating [59, 60], indirect heating [61] and trauma [62]. Diabetic sensory neuropathy typically affects unmyelinated primary afferent fibres and impairs vasodilatation related to unmyelinated C fibres [63–65]. Pressure-induced vasodilation (PIV) is the relationship between cutaneous mechano-sensitivity and vasodilation [66]. This allows augmentation of skin blood flow and delay in the development of ischaemia in response to pressure. Mechanistically, PIV is NO-mediated and involves capsaicin-sensitive afferent nerve fibres releasing calcitonin gene-related peptide in the endothelium [67]. PIV is absent in subjects [66] and animals [68] with diabetes. Thus, increased plantar pressures may result in a greater degree of perfusion impairment in diabetes. In skin with impaired circulation, increased oxidative stress also decreases glutathione (GSH) reductase activity leading to GSH depletion which may in turn contribute to impaired cellular proliferation [37], decreased synthesis of collagen and proteoglycans and enhanced protease activity [69].

However, despite better understanding of the causes of diabetes-related foot ulcers and proven prevention modalities, lower extremity amputation from diabetes remain very prevalent [70]. It has been reported that patients with diabetes were 9 times more likely to have a major amputation based on local practice styles after accounting for people's age, sex, and race.

STRATEGIES FOR PREVENTION OF DIABETIC FOOT ULCERS AND AMPUTATIONS

Success in treatment and prevention of lower extremity diabetes-related complications is only achieved with a motivated multidisciplinary approach where communication and collaborative efforts are at a high level with the goal of providing the right care to the right people at the right time and in the right amount. An example of this is the Limb Preservation Service Model at the Madigan Army Medical Center where an intensive programme of screening, education, treatment and timely appropriate referrals lead to an 82% reduction in amputation rates despite a 48% increase in patients diagnosed with diabetes [71]. This and similar studies have led to the understanding that the pathway to diabetic foot complications is multifactorial. Prevention strategies should include a multidisciplinary approach for both improved patient outcomes and short- and long-term cost-effectiveness [72]. A multidisciplinary approach is recommended for individuals with high-risk feet and foot ulcers, especially those with a history of prior ulcer or amputation [73]. One of the reasons is that diabetic patients have a complex comorbid status associated with the presence of progressive peripheral neuropathy and sensitivity loss, poor vascular supply due to arterial disease involving small and large vessels, and a compromised immune system. As a consequence, these patients require additional comprehensive testing and evaluations in order to establish the most appropriate plan of care.

This will be achieved by annual examinations, baseline testing, intervention and education which include:

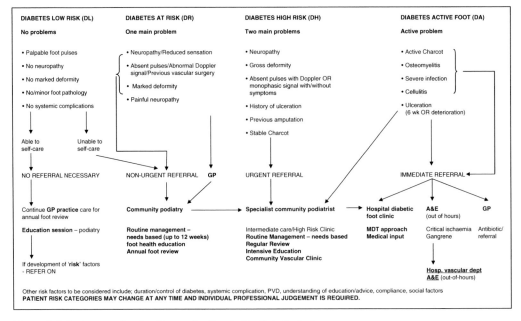

Figure 9.1 Foot care referral pathways for the at-risk diabetic foot.

1. Evaluation of diabetic peripheral neuropathy and peripheral arterial disease.
2. Treatment and care for patients at high risk or with current wounds and ulcers, including podiatric care, debridement, wound and infection care, footwear, off-loading devices.
3. Providing patient education.
4. Creating a database across the continuum of outpatient, inpatient and rehabilitative care.
5. Following outcome measures longitudinally that can be used to determine the effectiveness of the programme and to detect areas that require further improvement.

Once the diagnosis of diabetic peripheral neuropathy and/or peripheral arterial disease is established, a multispecialty approach to foot care is appropriate and recommended at 3- to 6-month intervals [73].

A comprehensive foot examination should comprise the following components: a general evaluation of the patient's past medical history; assessment of diabetes control; a comprehensive lower extremity physical examination. Peripheral neuropathy evaluation should comprise clinical examination (including ankle reflexes), Semmes-Weinstein monofilament and tuning fork examination, and/or quantitative sensory testing and electrophysiology if needed. Lower extremity vascular status should be assessed by clinical examination of peripheral pulses, arterial Doppler studies and ankle and/or toe brachial pressure indices (but bearing in mind these can be falsely elevated by the presence of arterial calcification). A musculoskeletal examination should focus on identifying structural foot deformities, including Charcot arthropathy using various imaging procedures (see below) and measurements of peak foot pressures (if available).

A specific risk-based protocol should be established and agreed upon with local healthcare providers and either preventative or acute care provided based on the risk score (Figure 9.1). Low-risk patients can be re-screened annually. High-risk patients should be scheduled

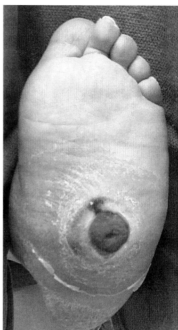

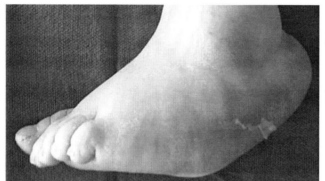

Figure 9.2 The Charcot foot: (A) Side view (B) Sole.

for regular podiatry evaluation at least once a quarter. In addition, a certified pedorthist should evaluate patients for therapeutic shoes and insoles at the conclusion of their initial evaluation by the podiatrist. Protocols for wound care consistent with standard wound care practices should be implemented including off-loading with total contact casts, customized removable cast walkers, and healing sandals, wound debridement, glycaemic control, infection control and lower extremity revascularization.

A DIAGNOSTIC CONUNDRUM: DIFFERENTIATING CHARCOT ARTHROPATHY FROM OSTEOMYELITIS

A key issue with regard to preventing complications of the foot is being able to differentiate neuroarthropathy from infection at an early stage. The authors have experienced patients who were sent to the clinic having been informed that an 'amputation was absolutely necessary because the foot was destroyed by infection' when the correct diagnosis was a Charcot foot. Neuropathic arthropathy (Figure 9.2) is more common than often perceived, and has a prevalence of 0.8–7.5% (in diabetic patients with neuropathy) and in up to 35% of cases it may become bilateral [74, 75]. Patients typically have suffered from previous poor diabetes control. In a report from Manchester, United Kingdom, 9% of randomly selected neuropathic diabetic patients were found to have changes consistent with Charcot arthropathy on foot radiographs [76]. Clinical suspicion is paramount. However, one also must appreciate that episodes of recurrent foot swelling are common in patients with diabetes and that these are often associated with negative X-rays but positive bone scans. All patients with diabetes and redness, swelling and increased foot temperature should be considered to be at risk of Charcot arthropathy and undergo an initial radiological assessment (Table 9.1). In Charcot arthropathy, there are no signs of systemic inflammation, i.e. the white cell count and erythrocyte

Table 9.1 When should an X-ray be performed?

In a Charcot foot
▩   At presentation of a hot, red, swollen foot
▩   At 6 months to assess the efficacy of off-loading
▩   Prior to the transition from an air cast to bespoke shoes
▩   Subsequently if reactivation is suspected
In osteomyelitis
▩   At presentation in a Wagner Stage 2 ulcer
▩   On reactivation of infection in previous osteomyelitis

sedimentation rate (ESR) are not elevated. Reduced bone density of the lower limb is also a feature of diabetic neuropathy and has been identified in patients with Charcot arthropathy [76]. However, asymptomatic fractures are discovered in 22% of diabetic patients with neuropathy. Often it is impossible to know whether patients presenting with traumatic foot fractures are at risk of developing Charcot arthropathy. All should be vigorously managed with off-loading until the signs of acute inflammation have resolved [77].

Healthcare providers can be misled by the relatively mild extent of peripheral neuropathy; Charcot feet can develop in the presence of minimal evidence of peripheral neuropathy and, indeed, light touch sensation can be intact. Charcot arthropathy is, however, unusual in patients with peripheral vascular disease and it has been proposed that the presence of reduced peripheral perfusion is protective against this complication of diabetes. In the presence of vascular insufficiency, bone resorption and periosteal new bone formation are inhibited.

THE PATHOPHYSIOLOGY OF THE DIABETIC CHARCOT FOOT

Small fibre neuropathy may be a prerequisite to the development of a Charcot foot, i.e. autonomic > pain fibres affected. There are two principal mechanistic processes that have been invoked in the pathogenesis of the Charcot foot: the neurovascular theory and the neurotraumatic theory [78]. The neurovascular theory invokes an increase in bone blood flow, perhaps including increased arterio-venous shunting due to a reduction in tone of vasoconstrictor innervations, resulting in bone resorption ultimately leading to fracture and deformities [79]. Clinically, arterio-venous shunting may be associated with prominent veins on the lower leg. In contrast, the neurotraumatic theory implicates repetitive trauma with fractures and progressive destruction of the architecture of the foot [80]. Precipitating causes for Charcot arthropathy that have been identified by a careful clinical history include trauma, infection, amputation and recent revascularization.

Most recent data indicate that bone remodeling is increased in subjects with Charcot arthropathy. For example, levels of urinary cross-linked N-telopeptides of type I collagen are increased in Charcot arthropathy [81] consistent with increased bone resorption. In concert, levels of pyridinoline cross-linked carboxy-terminal telopeptide domain of type I collagen (ICTP) and urinary deoxypyridinoline (DPD) (both markers of increased osteoclastic activity bone resorption) and alkaline phosphatase (a marker of osteoblast activity) have been shown to be increased in patients with acute Charcot arthropathy [82, 83].

The location of the radiological bony changes can give good clues as to the underlying diagnosis. For example, neuropathic osteoarthropathy is primarily an articular disease and is most common at the Lisfranc (tarsometatarsal) joint which can lead to lateral and superior subluxation of the metatarsal heads and the development of a rocker bottom foot deformity (Figure 9.3). Involvement of Chopart (transverse tarsal) joints is also common and initial

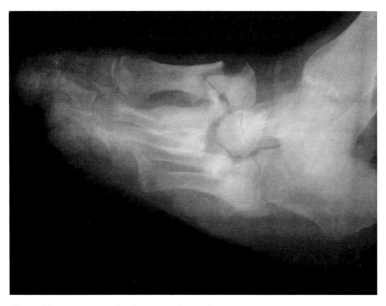

Figure 9.3 Radiographic appearances in Charcot arthropathy.

pathology often affects the medial column of the foot. Finally, neuropathic arthropathy tends to involve several joints in a region whereas infection tends to remain localized or spread contiguously. However, secondary ulceration and infection of the Charcot foot is common and can create considerable difficulties in distinguishing osteomyelitis from neuroarthropathy. In Charcot arthropathy, in approximately 70% of subjects, the destructive processes primarily affects the midfoot and in 15% the forefoot or rearfoot is mainly affected [84]. The destructive process is usually contained in one area and has been described as being atrophic or hypertrophic. The forefoot is the commonest site for atrophic changes and may present as osteolysis of distal metatarsals which can resemble a pencil point. Hypertrophic disease affects midfoot distally and has been defined according to Eichenholtz's classification system (Table 9.2). The 'Ds' of Charcot arthropathy have been described:

- Dislocation.
- Debris.
- Disorganization.
- Changes of bone Density.

Radiographic findings in the acute Charcot foot may be very subtle and include malalignment and subluxation. The articular surface is often affected in subacute stages and may become fragmented and develop subchondral cysts and marginal erosions. With progression of the disease, subluxation becomes more marked, joint surface incongruity develops and osteoarticular destruction becomes severe [84]. The X-ray findings of sclerosis, collapse, and fragmentation of the metatarsal heads have been reported to be similar to those observed in Freiberg's infarction [84, 85] but are more aggressive and extensive. Fractures of the calcaneus are common as well as avulsion of the Achilles tendon which may be an early finding on radiological examination. Although less common, the metatarsal ends and phalanges can shorten and demonstrate resorption [86].

Table 9.2 Eichenholzt Classification System [83]

■ Stage 0: Clinical stage: (prefragmentation): hot red, swollen foot
■ Stage 1: Developmental/fragmentation stage: periarticular fracture and joint dislocation (acute Charcot)
■ Stage 2: Coalescence stage: bone debris resorption (Subacute Charcot)
■ Stage 3: Consolidation stage: restabilization and fusion (Chronic Charcot)

Osteomyelitis rarely occurs in the absence of a skin source of sepsis: indeed, most (90%) result from spread from adjacent skin ulceration, cellulitis or abscess, together with a sinus tract [84, 87]. Therefore, osteomyelitis is found associated with skin ulceration which is most frequent at sites such as the metatarsal heads and the distal phalanges. In practice, osteomyelitis most frequently occurs on plantar aspects of the first and fifth metatarsal heads as well as the distal phalanx of the great toe. About 25% of ulcers on the toes are dorsally situated. When osteomyelitis occurs in the hindfoot, the heel is most frequently affected [88].

GOLD STANDARD IMAGING MODALITIES

When X-ray evaluation has not revealed any abnormality, or when differentiation of Charcot changes from osteomyelitis is required, additional imaging procedures are often performed. Magnetic resonance (MR) imaging has emerged as the best method for the detection of osteomyelitis with a specificity of up to 80% [84]. This technique also allows determination of the extent of soft tissue infection, which can be very helpful in the planning of surgical approaches. Alterations of the bone marrow signal provide the basis for the diagnosis of osteomyelitis using MR imaging [84]. In bone marrow infection, there is loss of the normal fatty marrow signal on T1-weighted images, a hyperintense signal on T2-weighted or short tau inversion recovery (STIR) images, and post gadolinium T1-weighted images are enhanced [84]. Other procedures that may also be useful include a triple phase bone scan (although this may not help distinguish infection from arthropathy but will give an evaluation of progression/regression) and white cell scans.

THERAPEUTIC APPROACHES

The pathway to diabetic foot ulceration is multifactorial. It is the culmination of deleterious events such as repetitive or overt trauma in the setting of peripheral neuropathy and/or peripheral arterial disease. The pathway to prevention of these complications relies on early identification, education and implementation of a complete multidisciplinary management programme [89].

Identification of risk factors that lead to amputation

The first step in prevention is identification of causal pathways that lead to diabetic foot ulceration. Diabetic peripheral neuropathy is still the major risk factor for diabetic foot ulceration. Other factors include limited joint mobility, repetitive stress and deformity. Once an ulceration occurs in the setting of the aforementioned conditions, the likelihood of a poor and prolonged healing process is increased. Factors contributing to poor wound healing include anaemia, infection, hyperglycaemia, hypoxia, pressure, environmental and psychosocial factors. The influence of lack of compliance to prescribed footwear cannot be underestimated. These factors are further complicated by the presence of peripheral arterial disease. The cycle of repetitive stress as described by Paul Brand has three mechanisms of escape:

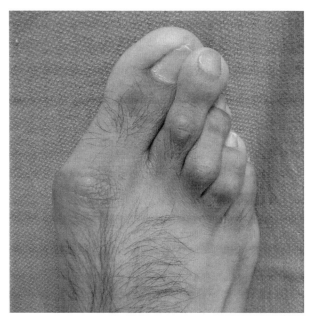

Figure 9.4 Characteristic foot deformities contributing to the development of ulceration in the insensate foot.

1. Stress correction.
2. Healing of wounds.
3. Decrease of inflammation.

WOUND HEALING IN DIABETIC SKIN

The optimal approach to the management of the diabetic foot ulcer lies in its prevention through the implementation of screening programmes aimed at the early detection of neuropathy, ischaemia, deformity and oedema. These programmes have been demonstrated to prospectively reduce the need for subsequent amputations [15, 90]. However, even with aggressive screening, chronic lower limb ulceration remains a common and serious consequence of diabetes.

ASSESSMENT AND CORRECTION OF FOOT DEFORMITIES IN THE DIABETIC POPULATION

Foot deformities have long been identified as risk factors for foot ulceration (Figure 9.4). The origin of the deformities may be congenital, idiopathic or traumatic. Atrophy of the intrinsic and extrinsic musculature of the lower extremity has been linked to motor neuropathy. This leads to biomechanical imbalances in the foot and resultant rigid or flexible deformities such as hammer toes and claw toes. Increase in glycosylation products has been linked to the development of equinus. All of these factors contribute to an increase in plantar foot pressures and, with repetitive stress, the development of foot ulceration. The University of Texas diabetic foot risk classification system [90–93] places patients in risk group categories based on the presence of neuropathy, deformity and history of pathology, presence of wound, acute Charcot, infection and ischaemia. A bunion deformity in the presence of neuropathy results in a twelve-fold increase in risk of development of an ulcer. Having a history of ulceration further increases the risk 36-fold. Patients without evidence of peripheral arterial disease and poor blood glucose control are potential candidates for corrective procedures. Intervention at this level should occur after conservative measures have been exhausted and assessed by the individual risk verses benefit ratio. Once ulceration occurs, elimination of the abnormal plantar pressures becomes crucial. The utilization of shoes, insoles and other modalities to off-load plantar pressure sites is still the gold standard of care and maintenance, while total contact casting continues to be a more effective off-loading device in the setting of healing ulcers [93].

The treatment of the acute Charcot foot is challenging and made worse by late presentation with deformity. Essentially, the optimal treatment lies in early detection and effective off-loading of the foot using either plaster casts or removable air casts worn for periods often in excess of 1 year. This is then followed by a period of variable duration of transition into bespoke footwear. Surgical realignment may be necessary for severely deformed feet which predispose to foot ulceration [94]. However, surgery is often challenging and its success is highly variable.

Bisphosphonates are potent inhibitors of osteoclast-mediated bone resorption and have been shown to reduce discomfort, swelling, skin temperature [95, 96] and biochemical markers of bone turnover and bone loss [95]. Clinical trials are currently underway exploring the efficacy of intravenous and oral bisphosphonates in the acute management of the Charcot foot.

POSSIBLE FUTURE THERAPEUTIC OPTIONS TO PREVENT FOOT ULCERATION AND ACCELERATE WOUND HEALING

Treatment with topical retinoic acid

Topical retinoid treatment improves histological structure and biochemical function of skin damaged by diabetes [27, 97]. Treatment of skin from subjects with diabetes with retinoic acid has been shown to reduce active MMP-1 and MMP-9 by 75% and by 81%, respectively [27]. Type I procollagen production is increased by 2- to 3-fold in retinoic acid-treated skin relative to control skin. The time-course for increased type I procollagen generation is the same as the time-courses for inhibition of MMP elaboration production. Levels of total (soluble) collagen also increase, with a time-course slightly delayed relative to the rise in procollagen. Thus, treated skin has an overall improvement in structure and function which should make it more resistant to ulcer formation and exhibit improved healing after wounding.

Treatment with alpha-lipoic acid

Recent studies have identified a second, potentially useful therapeutic – i.e. α-lipoic acid – for prevention of ulcers in diabetic skin [98]. In a model of experimental diabetes, α-lipoic acid was found to restore wound healing in diabetic rats to rates observed in healthy non-diabetic animals. At the histological level, α-lipoic acid induced a denser provisional matrix, a more luxuriant vasculature and fewer inflammatory cells in the matrix.

These findings suggest that, like the biologically active retinoids [27], α-lipoic acid results in enhanced healing of subsequently induced superficial skin wounds [98]. Of interest, the targets of retinoids and α-lipoic acid action, as well as the mechanisms by which these agents act, appear to be complementary, since the effects of the antioxidant appear to be mediated via improving skin microcirculation [99] and/or increased availability of NO. Therefore, the combination of retinoic acid with an antioxidant may ultimately prove to be the optimum therapeutic approach to improved overall skin quality and function. Clinical trials are underway to test the efficacy of these treatment approaches.

COSTS OF FOOT ULCERATION

In the United Kingdom, diabetes and its complications consume 9% of the National Health Service budget (£5.2 billion/year). People with diabetes are admitted twice as often and stay twice as long as others, using 10% of hospital inpatient resources. In the next 30 years, the economic burden of diabetes will rise by 40–50%. Up to 20% of total expenditure in diabetes is on foot complications. The total cost of diabetic foot problems is about £252 million/year (only direct costs and excluding the costs of amputations). The cumulative lifetime incidence of foot ulcers is high at 25%. Average inpatient costs (1997) for ulcers have been reported to be $16 580; major amputations, $31 436. The average outpatient cost for an ulcer episode is about $28 000 over 2 years. There are also indirect costs due to loss of productivity, individual and family costs, and loss of quality of life.

Preventing ulcers and amputations is cost-effective and skin fragility is a key cause. Based upon cost–utility analysis (Markov model), if an intervention reduces the incidence of ulcers and amputations by 25%, it is cost-effective and saves money. Improving skin structure and function is likely to reduce risk by more than 25% and will be highly cost-effective.

SUMMARY

Lower extremity complications continue to be a leading cause of hospitalizations for persons with diabetes. The financial burden on the population as a whole remains in the millions and rises with each year. The optimal approach to the management of diabetic foot complications lies in prevention through the implementation of screening programmes aimed at the early detection of neuropathy, ischaemia, infection, deformity and oedema. Improved understanding of the pathogenesis of this complex problem is giving new insights and hopes for the development of mechanism-based preventative treatments.

The patient–doctor relationship is often strained by the innate multifaceted complexity of diabetic foot conditions, a history of poor outcomes and a perceived lack of compliance. There is evidence to support that many practitioners do not fully understand the key psychological factors and impact associated with this chronic condition. Consider a patient with a non-healing wound with months of stringent wound care instructions and large off-loading devices. Hayland and colleagues [100] reported that patients spend an average of 1.5–2 h a day thinking about their leg ulcers. Patients with chronic wounds consistently view themselves and the wound negatively. Wounds that can be concealed tend to have less emotional impact. The diabetic foot is almost always recognized by the presence of bulky off-loading devices or custom-moulded shoes which have a perceived decreased cosmetic appearance. Even when the result is favourable and limb loss is prevented, often there is still physical manifestation of the disease. For many diabetic patients their foot condition is the only outward evidence of their chronic condition. A key aspect therefore of prevention and treatment of diabetic foot complications is empathy, and constant assessment and discussion with patients about the impact of the complication on their quality of life [101] and evaluation for coexistent depression. Careful consideration of these issues is vital in the development of effective and personalized treatment plans.

Acknowledgements
The authors are supported by the National Institute of Health (NINDS-NS047653–03 to RPB and R01AT002146 to MJS) and Eli Lilly (MJS).

REFERENCES

1. Edmonds ME. The diabetic foot. *Diab Metab Res Rev* 2004; 20(suppl 1):S9–S12.
2. Boulton AJ, Kirsner RS, Vileikyte L. Clinical practice. Neuropathic diabetic foot ulcers. *N Engl J Med* 2004; 351:48–55.

3. Pecoraro RE, Reiber GE, Burgess EM. Pathways to diabetic limb amputation. Basis for prevention. *Diabetes Care* 1990; 13:513–521.

4. Reiber GE. The epidemiology of diabetic foot problems. *Diabet Med* 1996; 13(suppl 1):S6–S11.

5. Lavery LA, Armstrong DG, Wunderlich RP et al. Diabetic foot syndrome: evaluating the prevalence and incidence of foot pathology in Mexican Americans and non-Hispanic whites from a diabetes disease management cohort. *Diabetes Care* 2003; 26:1435–1438.

6. Reiber GE. The epidemiology of foot ulcers and amputations in the diabetic foot. In: Bowker JH, Pfeifer MA (eds). *Levin and O'Neal's The Diabetic Foot*, 6th edition. Mosby, St. Louis, 2001, pp 13–32.

7. Gregg EW, Sorlie P, Paulose-Ram R et al. Prevalence of lower-extremity disease in the US adult population >=40 years of age with and without diabetes: 1999–2000 national health and nutrition examination survey. *Diabetes Care* 2004; 27:1591–1597.

8. Vileikyte L. Diabetic foot ulcers: a quality of life issue. *Diab Metab Res Rev* 2001; 17:246–249.

9. Boulton AJ, Kirsner RS, Vileikyte L. Clinical practice. Neuropathic diabetic foot ulcers. *N Engl J Med* 2004; 351:48–55.

10. Siitonen OI, Niskanen LK, Laakso M et al. Lower-extremity amputations in diabetic and nondiabetic patients. A population-based study in eastern Finland. *Diabetes Care* 1993; 16:16–20.

11. Trautner C, Haastert B, Giani G, Berger M. Incidence of lower limb amputations and diabetes. *Diabetes Care* 1996; 19:1006–1009.

12. Carrington AL, Mawdsley SK, Morley M et al. Psychological status of diabetic people with or without lower limb disability. *Diabetes Res Clin Pract* 1996; 32:19–25.

13. Singh N, Armstrong DG, Lipsky BA. Preventing foot ulcers in patients with diabetes. *JAMA* 2005; 293:217–228.

14. Pomposelli FB Jr, Jepsen SJ, Gibbons GW et al. Efficacy of the dorsal pedal bypass for limb salvage in diabetic patients: short-term observations. *J Vasc Surg* 1990; 11:745–752.

15. Edmonds ME. Experience in a multidisciplinary diabetic foot clinic. In: Connor H, Boulton AJM, Ward JD (eds). *The foot in diabetes: proceedings of the First National Conference on the Diabetic Foot, Malvern, England, May 1986*, John Wiley, Chichester, England, 1987, pp 121–134.

16. Boulton AJM. The diabetic foot: neuropathic in aetiology? *Diabet Med* 1990; 7:852–858.

17. Ctercteko GC, Dhanendran M, Hutton WC, Le Quesne LP. Vertical forces acting on the feet of diabetic patients with neuropathic ulceration. *Br J Surg* 1981; 68:608–614.

18. Brand PW. Repetitive stress in the development of diabetic foot ulcers. In: Levin ME, O'Neal LW (eds). *The diabetic foot*, 4th edition. CV Mosby, St. Louis, 1998, pp 83–90.

19. LoGerfo FW, Coffman JD. Current concepts. Vascular and microvascular disease of the foot in diabetes. Implications for foot care. *N Engl J Med* 1984; 311:1615–1619.

20. Luo J-D, Wang Y-Y, Fu W-L, Wu J, Chen AF. Gene therapy of endothelial nitric oxide synthase and manganese superoxide dismutase restores delayed wound healing in type 1 diabetic mice. *Circulation* 2004; 110:2484–2493.

21. Goova MT, Li J, Kislinger T et al. Blockade of receptor for advanced glycation end-products restores effective wound healing in diabetic mice. *Am J Pathol* 2001; 159:513–525.

22. Galeano M, Torre V, Deodata B et al. Raxofelast, a hydrophilic vitmain E-like antioxidant, stimulates wound healing in genetically diabetic mice. *Surgery* 2001; 129:467–477.

23. Liu R, Bal HS, Desta T, Graves DT. Tumor necrosis factor-alpha mediates diabetes-enhanced apoptosis of matrix-producing cells and impairs diabetic healing. *Am J Pathol* 2006; 168:757–764.

24. Gibbons GW, Eliopoulos GM. Infection of the diabetic foot. In: Kozak GP, Hoar CS Jr, Rowbotham JL, Wheelock FC Jr, Gibbons GW, Campbell D (eds). *Management of diabetic foot problems: Joslin Clinic and New England Deaconess Hospital*. WB Saunders, Philadelphia, 1984, pp 97–102.

25. Teno S, Kanno H, Oga S et al. Increased activity of membrane glycoprotein PC-1 in the fibroblasts from non-insulin-dependent diabetes mellitus patients with insulin resistance. *Diabetes Res Clin Pract* 1999; 45:25–30.

26. Loots MA, Lamme EN, Mekkes JR et al. Cultured fibroblasts from chronic diabetic wounds on the lower extremity (non-insulin-dependent diabetes mellitus) show disturbed proliferation. *Arch Dermatol Res* 1999; 291:93–99.

27. Lateef H, Stevens MJ, Varani J. All-trans-retinoic acid suppresses matrix metalloproteinase activity and increases collagen synthesis in diabetic human skin in organ culture. *Am J Pathol* 2004; 165:167–174.

28. Varani J, Warner RL, Gharaee-Kermani M et al. Vitamin A antagonizes decreased cell growth and elevated collagen-degrading matrix metalloproteinases and stimulates collagen accumulation in naturally aged human skin. *J Invest Dermatol* 2000; 114:480–486.

29. Ricciarelli R, Maroni P, Ozer N *et al.* Age-dependent increase of collagenase expression can be reduced by alpha-tocopherol via protein kinase c inhibition. *Free Radic Biol Med* 1999; 27:729–737.

30. Varani J, Perone P, Fligiel SE *et al.* All-trans-retinoic acid preserves viability of fibroblasts and keratinocytes in full-thickness human skin and fibroblasts in isolated dermis in organ culture. *Arch Dermatol Res* 1994; 286:443–447.

31. Margolis D, Hoffstad O. Diabetic neuropathic foot ulcers. *Diabetes Care* 2002; 25:10–15.

32. Spravchikov N, Sizyakov G, Gartsbein M *et al.* Glucose effects on skin keratinocytes: implications for diabetes skin complications. *Diabetes* 2001; 50:1627–1635.

33. Griffiths CE, Russman AN, Majmudar G *et al.* Restoration of collagen formation in photodamaged human skin by tretinoin (retinoic acid). *N Engl J Med* 1993; 329:530–535.

34. Varani J, Perone P, Fligiel SE *et al.* Inhibition of type 1 procollagen production in photodamage: correlation between presence of high molecular weight collagen fragments and reduced procollagen synthesis. *J Invest Dermatol* 2002; 119:122–129.

35. Pop-Busui R, Sima AAF, Stevens MJ. Diabetic neuropathy and oxidative stress. *Diab Metab Res Rev* 2006; 22:257–273.

36. Wolff SP. Diabetes mellitus and free radicals. *Br Med Bull* 1993; 49:642–652.

37. Rees RS, Smith DJ Jr, Adamson B *et al.* Oxidant stress: the role of the glutathione redox cycle in skin preconditioning. *J Surg Res* 1995; 58:395–400.

38. Shukla A, Rasik A, Dhawan B. Asiaticoside-induced elevation of antioxidant levels in healing wounds. *Phythother Res* 1999; 13:50–54.

39. Guzik TJ, Mussa S, Gastaldi D *et al.* Mechanisms of increased vascular superoxide production in human diabetes mellitus: role of NAD(P)H oxidase and endothelial nitric oxide synthase. *Circulation* 2002; 105:1656–1662.

40. Frank S, Kampfer H, Wetzler C *et al.* Nitric oxide drives skin repair: novel function of an established mediator. *Kidney Int* 2002; 61:882–888.

41. Ziche M, Morbidelli L, Masini E *et al.* Nitric oxide mediates angiogenesis in vivo and endothelial cell growth and migration in vitro promoted by substance P. *J Clin Invest* 1994; 94:2036–2044.

42. Schaffer MR, Efron PA, Thornton FJ *et al.* Nitric oxide, an autocrine regulator of wound fibroblast synthetic function. *J Immunol* 1997; 158:2375–2381.

43. Noiri E, Peresleni T, Srivastava N *et al.* Nitric oxide is necessary for a switch from stationary to locomoting phenotype in epithelial cells. *Am J Physiol* 1996; 170: C794–C802.

44. Witte MB, Thornton FJ, Tantry U *et al.* L-arginine supplementation enhances diabetic wound healing: involvement of the nitric oxide synthase and arginase pathways. *Metabolism* 2002; 51:1269–1273.

45. Yu Y, Thorpe SR, Jenkins AJ *et al.* Advanced glycation end-products and methionine sulphoxide in skin collagen of patients with type 1 diabetes. *Diabetologia* 2006; 49:2488–2498.

46. Wear-Maggitti K, Lee J, Conejero A *et al.* Use of topical sRAGE in diabetic wounds increased neovascularization and granulation tissue formation. *Ann Plast Surg* 2004; 52:519–522.

47. Meerwaldt R, Links TP, Graaff R *et al.* Increased accumulation of skin advanced glycation end-products precedes and correlates with clinical manifestation of diabetic neuropathy. *Diabetologia* 2005; 48:1637–1644.

48. Schmidt AM, Shi DY, Shi FY *et al.* The multiligand receptor RAGE as a progression factor amplifying immune and inflammatory responses. *J Clin Invest* 2001; 108:949–955.

49. Schmidt AM, Yan SD, Wautier JL *et al.* Activation of receptor for advanced glycation end products: implications for induction of oxidant stress and cellular dysfunction in the pathogensis of vascular lesions. *Arterioscler Thromb* 1994; 10:1521–1528.

50. Owen WF, Hou FF, Stuart Ro *et al.* Beta 2-microglobulin modified with advanced glycation end products modulates collagen synthesis by human fibroblasts. *Kidney Int* 1998; 53:1365–1373.

51. Berlanga J, Cibrian D, Guillen I *et al. Clin Sci* 2005; 109:83–95.

52. Ilnytska O, Lyzogubov VV, Stevens MJ *et al.* Bly (ADP-ribose polymerase) inhibition alleviates experimental diabetic sensory neuropathy. *Diabetes* 2006; 55:1686–1694.

53. Hattori Y, Kawasaki H, Kazuhiro A, Kanno M. Superoxide dismutase recovers altered endothelium-dependent relaxation in diabetic rat aorta. *Am J Physiol* 1991; 261: H1086–H1094.

54. Kunisaki M, Bursell S-E, Umeda F *et al.* Normalization of dicaylglycerol-protein kinase C activation by vitamin E in aorta of diabetic rats and cultured rat smooth muscle cells exposed to elevated glucose levels. *Diabetes* 1994; 43:1372–1377.

55. Moncada S, Gryglewski RJ, Bunting S, Vane JR. A lipid peroxide inhibits the enzyme in blood vessel microsomes that generates from prostaglandin endoperoxides the substance (prostaglandin X) which prevents platelet aggregation. *Prostaglandins* 1976; 12:715–737.

56. Kellogg AP, Wiggin T, Larkin D et al. Protective effects of cyclooxygenase-2 gene inactivation against peripheral nerve dysfunction and intraepidermal nerve fiber loss in experimental diabetes. *Diabetes* 2007; 56:2997–3005.

57. Ward KK, Low PA, Schmelzer JD, Zochodne DW. Prostacyclin and noradrenaline in peripheral nerve of chronic experimental diabetes in rats. *Brain* 1989; 112:197–208.

58. Tur E, Yosipovitch G, Bar-On Y. Skin reactive hyperemia in diabetic patients: a study by laser Doppler flowmetry. *Diabetes Care* 1991; 14:958–962.

59. Stevens MJ, Edmonds ME, Douglas SLE, Watkins PJ. Influence of neuropathy on the microvascular response to local heating in the human diabetic foot. *Clin Sci* 1991; 80:249–256.

60. Rendell M, Bamisedun O. Diabetic cutaneous microangiopathy. *Am J Med* 1992; 93:611–618.

61. Bornmyr S, Svensson H, Lilja B, Sundkvist G. Cutaneous vasomotor responses in young type I diabetic patients. *J Diabetes Complications* 1997; 11:21–26.

62. Rayman G, Williams SA, Spencer PD et al. Impaired microvascular response to minor skin trauma in type 1 diabetes. *BMJ (Clin Res Ed)* 1986; 292:1295–1298.

63. Vinik AI, Holland MT, Le Beau JM et al. Diabetic neuropathies. *Diabetes Care* 1992; 12:1926–1975.

64. Feldman EL, Stevens MJ, Russell JW. Diabetic peripheral and autonomic neuropathy. In: Sperling MA (ed.). *Contemporary Endocrinology: Type I Diabetes: Etiology and Treatment*. Humana Press, Totowa, NJ, 2003, pp 437–461.

65. Anand P, Terenghi G, Warner G et al. The role of endogenous nerve growth factor in human diabetic neuropathy. *Nat Med* 1996; 2:703–707.

66. Fromy B, Abraham P, Bouvet C et al. Early decrease of skin blood flow in response to locally applied pressure in diabetic subjects. *Diabetes* 2002; 51:1214–1217.

67. Fromy B, Merzeau S, Abraham P, Saumet JL. Mechanisms of the cutaneous vasodilator response to local external pressure application in rats: involvement of CGRP, neurokinins, prostaglandins and NO. *Br J Pharmacol* 2000; 131:1161–1171.

68. Sigaudo-Roussel D, Demiot C, Fromy B et al. Early endothelial dysfunction severely impairs skin blood flow response to local pressure application in streptozotocin-induced diabetic mice. *Diabetes* 2004; 53:1564–1569.

69. Habuchi O, Miyachi T, Kaigawa S, Nakashima S, Fujiwara C, Hisada M. Effects of glutathione depletion on the synthesis of proteoglycan and collagen in cultured chrondrocytes. *Biochim Biophys Acta* 1991; 1093:153–161.

70. Centers for Disease Control and Prevention. State-specific prevalence of obesity among adults – United States, 2005. *MMWR* 2006; 55:985–988.

71. Driver VR, Madsen J, Goodman RA. Reducing amputation rates in patients with diabetes at a military medical center: the limb preservation service model. *Diabetes Care* 2005; 28:248–253.

72. Apelqvist J, Larsson J. What is the most effective way to reduce incidence of amputation in the diabetic foot? *Diabetes Metab Res Rev* 2000; 16(suppl 1):S75–S83.

73. American Diabetes Association. Standards of medical care in diabetes—2007. *Diabetes Care* 2007; 30(suppl 1):S4–S41.

74. Armstrong DG, Todd WF, Lavery LA et al. The natural history of acute Charcot's arthropathy in the diabetic foot speciality clinic. *Diabet Med* 1997; 14:357–363.

75. Harrelson JM. The diabetic foot: Charcot arthropathy. *Instr Course Lect* 1993; 42:141–146.

76. Young MJ, Marshall A, Adams JE, Selby PL, Boulton AJM. Osteopenia, neurological dysfunction, and the development of Charcot neuroarthropathy. *Diabetes Care* 1995; 18:34–38.

77. Rajbhandari SM, Jenkins RC, Davies C, Tesfaye S. Charcot neurarthopathy in diabetes mellitus. *Diabetologia* 2002; 45:1085–1096.

78. Edelman SV, Kosofsky EM, Paul RA, Kosak GP. Neuroarthropathy (Charcot's joint) in diabetes mellitus following revascularization surgery. Three case reports and a review of the literature. *Arch Intern Med* 1987; 147:1504–1508.

79. Myerson MS. Diabetic neuroarthopathy. In: Myerson MS (ed.). *Foot and Ankle Disorders*. W.B. Saunders Company, Philadelphia, 1999, pp 439–465.

80. Edelson GW, Jensen JL, Kaczynski R. Identifying acute Charcot arthropathy through urinary cross-linked N-telopeptides. *Diabetes* 1996; 45(suppl 2):108A.

81. Gough A, Abraha H, Purewal TS et al. Measurement of markers of osteoclast and osteoblastic activity in patients with acute and chronic diabetic Charcot neuroarthropathy. *Diabet Med* 1997; 14:527–531.

82. Selby PL, Jude EB, Burgess J *et al.* Bone turnover markers in acute Charcot neuroarthropathy. *Diabetologia* 1998; 41(suppl 1): A275.

83. Sommer TC, Lee TH. Charcot foot: the diagnostic dilemma. *Am Fam Physician* 2001; 64:1591–1598.

84. Ledermann HP, Morrison WB. Differential diagnosis of pedal osteomyelitis and diabetic neuroarthropathy: MR imaging. *Semin Musculoskelet Radiol* 2005; 9:272–283.

85. Nguyen VD, Keh RA, Dachler RW. Freiberg's disease in diabetes mellitus. *Skeletal Radiol* 1991; 20:425–428.

86. Zlatkin MB, Pathria M, Sartoris DJ, Resnick D. The diabetic foot. *Radiol Clin North Am* 1987; 25:1095–1105.

87. Bamberger DM, Daus GP, Gerding DN. Osteolyelitis in the feet of diabetic patients. Long-term results, prognostic factors, and the role of antimicrobial and surgical therapy. *Am J Med* 1987; 83:653–660.

88. Ledermann HP, Morrison WB, Schweitzer ME. Pedal abcesses in patients suspected of having pedal osteomyelitis: analysis with MR imaging. *Radiology* 2002; 224:649–655.

89. Edmonds ME. Progress in the care of the diabetic foot. *Lancet* 1999; 354:270–272.

90. Armstrong DG, Lavery LA, Harkless LB. Treatment-based classification system for assessment and care of diabetic feet. *J Am Podiatr Med Assoc* 1996; 86:311–316.

91. Armstrong DG, Lavery LA, Harkless LB. Who is at risk for diabetic foot ulceration? *Clin Pod Med Surg* 1998; 15:11–19.

92. Lavery LA, Armstrong DG, Vela SA *et al.* Practical criteria for screening patients at high risk for diabetic foot ulceration. *Arch Intern Med* 1998; 158:157–162.

93. Armstrong DG, Nguyen HC, Lavery LA *et al.* Off-loading the diabetic foot wound: a randomized clinical trial. *Diabetes Care* 2001; 24:1019–1022.

94. Daniels T, Waddell JP. Musculoskeletal images: Charcot arthropathy. *Can J Surg* 2002; 45:363–364.

95. Jude EB, Selby PL, Burgess J *et al.* Bisphosphonates in the treatment of Charcot neuroarthropathy: a double-blind randomised controlled trial. *Diabetologia* 2001; 44:2032–2037.

96. Selby PL, Young MJ, Adams JE, Boulton AJM. Bisphosphonate: a new treatment for diabetic Charcot neuroarthropathy. *Diabet Med* 1994; 11:14–20.

97. Varani J, Perone P, Merfert MG *et al.* All-trans retinoic acid improves structure and function of diabetic rat skin in organ culture. *Diabetes* 2002; 51:3510–3516.

98. Lateef H, Aslam MN, Stevens MJ, Varani J. Pretreatment of diabetic rats with lipoic acid improves healing of subsequently-induced abrasion wounds. *Arch Dermatol Res* 2005; 297:75–83.

99. Demiot C, Fromy B, Saumet JL, Sigaudo-Roussel D. Preservation of pressure-induced cutaneous vasodilation by limiting oxidative stress in short-term diabetic mice. *Cardiovasc Res* 2006; 69:245–252.

100. Hyland ME, Lay A, Thomson B. Quality of life of leg ulcer patients: questionnaire and preliminary findings. *J Wound Care* 1994; 3:294–298.

101. Schipper H, Clinch JJ, Olweny CLM. Quality of life studies: definitions and conceptual issues. In: Spilker B (ed.). *Quality of Life and Pharmacoeconomics in Clinical Trails*, 2nd edition. Lippincott-Raven, Philadelphia, 1996, pp 11–24.

10

How should we manage the pregnant patient with type 2 diabetes?

F. Dunne

BACKGROUND

Type 2 diabetes is an ongoing concern with the number of new cases increasing explosively and at a younger age due to obesity. As a result, the number of cases arising in women of child-bearing age is also increasing at an alarming rate and will be encountered more frequently in antenatal clinics. At present, approximate 25% of pregnant women with pregestational diabetes have type 2 disease and the number is likely to continue to rise. Until very recently, type 2 diabetes was perceived as a benign form of diabetes but this is not the case when one examines pregnancy outcomes. Perinatal mortality and congenital malformations are significantly greater than those in background populations and at least as poor as those identified in women with type 1 diabetes. In addition, the rates of hypertension, preeclampsia and post-partum haemorrhage are greater than in the general obstetric population as is the rate of operative delivery. To improve outcomes we need to recognize that type 2 diabetes is a serious condition. Through educational programmes, population and target screening, and strategies to help vulnerable groups e.g. ethnic minorities, we have the ability to identify and counsel women with type 2 diabetes early enough to make a difference.

RELATIONSHIP OF DIABETES TO PREGNANCY

The most prevalent medical condition in the pregnant population is diabetes [1]. The proportion of type 1 diabetes, type 2 diabetes and gestational diabetes (GDM) is dependent on the background population. Type 1 diabetes (primarily insulin deficiency) is more common in a Caucasian population. On the other hand, type 2 and gestational diabetes (associated with both insulin resistance and impaired insulin secretion [2, 3] are more common in ethnic minority groups. Type 2 diabetes and gestational disease share the same risk factors, have a corresponding prevalence within a given population, and have the same genetic susceptibility. They are assumed to be aetiologically indistinct with one preceding the other.

Diabetes in relation to pregnancy continues to pose problems. Large observational studies have demonstrated an increased risk of fetal and neonatal death, congenital malformations, preterm delivery, macrosomia, pre-eclampsia and increased need for Caesarian section [4–10].

Women with type 2 diabetes have at least as poor and often worse pregnancy outcomes when compared to women who have type 1 diabetes. They are usually older, more

Fidelma Dunne, MD, PhD, MMedEd, Consultant Endocrinologist, Head of School of Medicine, School of Medicine, National University of Ireland, Galway and Galway University Hospitals, Galway, Ireland.

obese, from a non-Caucasian background, and a significant number are from a lower socioeconomic group [4, 10–13]. Additionally, they are frequently of higher parity, are more likely to have pre-existing hypertension and to be treated with medications associated with congenital malformations. Many women with type 2 diabetes receive care in the community and may be unaware of the importance of glycaemic control at the time of conception. As outlined in the CEMACH report, women with type 2 diabetes are less likely to have had a HbA1C measurement prior to pregnancy, are less likely to attend pre-pregnancy care (PPC) and are less likely to receive folic acid when compared to women with type 1 diabetes [14].

In 1989 the St Vincent Joint Task Force for Diabetes set as one of its targets the improvement in pregnancy outcome for women with diabetes so that the risks approached that of the non-diabetic population [15, 16]. To achieve this target, strategies were developed to improve pre-pregnancy care, encourage the uptake of folic acid, and refine blood glucose testing and insulin therapy. These strategies have helped and improvements have been demonstrated. The Diabetes Control and Complications Trial (DCCT) has shown that women with type 1 diabetes receiving intensive management have a reduction in congenital anomalies and miscarriages [17]. Published studies on pre-pregnancy care have demonstrated its importance in terms of miscarriage and congenital malformation rates [18–20]. Despite these advances, the targets of the St Vincent Task Force have not been achieved, as illustrated by recent publications [10, 11, 21–23].

TYPE 2 DIABETES PREGNANCY AND ETHNICITY

Type 2 diabetes in pregnancy is often perceived as a less serious condition as it is controlled by diet and oral hypoglycaemic agents before pregnancy and looked after almost exclusively in primary care [10]. However, in defined locations with mixed populations, women with type 2 diabetes form a significant proportion of those attending pre-pregnancy/antenatal clinics. In addition, type 2 diabetes is an emerging problem in the paediatric and adolescent population [24–27], as is childhood obesity [28], which predisposes to the disease. Consequently, the occurrence of type 2 diabetes in pregnancy will continue to be a significant and increasing problem in the coming decades.

The prevalence of type 2 diabetes has been estimated in a number of specific populations and may not be generalizable. The prevalence in the Pima Indians is 6.3% [29]. A large population-based survey carried out in the USA suggested an increasing prevalence of type 2 diabetes in the pregnant population [30]. Women with type 2 diabetes in pregnancy tend to be older, heavier and of greater parity when compared to women with type 1 diabetes or non-diabetic women drawn from the same geographical location [12]. They are more likely to be from an Indo-Asian or Afro-Caribbean background [10]. Type 2 diabetes frequently develops in women with previous GDM. In one large UK study, 35% of Indo-Asian women with GDM in the index pregnancy had persistent postpartum glucose intolerance [31]. Where GDM appears early in pregnancy (before 20 weeks), the diagnosis often represents previously undiagnosed type 2 disease [31]. Type 2 diabetes is also common in women with polycystic ovarian syndrome.

What are the risks for the baby?
As in all diabetic pregnancies, infants born to mothers with type 2 diabetes are at increased risk of congenital malformations, both major and minor. In a large UK study describing the outcomes in 182 singleton pregnancies complicated by type 2 diabetes, 18 congenital anomalies occurred, mainly in women with poor control [10] (Table 10.1). Only 2 abnormalities occurred in women with normal control at booking. These infants had an 11-fold greater risk of a congenital malformation when compared with national statistics. Although 15/18

Table 10.1 Fetal/neonatal outcomes in Type 2 diabetes (with permission from [10])

	Normal control (n = 60)	Average control (n = 69)	Poor control (n = 53)
Miscarriage	4	3	9
Malformations	2	6	13
Stillbirths	2	0	0
Neonatal deaths	0	3	2
Total events	8 (13%)	12 (17%)	24 (45%)

Table 10.2 Does pre-pregnancy care help? (with permission from [20])

	Attenders	Non-attenders	P-value
Stable relationship	100%	57%	0.004
Current smokers	8%	28%	0.03
Mean HbA1c	7.5%	9.0%	0.008
Week of booking	7	9	0.09
Macrosomia	25%	40%	0.09
Neonatal deaths	0	2	
Neonatal unit care	17%	34%	0.04

resulted in a live outcome, infant mortality was high with four deaths occurring. The most common malformations were cardiac (53%) followed by musculoskeletal (27%). These findings are similar to those reported in Hispanic women in southern California where 11.7% of babies were born with major congenital anomalies compared to 2% in the background non-diabetic population [32]. Like the UK study, the majority of malformations occurred in those with poor glycaemic control who did not receive pre-pregnancy care. As highlighted previously, poorer attendance for pre-pregnancy care, later booking for antenatal care and poorer glycaemic control during organogenesis contribute to the higher malformation rate [10, 13, 21] (Table 10.2). The congenital malformation rate may also be influenced by uptake of folic acid but it is difficult to obtain accurate information on this. In the normal population, the uptake of folic acid is still below 50% [33] and in diabetic women it is approximately 30% [4]. The miscarriage rate in type 2 diabetes in the UK study was high at 8.8%, almost doubling to 15.7% in those with poor glycaemic control [10], and 56% occurred in the first trimester.

Perinatal mortality is, at best, as good as type 1 diabetes [21] but reported by some authors to be far greater [34]. The latter study reported four perinatal deaths in 113 type 2 diabetic patients and none in 46 type 1 diabetic patients. There were no differences in neonatal morbidities between the groups. Cundy and colleagues have shown a very high perinatal mortality in women with type 2 diabetes, mainly due to late stillbirths [11]. In the large UK series, there were two stillbirths (1.2%), two early and one late neonatal death and two further deaths in the postnatal period out of a total of 182 singleton pregnancies. The perinatal mortality rate was 25/1000, 2.5-fold greater than regional or national figures and occurring mainly in infants with congenital heart disease [10]. More recently, Clausen and colleagues demonstrated perinatal mortality to be four times and congenital malformations two times greater than women with type 1 diabetes [13].

Table 10.3 PPC checklist

Plan pregnancy, this will take 3–6 months
Use contraception until HbA1c is normal (<7%)
Smoking status and advice
Alcohol status and advice
Dietetics review
Blood glucose monitoring at least four times per day
Blood glucose targets of F <5.3; 1-h PP <7.8; 2-h PP <6.7 mmol/l
Weight, height, BMI
Review diabetes control (HbA1c)
Review renal function (albumin:creatinine ratio [ACR], blood biochemistry)
Retinal screen/digital photography
Rubella screen
Review medications: stop statins, fibrate, angiotensin-converting enzyme
(ACE) inhibitors, angiotensin receptor blockers (ARB)
If blood pressure control is necessary, use methyldopa/nifedipine
Folic acid 5 mg once daily for at least 12 weeks
If taking oral hypoglycaemic agents, transfer to insulin
Discuss hypoglycaemia and management /glucagon kit
Encourage early booking to antenatal clinic as soon as pregnancy test is positive
If GDM was present in previous pregnancy, re-screen with oral glucose tolerance test

What are the risks for the mother?

In any diabetic pregnancy the risk of a maternal complication developing is high compared to background non-diabetic figures. Polyhydramnios was 3-fold greater compared to non-diabetics (9% compared to 3%) in the UK series, with infant mortality more likely in pregnancies affected by polyhydramnios. Postpartum haemorrhage was also much more common but appeared unrelated to macrosomia. Pregnancy-induced hypertension and/or pre-eclampsia was twice as common (20% compared to 10% in the background group) and, again, an infant death was more likely in this group [10]. Delivery by Caesarian section is common in women with type 2 diabetes with a rate of 53% reported [10] and confirmed in other series [11]. Diabetes complications in women with type 2 diabetes are not well documented. Omori and colleagues identified a high rate of retinopathy (32%) and overt nephropathy (1.4%) in their series [35].

PREPARATION FOR PREGNANCY, PRE-PREGNANCY CARE (PPC)

Over the last two decades the literature has cast little doubt on the importance of PPC for women with both type 1 and type 2 diabetes [18–20, 36, 37] (Table 10.3). Intensive glucose management at this time confers significant benefits to the health of the mother and her baby. A minimum of 3 months PPC is advised. PPC seeks to assist women in achieving excellent glycaemic control prior to conception (HbA1c <7%) and to maintain this during the critical period of organogenesis. This is achieved through motivation and manipulation of diet and exercise. A systematic review included data from thirteen observational studies comparing poor versus optimal glycaemic control in relation to maternal fetal and neonatal outcomes and involved 5480 women. Poor glycaemic control increased the likelihood of miscarriage (odds ratio [OR] 3.23) and perinatal mortality (OR 3.03) [38]. In addition, poor glycaemic control increased the likelihood of congenital malformations (OR 3.4) for each 1 per cent point increase in HbA1c [38].

Overall, the risk of an adverse outcome is halved with each percentage point HbA1c reduction achieved before pregnancy [36]. This information can act as a powerful motivator for women to achieve glucose targets during PPC and to reassure women and their health-care providers that all improvements in blood glucose are helpful.

In some women insulin *de novo* is needed, while in others it is the opportune time to change from oral hypoglycaemic agents to insulin. High-dose folic acid is commenced to reduce the incidence of neural tube defects and a minimum of 12 weeks of treatment is recommended. Antihypertensive medication with angiotensin-converting enzyme (ACE) inhibitors and angiotensin receptor blockers (ARB) are stopped. This class of drugs have been associated with fetopathy including renal tubular dysplasia, intrauterine growth restriction, hypocalvaria, patent ductus arteriosus, fetal anuria and neonatal death [39, 40]. Instead, methyldopa nifedipine or labetalol can be used.

Statins are contraindicated in pregnancy and should be discontinued [41]. HMG-CoA reductase is important for development of the embryo. If it is inhibited, there is a decrease in mevalonate and other growth-regulating proteins. This has implications for membrane synthesis, DNA replication, cellular proliferation and protein glycation, all critical for embryonic and placental development [42]. Contraception should continue until the HbA1c is within the normal range.

For a woman with type 2 diabetes, this is the time to initiate seven-point glucose testing, to have a consultation with a dietitian, and to start insulin if diet and exercise do not maintain glucose levels within a normal range. This is frequently a basal-bolus regime with a bolus of short-acting insulin with each meal and a basal insulin at bedtime. Time needs to be devoted to recognition and treatment of hypoglycaemia with the woman and her partner, and the latter should be advised on the administration of glucagon. Hypoglycaemic unawareness is common in pregnancy and maternal mortality occurs as a result of hypoglycaemia.

One should also take the opportunity to screen for diabetic complications. Retinal examination should be carried out through dilated pupils with retinal photography or use of a slit lamp. If unsure, always refer the patient to an ophthalmologist for a baseline assessment. Check blood pressure and if borderline do a 24-h ambulatory assessment. Renal status needs to be assessed by a baseline 24-h urinary protein excretion and serum creatinine. PPC is strongly recommended by the recent National Institute for Health and Clinical Excellence (NICE) guidelines on Diabetes in Pregnancy [43].

Are oral hypoglycaemic agents safe?

Oral hypoglycaemic agents (sensitizers and secretogogues) are the main treatment modalities for type 2 diabetes. Consequently, these women usually attend PPC or their first antenatal clinic still taking these medications. While there have been some recent encouraging articles on the use of some oral agents in pregnancy, professionals are still advised (at least in Europe) to switch all patients with established type 2 diabetes to insulin [44]. This recommendation is for all classes of drugs (sulphonylureas, meglitinides, thiazolidinediones (TZDs) and modulators of the incretins).

A recent retrospective analysis of the outcomes of 379 pregnancies in women with type 2 diabetes exposed to oral hypoglycaemic agents or insulin has shown that sulphonylureas are inferior to insulin treatment in women with type 2 diabetes during pregnancy [45]. The perinatal mortality rate was higher at 125/1000 in women exposed to a sulphonylurea throughout pregnancy compared to 28/1000 for those switched from sulphonylurea to insulin in early pregnancy and 33/1000 in those never exposed to a sulphonylurea in pregnancy.

There are also concerns regarding metformin as it crosses the placenta [46]. Metformin used in late pregnancy in women with type 2 diabetes has been associated with stillbirths [45, 47]. More recently, a large prospective study in Australia examined the efficacy and safety of metformin in women with gestational diabetes. It showed that the pregnancy outcome among women treated with metformin is comparable to women receiving insulin [48]. However, a large prospective trial in women with type 2 diabetes is needed before a change in current practice is recommended.

Thiazolidinediones are insulin sensitizers that work via activation of the nuclear peroxisome proliferator-activated receptor gamma (PPARγ). They are used in type 2 diabetes and increasingly in polycystic ovary syndrome (PCOS) [49]. As a consequence, we are likely to encounter more women conceiving on these drugs. PPARγ plays a role in placental maturation and implantation of the embryo [50]. TZDs cross the placenta and have been associated with fetal death and growth retardation in animal studies [51]. There is a lack of evidence on the use of PPARγ agonists in pregnancy. This in combination with their documented toxicity in animals would advocate their immediate withdrawal in a confirmed pregnancy and their stoppage if a woman is actively planning a pregnancy or attending PPC.

First antenatal visit

If a woman has not attended PPC, her first encounter with a diabetologist may be at her first antenatal visit. At this visit it is important to establish length of diabetes, presence or absence of retinopathy, nephropathy or hypertension. A retinal screen through dilated fundoscopy is mandatory. Baseline HbA1c, thyroid function tests (TFT), serum creatinine and a urine protein to creatinine ratio should be carried out. All antihypertensive and lipid-lowering agents are discontinued. If required, methyldopa, labetalol or nifedipine can be started for blood pressure (BP) control.

A review of home blood glucose monitoring readings is necessary and glycaemic targets given (preprandial 4–6 mmol/l; postprandial 4–8 mmol/l). If the patient is not already self-monitoring, then this is initiated. Oral hypoglycaemic agents are stopped and insulin commenced. The importance of avoiding hypoglycaemia is emphasized and tools to deal with it such as dextrose tablets and glucagon given. Hypoglycaemia is more common in trimester 1 and highest in weeks 10–15 [52, 53]. Although hypoglycaemia occurs less frequently in women with type 2 compared to type 1 diabetes, 24-h continuous glucose monitoring (CGMS) shows significant episodes not identified by standard self-monitoring [54].

Medical nutritional therapy (MNT) is the cornerstone of treatment in all pregnancies complicated by diabetes and all women will need a detailed consultation with a dietitian. If this is not available, then the woman should be instructed to avoid single meals and foods with simple carbohydrates. In particular, a small meal at breakfast with limited carbohydrate is advised as this is the time associated with the greatest insulin resistance. Three small meals and three additional snacks are usually required. This limits the glucose level presented to the bloodstream at any one time. In addition, exercise is an important factor in improving glycaemic control in pregnancies complicated by diabetes. Activities such as swimming and walking are appropriate. Exercise reduces insulin resistance, a central component of the aetiology of type 2 diabetes. During exercise there is preferential carbohydrate utilization and this has an impact on insulin and food requirements. There is a low risk of pregnancy-induced hypoglycaemia in pregnant women with type 2 diabetes [55].

From an obstetric perspective a dating ultrasound scan is necessary, as is normal antenatal screening. If still early in the pregnancy, folic acid can be commenced and continued until the end of the first trimester.

What insulin to choose?

Insulin is the treatment of choice for women with type 2 diabetes during pregnancy. It does not cross the placenta and its efficacy has been proven in many studies. A combination of short- (bolus) and long- (basal) acting insulins is frequently required. The goal of insulin therapy is to achieve glucose profiles similar to those of non-diabetic pregnant women and to confine postprandial glucose excursions to a tight range. The challenge is to achieve this goal whilst avoiding hypoglycaemia.

Traditionally, human insulins have been used, as allergic reactions occur in <1% and they are associated with low insulin antibody titres [56]. The latter is important as antibody-bound insulin crosses the placenta and may increase the level of insulin in the foetus, promoting macrosomia and fetal hypoglycaemia. Human insulins are available with various durations of action which allow flexibility for individualized regimes. After the first trimester, insulin requirements increase. As a result, increasing doses of short-acting insulin is required to control postprandial glucose excursions and increasing doses of long-acting insulin to maintain a euglycaemic basal state.

There has been one randomized trial comparing a twice-daily insulin regimen of regular and intermediate insulin at morning and bedtime compared to four times daily regimen of short-acting insulin before meals and intermediate insulin at bedtime [57]. Maternal glycaemic control and neonatal hypoglycaemia were significantly better in women receiving the four times a day regimen. The data support the use of a basal bolus regimen.

Short-acting insulin analogues provide a more accurate simulation of physiological insulin release. They reduce postprandial insulin excursions while preventing preprandial hypoglycaemia [58]. Short-acting insulin analogues have been shown to be both safe and effective in pregnant women with type 1 diabetes. In addition, these analogues confer benefits in relation to episodes of hypoglycaemia [59, 60]. Although not proven, it is highly likely that the same benefits would be observed in pregnant women with type 2 diabetes.

To date, there have been no randomized controlled trials of long-acting insulin analogues in pregnant women. Case reports have shown that insulin glargine is effective in controlling glucose with less nocturnal hypoglycaemia compared to NPH insulin [61, 62]. However, it did not show any benefits in terms of birth weight, fetal macrosomia or neonatal morbidity [63]. There are no published data on the use of insulin detemir in pregnancy but a randomized controlled study has been initiated, with results expected in 2010.

How much insulin is required?

Insulin requirements change throughout pregnancy, generally increasing from week 15 to term in women with type 1 diabetes [64]. This parallels the growth of the fetoplacental unit and is consistent with the increase in insulin resistance. There is a period of time in the late first trimester when requirements decrease and the woman is at increased risk of hypoglycaemia. One further study examined insulin requirements in women with type 2 diabetes. They showed that during pregnancy insulin requirements are greater in women with type 2 compared to those with type 1 diabetes. The requirements increase from 0.86 units/kg in trimester 1, to 1.18 units/kg in trimester 2, to 1.62 units/kg in trimester 3 [65]. Insulin requirements tend to decline prior to delivery as the function of the placenta declines.

MANAGEMENT UP TO 20 WEEKS GESTATION

Early pregnancy care focuses on maintaining normoglycaemia especially during the first seven gestational weeks coinciding with organogenesis. During this time insulin dosing adjustments are frequent because of the physiological tendency to early morning hypoglycaemia. If unrecognized, this may lead to rebound hyperglycaemia. Characteristically, insulin doses drop in the late first trimester and then rise slowly to 20 weeks. During the first trimester folic acid is continued. A booking ultrasound scan confirms gestational age and a detailed anomaly scan is scheduled for 20 weeks' gestation. Screening with α-fetoprotein is offered and nuchal fold thickness and amniocentesis should be offered when necessary. With reference to diabetes complications, dilated retinal examinations should be scheduled once in each trimester for those without retinopathy at booking, but more frequently every six weeks for those with established retinopathy at the booking visit. Urinalysis should be carried out at each visit for protein. If incipient (microproteinuria) or established (proteinuria and/or abnormal creatinine) nephropathy is present at booking, then monthly estimations of albumin excretion and serum creatinine should be made. Patients should be seen every two weeks with ongoing open access to the multiprofessional diabetes team.

MANAGEMENT FROM 20 WEEKS TO TERM

The second half of pregnancy concentrates on fetal well-being. Ultrasound scans for fetal growth occur frequently as determined by local policy. If macrosomia develops, the findings from ultrasound may inform the decision about delivery. In later pregnancy biophysical profiles can provide useful information on fetal well-being [66]. For high-risk babies (in mothers who display evidence of vascular disease– retinopathy, nephropathy and hypertension) – Doppler studies are important [66]. For the mother, surveillance of the eyes continues and clinical monitoring for the development of pre-eclampsia and hypertension is important.

MANAGEMENT OF GLUCOSE AT LABOUR AND DELIVERY

The timing and mode of delivery is individualized. If mother and fetus are both well, then one should aim for a term vaginal delivery [16]. If early delivery is necessary, then glucocorticoids may be used for lung maturity. This will cause hyperglycaemia and insulin doses will need to be adjusted [67]. Normal glucose control (4–7 mmol/l) in the perinatal period is important to prevent neonatal hypoglycaemia. This can be achieved by glucose and insulin infusions adjusted frequently according to the maternal glucose values [68], or by continuous insulin infusion with alternating glucose/non-glucose fluids [69]. Preventing neonatal hypoglycaemia will reduce admission for neonatal care and promote improved mother–infant bonding. Immediately after delivery, insulin requirements diminish to pre-pregnancy levels. If not on insulin prior to pregnancy, insulin may be discontinued and diet continued. Breast-feeding should be encouraged as this will help to maintain good glycaemic control. Oral hypoglycaemic agents are not used while actively breast-feeding. During this time if glycaemic control is inadequate then insulin may need to be continued.

MANAGEMENT IN THE POST-NATAL PERIOD

Breast-feeding

Breast-feeding provides benefits for both the mother and her infant and should be actively encouraged [70, 71]. Education about breast-feeding should begin in the preconception period and continue throughout pregnancy. Women often find their diabetes more easily managed for the duration of lactation with lower insulin requirements [72]. Hypoglycaemic episodes may occur commonly within 1 h of breast-feeding [73]. These episodes can be avoided by eating a snack containing 15 g of carbohydrate and some protein before or during breast-feeding. Nocturnal episodes can occur and necessitate a reduction in basal insulin. Prospective studies of the interactions of short or prolonged breast-feeding on maternal weight and body composition are lacking in diabetic women. Due to the importance of obesity on health outcomes in women with diabetes, the effect of breast-feeding on body mass index (BMI) and waist circumference should be studied [74, 75]. Breast-feeding for 12 months confers protection against premenopausal breast cancer [76]. Epidemiological evidence also suggests protection against epithelial ovarian cancer [77] and arthritis [78].

Complete breast-feeding for 6 months has been consistently linked to a decreased incidence of a wide range of childhood infectious diseases in non-diabetic women [79]. There is also evidence that it reduces eczema [80], coeliac disease [81] and sudden infant death syndrome [82]. These infants also show higher neuro-developmental scores at follow-up surveillance [83] and have a lower degree of obesity in childhood and adolescence compared to bottle-fed infants [84]. Such an effect could have a large public health impact [85]. A relationship has been shown between breast-feeding and reduction of type 2 diabetes in Pima Indian offspring [74, 86] and this trend in other populations has been confirmed in a meta-analysis [87]. There are several epidemiological studies documenting the association between short or no breast-feeding and type 1 diabetes in childhood [88]. The association of excessive infant weight gain may increase the susceptibility of the β-cell to autoimmune damage or apoptosis [89]. Recent studies suggest that the timing and introduction of soy milk and cereals into the diet of high-risk infants may play a role in development of type 1 diabetes-related autoimmunity [90].

Contraception
Planning of further pregnancies is mandatory and the need for contraception is essential to reduce the risk of future miscarriage and congenital malformations. Early lactation amenor-rhoea (LAM) occurs with exclusive breast-feeding and can be started immediately, providing 98% efficacy in pregnancy protection [91, 92]. A woman must breast-feed every 4 hours during daytime and every 6 hours during night-time hours and avoid milk supplementation. Beyond 6 months postpartum, or if menses returns, another contraceptive method should be used [93]. Barrier methods provide no metabolic side-effects and have no contraindications to their use: again, they can be used immediately. Intrauterine devices are safe and effective and are metabolically neutral but should not be used until at least 4 weeks postpartum. Hormonal contraceptives containing either progestin alone, or progestin combined with an oestrogen can be started 6 weeks postpartum. Oestrogen has no effect on glucose tolerance but can increase triglyceride levels, whilst progestins increase insulin resistance and worsen glucose tolerance in addition to increasing low-density lipoprotein (LDL)-cholesterol. Consequently, the lowest dose and potency of progestin should be used to minimize adverse effects on glucose and lipid metabolism. Oestrogens increase BP and promote coagulation, and therefore should be avoided in patients with hypertension, micro-vascular and macrovascular disease. Any diabetic woman who smokes should avoid combined oral contraceptives (COCs). Currently no studies exist that examine the COC in women with type 2 diabetes. However, these women often have other cardiovascular risk factors and/or the metabolic syndrome. In such women with several risk factors for arterial and venous thromboembolic disease, an oestrogen-containing pill would not be a first choice contraceptive method as it could further increase thromboembolic risk and BP. If there is a strong reason to opt for a COC, then regular monitoring of lipids and BP should occur [94]. A safer option is a progestin-only pill. Hormonal contraception is safe to use while breast-feeding with <1% transferred to breast milk, similar to the hormone level observed during ovulatory cycles [93].

Long-term follow-up and inter-pregnancy care
Since the targets set by the St Vincent Task Force [15], combined antenatal diabetes clinics and PPC clinics are more common. Through public campaigns women are aware of the importance and benefits of folic acid. Glucose control is improving through the use of short-acting insulin analogues [59]. Despite these sustained efforts, we have been unable to achieve the level of glucose control required to prevent adverse pregnancy outcome in the majority of women with type 2 diabetes [8, 10, 11, 13]. Thus, outcomes which are related to poor glycaemic control (e.g. congenital abnormalities and perinatal mortality are still unacceptably poor). In addition, we are witnessing a substantial increase in the prevalence of type 2 diabetes, which is occurring on average at least 20 years earlier, with an increasing number of teens and young children being diagnosed [95, 96]. In the USA, 45% of new-onset diabetes in the paediatric age group is type 2 diabetes [95] and onset of type 2 diabetes is associated with obesity.

Improvements may happen if we address the areas of education and screening. We need to devise educational programmes that are culturally sensitive if the message regarding type 2 diabetes is to reach the right people. Such educational programmes need to be available in both rural and urban communities. The importance of family planning and benefits of folic acid in achieving a successful pregnancy outcome need to be emphasized and be part of a routine educational package in women with type 2 diabetes of childbearing age [10]. In non-Caucasian communities we need to dispel the myth that this form of diabetes is not serious. Type 2 diabetes frequently goes unnoticed for months or years before diagnosis and many women are diagnosed at their first antenatal visit around week 10 [10, 12]. Organogenesis is thus complete at the time of the initial consultation. Thus, screening for type 2 diabetes in a systematic way rather than opportunistically may benefit those at greatest risk.

There is evidence that glucose intolerance in pregnancy might play a role in the increasing prevalence of type 2 diabetes. *In utero* exposure to diabetes is thought to lead to fetal hyperinsulinaemia, which causes an increase in fetal fat cells, leading to obesity and insulin resistance in childhood. This, in turn, leads to impaired glucose tolerance and diabetes in adulthood. Therefore, diabetes begets diabetes as these glucose-intolerant adults develop diabetes in pregnancy [97–99]. National educational programmes on lifestyle changes to avoid obesity and reduce fat intake are vital to break the cycle. Large intervention studies based on lifestyle changes have been shown to decrease the risk of progression to type 2 diabetes by up to 50% [100, 101]. Women with previous gestational diabetes have an increased future risk of type 2 diabetes, this risk being greatest in south Asian women [31]. These women require a postnatal oral glucose tolerance test (OGTT) to establish glucose status, and annual recall thereafter in OGTT negative women for re-assessment [31]. This will accommodate early pick-up of type 2 disease.

For women with established diabetes (type 1 and type 2) or previous GDM, a programme of inter-pregnancy care should be offered. This should concentrate on lifestyle intervention with diet and exercise with the aim of reducing central obesity and BMI prior to the next pregnancy. Ultimately intrauterine prevention of type 2 diabetes is the goal. The first step in this process is to avoid intrauterine over-nutrition and macrosomia.

REFERENCES

1. Centers for Disease Control. Perinatal mortality and congenital malformations in infants born to women with insulin dependent diabetes: US Canada Europe 1940–1988. *JAMA* 1990; 264:437–440.
2. Ryan EA, O'Sullivan MJ, Skyler JS. Insulin action during pregnancy: studies with the euglycaemic clamp technique. *Diabetes* 1985; 34:380–389.
3. Catalano PM, Tyzbir ED, Wolfe RR *et al*. Carbohydrate metabolism during pregnancy in control subjects and women with gestational diabetes. *Am J Physiol* 1993; 264:E60–E67.
4. Confidential Enquiry into Maternal and Child Health. *Diabetes in Pregnancy: Are we providing the best care? Findings of a national enquiry: England, Wales and Northern Ireland*. CEMACH, London, 2007.
5. Hawthorne G, Robson S, Ryall EA *et al*. Prospective population based survey of outcome of pregnancy in diabetic women: results of the Northern Diabetic Pregnancy Audit 1994. *BMJ* 1997; 315:279–281.
6. Jensen DM, Damm P, Melsted-Pedersen *et al*. Outcomes in type 1 diabetic pregnancies: a nationwide population based study. *Diabetes Care* 2004; 27:2819–2823.
7. Penney GC, Mair G, Pearson DWM *et al*. Outcomes of pregnancies in women with type 1 diabetes in Scotland: a national population based study. *Br J Obstet Gynaecol* 2003; 110:315–318.
8. Macintosh MCM, Fleming KM, Bailey JA *et al*. Perinatal mortality and congenital anomalies in babies of women with type 1 or type 2 diabetes in England, Wales and Northern Ireland: population based study. *BMJ* 2006; 333:177–180.
9. Dunne F. Type 2 diabetes and pregnancy. *Semin Fetal Neonatal Med* 2005; 10:333–339.
10. Dunne F, Brydon P, Smith K, Gee H. Pregnancy in women with Type 2 diabetes. 12 years outcome data 1990–2002. *Diabet Med* 2003; 30:734–738.
11. Cundy T, Gamble G, Townend K *et al*. Perinatal mortality in type 2 diabetes mellitus. *Diabet Med* 2000; 17:33–39.
12. Brydon P, Smith T, Proffitt M, Gee H, Holder R, Dunne F. Pregnancy outcome in women with type 2 diabetes needs to be addressed. *Int J Clin Practice* 2000; 54:418–419.
13. Clausen TD, Mathiesen E, Ekbom P, Hellmuth E, Mandrup-Poulsen T, Damm P. Poor pregnancy outcome in women with type 2 diabetes mellitus. *Diabetes Care* 2005; 28:323–328.
14. Roland JM *et al*. The pregnancies of women with type 2 diabetes: poor outcomes but opportunities for improvement. *Diabet Med* 2005; 22:1774–1777.

15. World Health Organisation (Europe) and International Diabetes Federation (Europe). Diabetes care and research in Europe: the St Vincent Declaration. *Diabet Med* 1990; 7:360.

16. British Diabetic Accociation. *Pregnancy and neonatal care subgroup of the St Vincent Joint Task Force for Diabetes.* Report. London: UK, 1994.

17. Diabetes Control and Complications Trial Research Group. Pregnancy outcomes in the Diabetes Control and Complications Trial. *Am J Obstet Gynaecol* 1996; 174:1343–1353.

18. Kitzmiller JL, Gavin LA, Gin GD *et al*. Preconception care of diabetes. *JAMA* 1991; 265:731–736.

19. Steel JM, Johnstone FD, Hepburn DA *et al*. Can prepregnancy care of diabetic women reduce the risk of abnormal babies? *BMJ* 2000; 321:730–731.

20. Dunne F, Brydon P, Smith T *et al*. Pre-conception care in insulin dependent diabetes mellitus. *QJM* 1999; 92:175–176.

21. Boulot P, Chabbert-Buffet N, d'Ercole C *et al*. French multi-centre survey of outcome of pregnancy in women with pregestational diabetes. *Diabetes Care* 2003; 26:2990–2993.

22. Evers IM, de Valk HW, Visser GH. Risk of complications of pregnancy in women with type 1 diabetes: a nationwide prospective study in the Netherlands. *BMJ* 2004; 328:915.

23. Platt MJ, Stanisstreet M, Casson IF *et al*. St Vincent's Declaration 10 years on: outcomes of diabetic pregnancies. *Diabet Med* 2002; 19:216–220.

24. Ehtisham S, Barrett TG, Shaw NJ. Type 2 diabetes in UK children—an emerging problem. *Diabet Med* 2000; 17:867–871.

25. Ng GYT, Burren CP. Type 2 diabetes in adolescence–unearthed at the time of registration with the general practitioner (GP). *Pract Diabetes Int* 2000; 17:273–274.

26. Rosenbloom AL, Joe JR, Young RS *et al*. Emerging epidemic of type 2 diabetes in youth. *Diabetes Care* 1999; 22:345–354.

27. Pinhas-Hamiel O, Zeitler P. Type 2 diabetes in adolescents, no longer rare. *Paediatr Rev* 1998; 19:434–435.

28. Sherman PM, Buller H. Obesity recommendations. *J Ped Gastro Nutrition* 1999; 29:113–115.

29. Pettitt DJ, Knowler WC, Baird HR, Bennett PH. Gestational diabetes: infant and maternal complications of pregnancy in relation to third-trimester glucose tolerance in the Pima Indians. *Diabetes Care* 1980; 3:458–464.

30. Engelgau MM, Herman WH, Smith P. The epidemiology of diabetes and pregnancy in the US 1988. *Diabetes Care* 1995; 18:1029–1033.

31. Sinha B, Brydon P, Taylor RS *et al*. Maternal ante-natal parameters as predictors of persistent postnatal glucose intolerance: a comparative study between Afro-Caribbeans, Asians and Caucasians. *Diabet Med* 2003; 20:382–386.

32. Towner D, Kjos SL, Leung B *et al*. Congenital malformations in pregnancies complicated by NIDDM. *Diabetes Care* 1995; 18:1446–1451.

33. Sen S, Nanzoor A, Deviasumathy M *et al*. Maternal knowledge, aritude and practice regarding folic acid intake in the preconceptual period. *Public Health Nutr* 2001; 4:909–912.

34. Sacks DA, Chen W, Greenspoon JS *et al*. Should the same glucose values be targeted for type 1 as for type 2 diabetics in pregnancy. *Am J Obstet Gynaecol* 1997; 177:1113–1119.

35. Omori Y, Minei S, Testuo T. Current status of pregnancy in diabetic women: a comparison of pregnancy in IDDM and NIDDM mothers. *Diabetes Res Clin Pract* 1994; 24:S273–S278.

36. Nielsen GL, Moller M, Sorensen HT. HbA1C in early pregnancy and pregnancy outcomes: a Danish population-based cohort study of 573 pregnancies in women with type 1 diabetes. *Diabetes Care* 2006; 29:2612–2616.

37. Temple RC *et al*. Prepregnancy care and pregnancy outcomes in women with type 1 diabetes. *Diabetes Care* 2006; 29:1744–1749.

38. Inkster ME *et al*. Poor glycated haemoglobin control and adverse pregnancy outcomes in type 1 and type 2 diabetes mellitus: systematic review of observational studies. *BMC Pregnancy Childbirth*. 2006; 6:30.

39. Cooper WO, Hernandez-Diaz S, Arbogast PG *et al*. Major congenital malformations after first-trimester exposure to ACE inhibitors. *N Engl J Med* 2006; 354:2443–2451.

40. Alwan S, Polifka JE, Friedman JM. Angiotensin 11 receptor antagonist treatment during pregnancy. *Birth Defects Res A Clin Mol Teratol* 2005; 73:123–130.

41. *Physicians Desk Reference*, 55th edition. Medical Economics, Montvale, NJ, 2001.

42. Bellosta S, Ferri N, Bernini F *et al*. Non-lipid related effects of statins. *Ann Med* 2000; 32:164–176.

43. National Institute for Health and Clinical Excellence. Guideline 63. *Diabetes in Pregnancy. Management of diabetes and its complications from pre-conception to the postnatal period*. March 2008.

44. Joint Formulary Committee. *British National Formulary*, 55th edition. London: British Medical Association and Royal Pharmaceutical Society of Great Britain, London, 2008.

45. Ekpebegh CO, Coetzee EJ, van der Merwe L *et al*. A 10-year retrospective analysis of pregnancy outcome in pregestational type 2 diabetes: comparison of insulin and oral glucose-lowering agents. *Diabet Med* 2007; 24:253–258.

46. Nanovskaya T *et al*. Transfer of metformin across the dually perfused human placental lobule. *Am J Obstet Gynaecol* 2006; 195:1081–1085.

47. Hellmuth E, Damm P, Molsted-Pedersen L. Oral hypoglycaemic agents in 118 diabetic pregnancies. *Diabet Med* 2000; 17:507–511.

48. Rowan JA, Hague WM, Gao W *et al*. Metformin versus insulin for the treatment of gestational diabetes. *N Engl J Med* 2008; 358:2003–2015.

49. Pasquali R, Gambineri A. Insulin-sensitizing agents in polycystic ovary syndrome. *Eur J Endocrinol* 2006; 154:763–775.

50. Froment P, Gizard F, Staels B *et al*. A role of PPARgamma in reproduction? *Med Sci (Paris)* 2005; 21:507–511.

51. Briggs CG, Freeman RK, Yaffe SJ. *Drugs in Pregnancy and Lactation*, 6th edition. Williams & Wilkins Co, Baltimore, MD, 2002.

52. Evers IM, ter Braak EWMT, de Valk HW *et al*. Risk indicators predictive for severe hypoglycaemia during the first trimester of type 1 diabetic pregnancy. *Diabetes Care* 2002; 25:554–559.

53. Rosenn BM, Miodovnik M, Holcberg G *et al*. Hypoglycaemia: the price of intensive insulin therapy for pregnant women with insulin dependent diabetes mellitus. *Obstet Gynaecol* 1995; 85:417–422.

54. Murphy HR, Rayman G, Lewis K *et al*. Effectiveness of continuous glucose monitoring during pregnancy: results of a randomized clinical trial. *Diabetologia* 2008; 51:S12.

55. Harris GD, White RD. Diabetes management and exercise in pregnant patients with diabetes. *Clin Diab* 2005; 23:165–168.

56. Chertow BS, Baranetsky NG, Sivitz WI *et al*. The effects of human insulin on antibody formation in pregnant diabetics and their newborns. *Obstet Gynaecol* 1988; 72:724–728.

57. Nachum Z, Ben-Shlomo I, Weiner E, Shalev E. Twice daily versus four times daily insulin dose regimens for diabetes in pregnancy: randomized controlled trial. *BMJ* 1999; 319:1223–1227.

58. Lapolla A, Dalfra MG, Fedele D. Insulin therapy in pregnancy complicated by diabetes: are insulin analogs a new tool? *Diabetes Metab Res Rev* 2005; 21:241–252.

59. Mathiesen ER, Kinsley B, Amiel SA *et al*. Maternal glycaemic control and hypoglycaemia in type 1 diabetic pregnancy: a randomised trial of insulin aspart versus human insulin in 322 pregnant women. *Diabetes Care* 2007; 30:771–776.

60. Hod M, Damm P, Kaaja R *et al*. Fetal and perinatal outcomes in type 1 diabetes pregnancy: a randomised study comparing insulin aspart with human insulin in 322 subjects. *Am J Obstet Gynaecol* 2008; 198:1–7.

61. Devlin JT, Hothersall L, Wilkis JL. Use of insulin glargine during pregnancy in a type 1 diabetic woman. *Diabetes Care* 2002; 25:1095–1096.

62. Di Cianni G, Volpe L, Lencioni C *et al*. Use of insulin glargine during the first weeks of pregnancy in five type 1 diabetic women. *Diabetes Care* 2005; 28:982–983.

63. Price N, Bartlett C, Gillmer MD. Use of insulin glargine during pregnancy: a case-control study. *BJOG* 2007; 114:453–457.

64. Jovanovic L, Knopp RH, Brown Z *et al*. Declining insulin requirement in the late first trimester of diabetic pregnancy. *Diabetes Care* 2001; 24:1130–1136.

65. Langer O, Anyaegbunam A, Brustman L *et al*. Pregestational diabetes: insulin requirements throughout pregnancy. *Am J Obstet Gynecol* 1988; 159:616–621.

66. Johnstone FD, Prescott RJ, Steel JM *et al*. Clinical and ultrasonic prediction of macrosomia in diabetic pregnancy. *Br J Obstet Gynaecol* 1996; 103:747–754.

67. Kaushal K, Gibson JM, Railton A *et al*. A protocol for improved glycaemic control following corticosteroid therapy in diabetic pregnancies. *Diabet Med* 2003; 20:73–75.

68. Lean MEJ, Pearson DWM, Sutherland HW. Insulin management during labour and delivery in mothers with diabetes. *Diabet Med* 1990; 7:162–164.

69. Caplan RH, Pagliara AS, Beguin EA *et al*. Constant intravenous insulin infusion during labor and delivery in diabetes mellitus. *Diabetes Care* 1982; 5:6–10.

70. Gunderson EP. Breastfeeding after gestational diabetes pregnancy: subsequent obesity and type 2 diabetes mellitus in women and their offspring. *Diabetes Care* 2007; 30:S161–S168.

71. Gunderson EP, Lewis CE, Wei GS *et al*. Lactation and changes in maternal metabolic risk factors. *Obstet Gynaecol* 2007; 109:729–738.

72. Stage E, Norgard H, Damm P *et al*. Long term breast feeding in women with type 1 diabetes. *Diabetes Care* 2006; 29:771–774.

73. Bradley C. Managing diabetes while breast feeding. *Diabetes Self Manag* 2007; 24:87–89.

74. Pettitt DJ, Forman MR, Hanson RL *et al*. Breastfeeding and incidence of non insulin dependent diabetes mellitus in Pima Indians. *Lancet* 1997; 350:166–168.

75. Linné Y, Dye L, Barkeling B *et al*. Weight development over time in parous women— the SPAWN study— 15 years follow-up. *Int J Obes Relat Metab Disord* 2003; 27:1516–1522.

76. Ursin G, Bernstein L, Lord SJ *et al*. Reproductive factors and subtypes of breast cancer defined by hormone receptor and histology. *Br J Cancer* 2005; 93:364–371.

77. Rosenblatt KA, Thomas DB. WHO Collaborative Study of Neoplasia and Steroid Contraceptives: Lactation and the risk of epithelial ovarian cancer. *Int J Epidemiol* 1993; 22:192–197.

78. Karlson EW, Mandl LA, Hankinson SE, Grodstein F. Do breast-feeding and other reproductive factors influence future risk of rheumatoid arthritis? Results from the Nurses Health Study. *Arthritis Rheum* 2004; 50:3458–3467.

79. Chantry CJ, Howard CR, Auinger P. Full breastfeeding duration and associated decrease in respiratory tract infection in US children. *Paediatrics* 2006; 117:425–432.

80. Greer FR, Sicherer SH, Burks AW. The Committee on Nutrition and Secretion on Allergy and Immunology, American Academy of Paediatrics. Effects of early nutritional interventions on the development of atopic disease in infants and children: the role of maternal dietary restriction, breastfeeding, timing of introduction of complementary foods, and hydrolyzed formulas. *Paediatrics* 2008; 121:183–191.

81. Hummel S, Hummel M, Banholzer J *et al*. Development of autoimmunity to transglutaminase C in children of patients with type 1 diabetes: relationship to islet autoantibodies and infant feeding. *Diabetologia* 2007; 50:390–394.

82. Alm B, Wennergren G, Norvenius SG *et al*. Breast-feeding and the sudden infant death syndrome in Scandinavia, 1992–1995. *Arch Dis Child* 2002; 86:400–402.

83. Schack-Nielsen L, Michaelsen KF. Advances in our understanding of the biology of human milk and its effect on the offspring. *J Nutr* 2007; 137:503S–510S.

84. Schafer-Graf UM, Hartmann R, Pawliczak J. Association of breast feeding and early childhood overweight in children from mothers with gestational diabetes mellitus. *Diabetes Care* 2006; 29:1105–1107.

85. Arenz S, von Kries R. Protective effect of breast feeding against obesity in childhood. Can a meta-analysis of observational studies help to validate the hypothesis? *Adv Exp Biol Med* 2005; 569:40–48.

86. Pettitt DJ, Knowler WC. Long term effects of the intrauterine environment, birth weight and breast-feeding in Pima Indians. *Diabetes Care* 1998; 21:B138–B141.

87. Owen CG, Martin RM, Whincup PH *et al*. Does breast feeding influence risk of type 2 diabetes in later life? A quantitative analysis of published evidence. *Am J Clin Nutr* 2006; 84:1043–1054.

88. Rosenbauer J, Herzig P, Kaiser P. Early nutrition and risk of type 1 diabetes mellitus – a nationwide case-control study in preschool children. *Exp Clin Endocrinol Diabetes* 2007; 115:502–508.

89. Dabelea D, D'Agostino RB, Mayer-Davis EJ *et al*; SEARCH for diabetes in youth study group. Testing the accelerator hypothesis. Body size, B-cell function, and age at onset of type 1 (autoimmune) diabetes. *Diabetes Care* 2006; 29:290–294.

90. Wahlberg J, Vaarala O, Ludvigsson J; ABIS study group. Dietary risk factors for the emergence of type 1 diabetes-related autoantibodies in 2½ year old Swedish children. *Br J Nutr* 2006; 95:603–608.

91. Labbok M, Perez A, Valdes V *et al*. The lactational amenorrhea method (LAM): a postpartum introductory family planning method with policy and programme implications. *Adv Contracept* 1994; 10:93–109.

92. World Health Organization. Quality care in family planning. In: *Medical Eligibility Criteria for Contraceptive Use*. Geneva, Switzerland, World Health Organization Reproductive Health and Research, 2000.

93. Truit ST, Fraser AB, Grimes DA *et al*. Combined hormonal versus nonhormonal versus progestin-only contraception in lactation. *Cochrane Database Syst Rev* 2003; 2:CDC003988.

94. Inturrisi M, Kitzmiller JL. Postpartum management of women with preexisting Diabetes Mellitus. In: Kitzmiller JL, Jovanovic L, Brown F, Coustan D, Reader DM. *Managing Preexisting Diabetes and Pregnancy*. Alexandria, VA: American Diabetes Association, 2008, pp 687–752.

95. Alberti G, Zimmet P, Shaw J *et al*. Type 2 diabetes in the young: the evolving epidemic; the international diabetes federation consensus workshop. *Diabetes Care* 2004; 27:1798–1811.
96. Permutt MA, Wasson J, Cox N. Genetic epidemiology of diabetes. *J Clin Inv* 2005; 115:1431–1439.
97. Dabelea D, Hanson RL, Bennett PH *et al*. Increasing prevalence of type 2 diabetes in American Indian children. *Diabetologia* 1998; 41:904–910.
98. Silverman BL, Metzger BI, Cho NH *et al*. Fetal hyperinsulinism and impaired glucose tolerance in asolescent offspring of diabetic mothers. *Diabetes Care* 1995; 18:611–617.
99. Dabelea D, Hanson RL, Lindsay RS *et al*. Intrauterine exposure to diabetes conveys risks for type 2 diabetes and obesity: a study of discordant sibships. *Diabetes* 2000; 49:2208–2211.
100. Tuomilheto J, Lindstrom J, Eriksson JG *et al*. Prevention of type 2 diabetes by changes in lifestyle among subjects with impaired glucose tolerance. *N Engl J Med* 2001; 344:1343–1350.
101. Knowler WC, Barrett-Connor E, Fowle SE *et al*. Reduction in the incidence of type 2 diabetes with lifestyle intervention or metformin. *N Engl J Med* 2002; 346:393–403.

11

What can we do to improve adherence in patients with diabetes?

J. Rungby, B. Brock

BACKGROUND

In order to minimize the risk of long-term macro- and microvascular complications, treatment regimens for patients with type 1 or 2 diabetes must be tailored individually. The goals of any treatment cannot be achieved without the acceptance of the patient. Thus, patient involvement in strategies for treatment has become an important part of the treatment of all chronic diseases, including diabetes. Emphasis must be put on the fact that what is considered the ideal treatment by the care provider is not necessarily considered optimal treatment by patients, who may have to comply with treatments on a permanent basis. The challenge is thus to merge the patient's perspective with current guidelines to achieve concordance whenever treating diabetes. Here, we describe some of the obstacles as well as the possibilities for improved concordance.

DEFINITION OF TERMS

Compliance is a term used to describe the degree to which a patient is following the directions given by the health professional, both regarding dosing intervals and the doses themselves. Thus, 80% compliance to a given prescribed medication indicates that the patient takes their medication 8 times out of 10.

Persistence describes the accumulated time from the initiation of a treatment to the – unintentional – discontinuation of this therapy. Thus, persistence describes the time span in which the patient is compliant (or non-compliant).

Adherence encompasses both of the above, including compliance and persistence. Adherence both focuses on the behaviour associated with taking medication and addresses the relevance of factors that improve the patient's chance of adhering to a certain medication regime.

Concordance relates not to the patient or to the care provider but rather to the communicative process between the two of them when prescribing medication or other kinds of medical care. Concordance is thus based on partnership between the patient and the care provider.

Jørgen Rungby, MD, DMSc, Head of Department, Department of Endocrinology, Aarhus University Hospital, Aarhus, Denmark.

Birgitte Brock, MD, PhD, Head of Department, Department of Clinical Pharmacology, Aarhus University Hospital, Aarhus, Denmark.

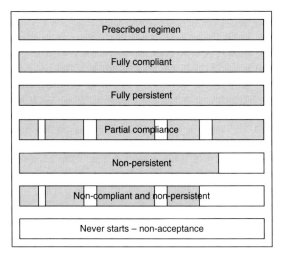

Figure 11.1 Patterns of adherence.

Due to this definition, concordance does not relate to the patient but instead relates solely to the consultation, which can be described as concordant when it involves two-way communication and informed, shared decision-making.

Medication possession ratio describes the number of filled prescriptions and is usually calculated as the number of days of medication dispensed as a percentage of 365 days.

Non-compliance, non-adherence and *non-concordance* can be divided into different categories. Thus, primary non-compliance occurs when the patient fails to take the medication prescribed by the health professional, while secondary non-compliance occurs when the patient fails to take the medication as instructed. Different sorts of non-compliance can also be related to the degree of intentionality. Intentional non-compliance may occur when the physician's diagnosis or treatment is rejected by the patient and, as a result, the patient decides not to follow the recommendations. On the other hand, unintentional non-compliance may be due to many different factors, including social, physiological and clinical variables, resulting in the patient not being *able* to follow recommendations. In order to provide the optimal care for the patient, it is essential to detect non-compliance. Adding a new drug to the treatment of hyperglycaemia, for example, has little, if any, effect with a non-compliant patient. Furthermore, adding new drugs to the non-compliant patient's list of prescribed medication increases the risk of serious adverse events due to overdosing, particularly when the patient is admitted from the primary healthcare system to an inpatient hospital setting.

ADHERENCE IN DIABETES

Most studies report adherence rates to oral antihyperglycaemic agents of 65–85% [1–14], with lower rates in complex regimens [11, 15, 16] and certain populations (34–54% reported in US Medicaid recipients) [17]. In a study comparing persistence with sulphonylurea monotherapy, metformin monotherapy or a combination of both, persistence with either monotherapy was 50% after 1 year, decreasing to 40% after 2 years. With the combination treatment, 30% were persistent after 1 year and just 16% after 2 years [18]. The pattern resembles that of other chronic diseases. Muszbek and colleagues reported a 12-month persistence varying

Table 11.1 Overall adherence in type 2 diabetes

Medication	Adherence rate (%)
Oral glucose-lowering agents	65–85 (average of 25 studies)
Insulin	60–80 (average of 2 studies)

Table 11.2 Barriers to adherence in diabetes

- Non-comprehension of the nature of the disease
- Non-comprehension of the treatment regimen
- Non-comprehension of positive drug effects as well as side-effects
- Regimen complexity, need to mix or split pharmaceuticals
- Dosing frequency
- Concomitant disease, particularly depression
- Economic factors

from 62–66% in dyslipidaemia, hypertension and diabetes with values for compliance being 67–76% after 12 months [19]. There appears to be room for improvement, bearing in mind that adherence in major clinical trials, which form the scientific background for treatment recommendations, is generally well above 80% (Table 11.1).

Factors affecting adherence

The factors identified as barriers to good adherence in diabetes differ little from those reported in other conditions. Two recent systematic reviews [1, 20] identify very similar patterns in the literature, with a number of potentially adjustable factors setting up barriers to adherence (Table 11.2). Often not recognized by care providers is the importance of communicating the 'whys and hows' of a treatment to the patient. In a study in type 2 diabetes, Schillinger and colleagues [21] found that patient comprehension was assessed during the consultation in just 12% of cases. Not assessing patient recall and comprehension was associated with a higher HbA1c. Understanding information given during a consultation may also be limited (in more than 50% of patients) both regarding the language used (e.g. understanding the meaning of 'stable blood glucose') and the instructions for dosing [22].

Since overt symptoms are often sparse with the three most vital components of the dysmetabolic syndrome (glucose, blood pressure and lipids), and since adherence is higher when treatment is perceived as alleviating symptoms or improving health [23], information and motivation become essential. The case in type 1 diabetes is of course very different, but adherence problems are also clinically relevant in this condition, particularly in paediatric or adolescent patients where concordance must be achieved not only between care providers and the patient but also between family members, the education system and the patient [24].

This is obvious for the care provider-to-patient interaction, but care provider-to-care provider communication and education appear to be equally important since there is a high degree of reluctance in physicians' attitudes to treatment, as documented by Peyrot and co-workers [25]. Thus, no patient should leave the consultation without an understanding of the disease component they are about to address with a new treatment plus information on, and comprehension of, the likely benefits of that treatment. Adherence problems are usually caused by under-use of medications. However, non-comprehension may also account for overdosing [13]. The continued education of diabetes care providers should be kept in mind.

Tolerability is rarely addressed during consultations in spite of the fact that adverse effects account for a substantial reduction in adherence [23].

The complexity and dosing frequency remain major determinants of adherence [5, 11, 16, 17]. As described by Paes and colleagues [5], adherence drops from 79% to 66% when dosing frequencies are increased from once- to twice-daily. Further increasing the frequency to three times daily reduced adherence to 38%.

The emotional well-being of type 2 diabetes patients is another important determinant of adherence [8, 26]. Thus, depression, often unrecognized in type 2 diabetes [27], must be addressed in order to ensure adherence.

The cost of treatment is also rarely discussed during consultations. There is, however, a significant impact of out-of-pocket costs on adherence. Patient reasons for not discussing costs with their clinicians were assessed by Piette and colleagues [28]. Common reasons for not bringing up this issue were:

- A lack of belief that the clinician was able to change matters.
- Embarrassment.
- Feeling that the subject was of minor importance.
- A lack of time during consultations.

Effects of adherence on outcome

Studies in hypertension [29, 30] and diabetes [31] demonstrate that poor adherence is associated with poorer outcome (blood pressure, hospitalization frequency and HbA1c). In a recent study aimed at patients with very poorly controlled type 2 diabetes (HbA1c higher than 9%), Odegaard and Gray [32] found specific adherence barriers associated with poor control, and the following were all reported as problems:

- Cost.
- Dosing regimens.
- Reading prescription labels.
- Obtaining refills.

Taking more than two daily doses and reading the prescriptions significantly affected HbA1c in a multivariate analysis in this particularly high-risk population.

Ways to improve adherence

Few trials have documented interventional effects on adherence. During adolescence, often a particularly difficult period for patients with type 1 diabetes and clinicians, intensive home-based psychological intervention may improve outcome [33]. Less intensive interventions have failed to do so [34, 35].

Unit dose packaging and refill reminders can improve adherence with sulphonylurea or metformin therapy [36, 37] and may improve outcomes (as measured by decreased use of healthcare services).

The use of fixed combination therapy (FCT) has been more extensively examined as FCT is becoming increasingly available in diabetes. Long-term use of insulins combining fast- and intermediate-acting agents has proven safe and efficacious, but little is known about the effects of these compounds on adherence when compared to standard injection regimens [38]. For insulin, the use of modern devices such as insulin pens most likely improves adherence [39].

With oral combinations becoming increasingly available, care providers need to evaluate their use. A number of considerations apply. Since the majority of the ever-increasing number of diabetic patients need treatment for both glycaemic control and a number of comorbidities, administration of multiple drugs will eventually become necessary. Often,

Table 11.3 Five ways to achieve concordance and improve adherence

■ Educate care providers and patient: information to the patient should comprise information about indication and expected outcome, as well as duration of treatment, discussion of ways to reduce fear of social stigmatization, information about tolerability, ideas for simplifying dosing regimens and ways to remember them, as well as information on how to renew prescriptions. ■ Consider adverse effects carefully ■ Reduce regimen complexity ■ Diagnose comorbidities affecting adherence, in particular depression ■ Reduce costs

there is a need for multi-step treatments with disease progression. Non-adherence increases with the number of drugs prescribed to the individual [19]. From a pharmacological viewpoint the compatibility of drugs in FCTs needs to be evaluated. The FCTs now commercially available have revealed no inter-drug problems concerning efficacy or safety.

The benefits that may be gained from FCTs include improvement in adherence, which in turn is likely to improve clinical outcomes [40]. Non-adherence rates are 15–35% for oral blood glucose-lowering agents, 20–40% for insulin and 10–25% for blood pressure- and cholesterol-lowering agents in type 2 diabetes. For some agents, this is even higher, depending on the measures available [1]. In a recent meta-analysis, Bangalore and co-workers found an overall improved adherence with FCT of 26% when studies in diabetes, hypertension and infectious diseases were compiled [41]. In diabetes, the combination of glibenclamide and metformin as an alternative to dual-tablet treatment increased the medication possession rate significantly (17–22%) [11].

SUMMARY

Even with clear evidence of poor adherence with diabetes therapies and some evidence for a negative outcome caused by this poor adherence, there is a paucity of clinical evidence guiding care providers towards better results when prescribing. Achieving concordance (i.e. a mutual agreement and understanding of the therapy) seems essential. There is, however, some evidence that addressing the factors listed in Table 11.3 will help to achieve concordance and improve adherence.

REFERENCES

1. Rubin RR. Adherence to pharmacologic therapy in patients with type 2 diabetes mellitus. *Am J Med* 2005; 118:27S–34S.
2. Schectman JM, Nadkarni MM, Voss JD. The association between diabetes metabolic control and drug adherence in an indigent population. *Diabetes Care* 2002; 25:1015–1021.
3. Mason BJ, Matsuyama JR, Jue SG. Assessment of sulfonylurea adherence and metabolic control. *Diabetes Educ* 1995; 21:52–57.
4. Matsuyama JR, Mason BJ, Jue SG. Pharmacists' interventions using an electronic medication-event monitoring device's adherence data versus pill counts. *Ann Pharmacother* 1993; 27:851–855.
5. Paes AH, Bakker A, Soe-Agnie CJ. Impact of dosage frequency on patient compliance. *Diabetes Care* 1997; 20:1512–1517.
6. Rosen MI, Beauvais JE, Rigsby MO, Salahi JT, Ryan CE, Cramer JA. Neuropsychological correlates of suboptimal adherence to metformin. *J Behav Med* 2003; 26:349–360.
7. Boccuzzi SJ, Wogen J, Fox J, Sung JC, Shah AB, Kim J. Utilization of oral hypoglycemic agents in a drug-insured U.S. population. *Diabetes Care* 2001; 24:1411–1415.
8. Ciechanowski PS, Katon WJ, Russo JE. Depression and diabetes: impact of depressive symptoms on adherence, function, and costs. *Arch Intern Med* 2000; 160:3278–3285.

9. Morningstar BA, Sketris IS, Kephart GC, Sclar DA. Variation in pharmacy prescription refill adherence measures by type of oral antihyperglycaemic drug therapy in seniors in Nova Scotia, Canada. *J Clin Pharm Ther* 2002; 27:213–220.

10. Evans JM, Donnan PT, Morris AD. Adherence to oral hypoglycaemic agents prior to insulin therapy in Type 2 diabetes. *Diabet Med* 2002; 19:685–688.

11. Melikian C, White TJ, Vanderplas A, Dezii CM, Chang E. Adherence to oral antidiabetic therapy in a managed care organization: a comparison of monotherapy, combination therapy, and fixed-dose combination therapy. *Clin Ther* 2002; 24:460–467.

12. Rajagopalan R, Joyce A, Smith D, Ollendorf D, Murray FT. Medication compliance in type 2 diabetes patients: retrospective data analysis. *Value Health* 2003; 6:328.

13. Spoelstra JA, Stolk RP, Heerdink ER *et al*. Refill compliance in type 2 diabetes mellitus: a predictor of switching to insulin therapy? *Pharmacoepidemiol Drug Saf* 2003; 12:121–127.

14. Venturini F, Nichol MB, Sung JC, Bailey KL, Cody M, McCombs JS. Compliance with sulfonylureas in a health maintenance organization: a pharmacy record-based study. *Ann Pharmacother* 1999; 33: 281–288.

15. Dezii CM, Kawabata H, Tran M. Effects of once-daily and twice-daily dosing on adherence with prescribed glipizide oral therapy for type 2 diabetes. *South Med J* 2002; 95:68–71.

16. Donnan PT, MacDonald TM, Morris AD. Adherence to prescribed oral hypoglycaemic medication in a population of patients with Type 2 diabetes: a retrospective cohort study. *Diabet Med* 2002; 19:279–284.

17. Dailey G, Kim MS, Lian JF. Patient compliance and persistence with antihyperglycemic drug regimens: evaluation of a medicaid patient population with type 2 diabetes mellitus. *Clin Ther* 2001; 23: 1311–1320.

18. Dailey G, Kim MS, Lian JF. Patient compliance and persistence with anti-hyperglycemic therapy: evaluation of a population of type 2 diabetic patients. *J Int Med Res* 2002; 30:71–79.

19. Muszbek N, Benedict A, Keskinaslan A, Khan Z. Economic consequences of non-compliance in the treatment of diabetes, hypertension and dyslipidemia – A systematic review. *J Hypertens* 2006; 24:S140.

20. Odegard PS, Capoccia K. Medication taking and diabetes: a systematic review of the literature. *Diabetes Educ* 2007; 33:1014–1029.

21. Schillinger D, Piette J, Grumbach K *et al*. Closing the loop: physician communication with diabetic patients who have low health literacy. *Arch Intern Med* 2003; 163:83–90.

22. Schillinger D, Grumbach K, Piette J *et al*. Association of health literacy with diabetes outcomes. *JAMA* 2002; 288:475–482.

23. Grant RW, Devita NG, Singer DE, Meigs JB. Polypharmacy and medication adherence in patients with type 2 diabetes. *Diabetes Care* 2003; 26:1408–1412.

24. Cameron FJ, Skinner TC, de Beaufort CE *et al*. Are family factors universally related to metabolic outcomes in adolescents with Type 1 diabetes? *Diabet Med* 2008; 25:463–468.

25. Peyrot M, Mathews DR, Snoek FJ. An international study of physiological resistance to insulin use among persons with diabetes. *Diabetologia* 2003; 46:A89.

26. Peyrot M, Rubin RR, Siminerio L. Physician and nurse use of psychosocial strategies and referrals in diabetes. *Diabetes* 2002; 51:A446.

27. Rubin RR, Ciechanowski P, Egede LE, Lin EH, Lustman PJ. Recognizing and treating depression in patients with diabetes. *Curr Diab Rep* 2004; 4:119–125.

28. Piette JD, Heisler M, Wagner TH. Problems paying out-of-pocket medication costs among older adults with diabetes. *Diabetes Care* 2004; 27:384–391.

29. Bramley TJ, Gerbino PP, Nightengale BS, Frech-Tamas F. Relationship of blood pressure control to adherence with antihypertensive monotherapy in 13 managed care organizations. *J Manag Care Pharm* 2006; 12:239–245.

30. Sokol MC, McGuigan KA, Verbrugge RR, Epstein RS. Impact of medication adherence on hospitalization risk and healthcare cost. *Med Care* 2005; 43:521–530.

31. Lawrence DB, Ragucci KR, Long LB, Parris BS, Helfer LA. Relationship of oral antihyperglycemic (sulfonylurea or metformin) medication adherence and hemoglobin A1c goal attainment for HMO patients enrolled in a diabetes disease management program. *J Manag Care Pharm* 2006; 12:466–471.

32. Odegard PS, Gray SL. Barriers to medication adherence in poorly controlled diabetes mellitus. *Diabetes Educ* 2008; 34:692–697.

33. Ellis DA, Frey MA, Naar-King S, Templin T, Cunningham P, Cakan N. Use of multisystemic therapy to improve regimen adherence among adolescents with type 1 diabetes in chronic poor metabolic control: a randomized controlled trial. *Diabetes Care* 2005; 28:1604–1610.

34. Lawson ML, Cohen N, Richardson C, Orrbine E, Pham B. A randomized trial of regular standardized telephone contact by a diabetes nurse educator in adolescents with poor diabetes control. *Pediatr Diabetes* 2005; 6:32–40.
35. Mendez FJ, Belendez M. Effects of a behavioral intervention on treatment adherence and stress management in adolescents with IDDM. *Diabetes Care* 1997; 20:1370–1375.
36. Skaer TL, Sclar DA, Markowski DJ, Won JK. Effect of value-added utilities on prescription refill compliance and Medicaid health care expenditures—a study of patients with non-insulin-dependent diabetes mellitus. *J Clin Pharm Ther* 1993; 18:295–299.
37. Rosen MI, Rigsby MO, Salahi JT, Ryan CE, Cramer JA. Electronic monitoring and counseling to improve medication adherence. *Behav Res Ther* 2004; 42:409–422.
38. Siminerio L. Challenges and strategies for moving patients to injectable medications. *Diabetes Educ* 2006; 32:82S-90S.
39. Valentine WJ, Palmer AJ, Nicklasson L, Cobden D, Roze S. Improving life expectancy and decreasing the incidence of complications associated with type 2 diabetes: a modelling study of HbA1c targets. *Int J Clin Pract* 2006; 60:1138–1145.
40. Simpson SH, Eurich DT, Majumdar SR *et al.* A meta-analysis of the association between adherence to drug therapy and mortality. *BMJ* 2006; 333:15.
41. Bangalore S, Kamalakkannan G, Parkar S, Messerli FH. Fixed-dose combinations improve medication compliance: a meta-analysis. *Am J Med* 2007; 120:713–719.

12

Organization of diabetes care and the multiprofessional team

J. Hill, R. Gadsby

BACKGROUND

Good diabetes management involves a co-ordinated team of different healthcare professionals (HCPs) with a variety of skills and competencies, working with the person with diabetes to support them in controlling the condition. Who makes up an individual's team varies, depending on where their diabetes care is located (primary or secondary care) and over time (as their condition progresses). With the challenge of managing the huge numbers of people with diabetes, limited traditional resources, and the recognition of skills of other HCPs, there has been a significant increase in the number of different disciplines involved in diabetes care. An example of this is the initiation of insulin therapy. In the past, insulin was initiated only by doctors in hospital clinics [1]. The development of the diabetes specialist nurse's role in the 1970s took on many of the practical aspects of insulin therapy [2], but this was still done in secondary care. Now, in response to the large numbers of people requiring insulin, more disciplines are involved in insulin initiation and titration. Most diabetes care in the UK and in a number of other countries, at least for type 2 diabetes, has moved out to primary care to practice nurses, primary care physicians, district nurses, pharmacists, dietitians and community diabetes teams.

For the person with diabetes, who they see will vary over time, as the condition progresses and through life events. The relatively well person with newly diagnosed type 2 diabetes may immediately meet a number of different people: a diabetes educator, dietitian, general physician/practitioner and practice nurse. This team aims to promote understanding and self-management skills, and to identify, treat and review risk factors for complications. The patient will also be seen for an annual retinal screening. They will see the pharmacist on a monthly visit to collect medication/education, and the podiatrist for foot care if required. As the condition progresses, many patients find their diabetes management becomes more complex, especially if they develop diabetes complications. They may be referred to secondary care specialists for more intensive treatments such as insulin therapy. Access will be needed to renal physicians and the dialysis team if they develop diabetic nephropathy; ophthalmologists and perhaps the low vision clinic team for laser treatment for diabetic retinopathy; and the vascular surgeon, orthotist and specialist podiatry services for diabetic foot problems.

Jill Hill, BSc(Hons), RGN, Diabetes Nurse Consultant, Community Diabetes Team, NHS Birmingham East and North, Birmingham, UK.

Roger Gadsby, MBE, BSc, MB ChB, DCH, DRCOG, FRCGP, General Practitioner and Associate Clinical Professor, Institute of Clinical Education, Warwick Medical School, University of Warwick, Coventry, UK.

It is not just the development of diabetic complications that leads to the patient's diabetes team becoming more specialized and complex. Life events, such as pregnancy, often need additional skills that the routine diabetes team are unable to manage. Women with diabetes who are pregnant, or planning a pregnancy, should have access to the specialist diabetes obstetric team, as recommended in the UK by standard 9 of the National Service Framework for Diabetes [3]. Children will be managed by a paediatric diabetes specialist team and then ideally progress through the young people's clinic to the adult service. As patients age and develop other comorbidities, other skills are required, and the HCPs managing their diabetes care may include district nurses, case managers, nursing and residential care staff.

The challenge for the team organizing diabetes management (usually the general practitioner and their nurse) is to ensure that the person with diabetes meets the appropriate healthcare professional at the relevant time, in the language required, and in an easily accessible location. That healthcare professional needs to be competent and adequately trained in diabetes management skills. There needs to be good communication between all the HCPs involved in the patient's diabetes care to prevent omissions and duplication of care. With the expansion of the diabetes team potentially involving so many healthcare professionals, this can be a considerable challenge.

The link between all these professionals, of course, is the patient at the centre of their diabetes care. One of the key features of a high quality diabetes service is that it delivers a patient-focused service in which people are empowered to manage their own care [4]. In the UK, the National Service Framework for Diabetes: Standards [3] emphasizes the importance of empowering people with diabetes. Standard 3 states:

'All children, young people and adults with diabetes will receive a service which encourages partnership in decision making, supports them in managing their diabetes, and helps them to adopt and maintain a healthy lifestyle. This will be reflected in an agreed and shared care plan in an appropriate format and language. Where appropriate, parents and carers should be fully engaged in this process.'

Providing equitable access to the healthcare professionals involved in diabetes care necessitates team working, and an integrated approach to service delivery. In the UK, the National Service Framework for Diabetes: Delivery Strategy recommends the development of diabetes networks covering a natural population served by a specialist diabetes service based within a NHS trust, to enable such an integrated service of diabetes care to be delivered to a population [5].

CONFUSING TITLES OF HCPs?

The increasing dissemination and delegation of the various components of diabetes care has contributed to the profusion of diabetes roles and titles now existing, which can be confusing for the patient and also to generalists wanting to refer patients for specialist help.

The doctor that most patients went to for diabetes management advice in the past was the diabetes specialist or diabetologist who was usually hospital based, and the patient was typically seen in a busy, crowded outpatient clinic. Nowadays, the doctor most likely to be managing the patient's diabetes care will be their primary care physician. Most primary care physician practices in the UK now run dedicated diabetes clinics which are staffed by practice nurses, usually with special training and experience in diabetes, and supervised by one partner who has special interest and experience in diabetes care. In a national questionnaire survey published in 2001, 71% of general practitioners surveyed held diabetes clinics [6]. In the UK, the contract for General Medical Services (or GP contract), introduced in 2004, had a 'pay for performance' element called the quality and outcomes framework. This initiative gives an incentive for the general practice to ensure that good quality care is delivered to its patients for a number of chronic conditions including diabetes. The diabetes clinical indicators include various measures of process and outcomes of diabetes care, for example, the number of people who have had an HbA1c measurement (process) and how many have a level at or below 7.5% (outcome) These form a significant proportion of the points that can be earned, and each point earns a small additional income to the practice. Local enhanced services for diabetes can allow practices to earn more by providing local high quality services that are over and above the routine care expected in the contract. This, for example, may encourage primary care physicians and their nurses to initiate insulin in the practice rather than refer to the hospital.

The UK government is encouraging more care for long-term conditions to be delivered in primary care nearer to the patient's home with their familiar local primary care team, and to reduce the use of expensive hospital-based services. A similar movement of services from secondary to primary care is also happening in a number of other developed countries. In the UK, these health policy changes are outlined in the white paper entitled *Our Health, Our Care, Our Say: A New Direction for Community Services* [7]. In 2006, for example, the aim was for an extra one million outpatient appointments to take place in primary care rather than in hospital. These significant changes in the delivery of care in a relatively short period of time encourage the development of innovative new posts. One idea in the UK is that a full-time GP may take up to 1 day a week to work as a GP with a special interest (GPwSI) in a specific clinical field. The development of the concept of the GPwSI in diabetes has helped to facilitate the move of diabetes hospital outpatient clinic appointments into the community. Framework documents for the work of GPwSIs have been published (www.doh.gov.uk/pricare/gp-specialinterests). GPwSIs in diabetes can fulfil a purely management function (for example, overseeing a diabetes network), or could fulfil a clinical function (for example, running diabetes clinics in the community for people with diabetes whose problems have not been able to be successfully managed in general practice, but who do not meet referral criteria for secondary specialist care).

There are now a number of positions that enable nurses to develop diabetes specialist practice, knowledge and skills. The diabetes specialist nurse (DSN) is probably the most recognized role. However, the title diabetes specialist nurse may include posts such as diabetes educator, diabetes research nurse, diabetes nurse facilitator, diabetes liaison nurse and clinical nurse specialist in diabetes. More recently, advanced nurse practitioners, lecturer practitioners and nurse consultants in diabetes have been appointed. The titles reflect a particular emphasis of their role, such as clinical practice, strategic management, research, case management or education. Although the numerous titles reflect the diversity of diabetes nursing services, there may be confusion about the core functions, level of qualification and area of practice.

The practice nurse is often the central figure in many patients' diabetes management, providing continuity and familiarity. Their role will encompass facilitating diagnosis (through identification of symptoms and proactive screening of at-risk people), education (by signposting to appropriate education programmes, giving initial and 'first-aid' information, and revising knowledge during reviews), monitoring (including phlebotomy services) and recording data, maintaining diabetes registers and calling patients for annual diabetes reviews. Some practice nurses are now independent prescribers and can initiate and titrate medication, following agreed guidance with the GP and local diabetes and medicine management teams, releasing GP time to focus on agreeing management plans with individual patients and to deal with any complex matters related to health.

NEW ROLES AND SERVICES IN DIABETES: INVOLVING PHARMACISTS

The role of the pharmacist in diabetes care has until recently been hardly recognized. In the UK, most patients would see their local pharmacist as the provider of medication prescribed by their diabetes doctor, a view probably shared by most HCPs. As pharmacists run businesses, they may find it difficult to attend diabetes network meetings or access diabetes training programmes and so their contribution to local diabetes care is not appreciated.

However, the new pharmacy contract which commenced in 2005 in England supported an extended role for community pharmacists, particularly in the support of patients with long-term conditions like diabetes. The pharmacist is well-placed to do this: they see the patient every month (when they collect regular prescriptions) and they are available on Saturdays and evenings when many conventional diabetes services are closed.

The Medicine Use Review (MUR) can be a particularly valuable service in supporting patients in understanding their often extensive list of medications, recognizing side-effects and potential contraindications or interactions, and advising patients on the correct way to take their medication. Patient concordance with taking medication is a recognized concern in diabetes care [8]. MURs are provided in pharmacies that fulfil clinical governance requirements and have a specified private area within their premises. Patients can refer themselves for an individual consultation with the pharmacist which typically will last for about 20 minutes.

Under the contract, community pharmacists can bid to contract with Primary Care Trusts to provide a range of enhanced services, similar to the local enhanced services in the GMS contract, where they are paid for high quality services that are over and above the routine services expected from a pharmacist. These can include diabetes screening, smoking cessation and weight management clinics.

Some pharmacists have qualified to be Independent or Supplementary Prescribers. This formalizes a prescribing relationship between the pharmacist and patient, with the agreement of the GP, to initiate and titrate medications for the various aspects of diabetes management. The pharmacist can prescribe, educate, monitor and review in a time and a locality that may be more convenient to the patient, particularly those that work. In some areas, where there is a large ethnic minority population, the pharmacist may even speak the same language as the patient. The potential for the community pharmacist is therefore considerable.

However, if pharmacists are extending their role in diabetes care, they have a responsibility to ensure they are competent to give diabetes advice. In particular, it is important that pharmacists give the same accurate evidence-based information and advice to patients that all health professionals should be giving. A report in *Which?* magazine (*Pharmacies get test of own medicine*) recently made headlines in the UK by suggesting some patients are being given inaccurate information by pharmacy staff [9].

COMMUNICATION BETWEEN HCPs INVOLVED IN DIABETES CARE

With increasing numbers of HCPs involved in delivering diabetes care, good communication between all parties is essential to avoid duplication of effort and to avoid giving mixed or contradictory messages. In many developed countries, medical notes are recorded on a clinical computer system or systems. Good communication is facilitated when these computer systems can talk to each other and where information technology (IT) can link up primary and secondary care records with community and pharmacy records.

In the UK, a huge IT project called *Connecting for Health* is seeking to provide such a 'joined-up' record system. When complete, this should enable all HCPs to link into a core set of clinical records to facilitate communication and to see and update the records in real time.

This system is also designed to handle the referral process from one HCP to another and so facilitate each HCP to see what others have done and what specific aspect of care they are being asked to undertake. As can be imagined, the project is running behind schedule. It remains to be seen whether its grand ambitions will be realized.

At present, the IT system in the NHS has a function called 'choose and book' which handles referrals from GPs to hospital specialists. A referral letter is written from the GP to the hospital specialist and is transferred, along with appropriate patient clinical details, electronically. The system then generates a letter to the patient containing a telephone number and password. The patient can then phone the hospital to make an appointment at a time and date that is convenient to them.

Referrals to other members of the multidisciplinary diabetes team are much less structured and fixed. These can occur through a telephone call or written referral note which is then posted to the relevant team member. In some intermediate clinics, several members of the multidisciplinary team may be consulting at the same time so referral between team members is facilitated and can be achieved by just knocking on a door and asking for an opinion.

Information back to the GP, whose clinical computer system holds the continuing medical record of the person with diabetes, from other members of the multidisciplinary team is usually by letter which is then scanned onto the clinical computer system. Some centres are beginning to pioneer the direct electronic transfer of records from secondary to primary care, which will be a feature of the integrated 'Connecting for Health' system in the UK once it is completely installed.

HEALTHCARE PROFESSIONAL EDUCATION

Adequate training in diabetes management is essential if healthcare professionals are to deliver a high quality diabetes service. In the UK, the Department of Health has recognized this and there has been an increasing emphasis on ensuring that HCPs are competent to work at the appropriate level in whatever their speciality is. In diabetes, this has led to the adoption of a competency-based framework for healthcare professionals which outlines the skills and competencies required to deliver various aspects of diabetes care [10]. The competencies are generic and not profession-specific. This may facilitate the future development of the role a more generic diabetes healthcare worker who can deliver much of the routine review care needed by people with diabetes. This 'blurring of the edges' between traditional roles can provide more flexibility in the diabetes team (e.g. to cover sickness and annual leave) and reduce the number of different people involved in the care of an individual, but may generalize diabetes care if the worker does not have sufficient depth of knowledge in enough aspects of diabetes management. In the UK, the relatively recent review of NHS job and salaries (entitled *Agenda for Change*) may also facilitate such developments. Posts and salary levels of staff will be determined by the needs of the diabetes service, not necessarily by the experience and qualifications of staff.

The division of labour in diabetes management and the dissemination of diabetes care to a much wider number of disciplines has had an impact on the roles of the diabetes specialist nurse and the diabetologist. Less of their time is spent providing clinical care to patients with diabetes. An increasing proportion of their working time is spent teaching other healthcare professionals to provide a good standard of up-to-date evidence-based diabetes care, usually linked into local practice and guidelines. This dissemination of skills means specialist staff can focus on patients with complex needs, while those requiring routine diabetes management can usually be managed by the general practitioner and practice nurse. Warwick University (www.warwick.ac.uk) has formalized this sharing of knowledge and skills with courses being delivered locally by local diabetes specialists, using the teaching materials and support provided by the university. This can facilitate a uniform diabetes plan in a local area and promote networking between all involved in diabetes care.

MANAGING THE WORKLOAD

With the large numbers of people with diabetes, how can all these patients get access to the limited numbers of healthcare professionals and the services they provide?

Traditionally, the patient has been seen in individual appointments in outpatients or Primary Care practices. Now, the large numbers of people with diabetes and the predicted rise in numbers worldwide [11] mean that this one-to-one approach is increasingly not feasible. Many of these patients have similar needs and seeing them in a group session not only gives economies of scale, but also means that each patient has more time, can learn more through interactive discussion and from each other and will get support from knowing they are not alone in living with diabetes [12]. In the UK, the National Institute of Clinical Excellence has produced guidelines for the provision of structured patient education for people with diabetes [13], which have been further recommended by the Patient Education Working Group [14].

People with diabetes should be able to access structured education, preferably in an interactive group. In the UK, the Dose Adjustment for Normal Eating (DAFNE) is an example of a structured education programme recommended for groups of up to 8 patients with type 1 diabetes [15]. The course runs for a complete week and covers a comprehensive programme of interactive learning about all aspects of living with type 1 diabetes. It was based on models from Germany.

For people with type 2 diabetes, the Diabetes Education in Self-Management for Newly Diagnosed and Ongoing Diabetes (DESMOND) [16] and X-PERT are examples of group education. In the UK, X-PERT is a 6-week programme consisting of sessions lasting about 150 minutes, for up to 18 patients with accompanying partners or carers [17]. To provide this depth of information in an interactive learning environment would be extremely difficult to achieve in the traditional clinic situation. These accredited national programmes may be time-consuming and relatively costly for some centres to deliver, so many diabetes teams run their own programmes. The author (JH) runs 2-hour introductory sessions for patients with newly diagnosed diabetes as there is insufficient capacity in the diabetes team to be able to offer X-PERT or DESMOND for the numbers of patients being diagnosed in the area. Each patient has 2 hours of learning opportunities. As up to 10 patients can be seen in a group, to give each patient 2 hours individual attention would be 20 hours of educator time!

HARD-TO-REACH GROUPS

In the UK, an Audit Commission report on diabetes services in England and Wales in the late 1990s highlighted that not all patients can access healthcare professionals equally. Certain groups, especially the housebound, those in residential homes, and ethnic minorities who do not speak English were identified particularly as missing out on services available to others [18]. South Asian people have a higher risk of developing diabetes [19], yet if they do not speak English, they are less likely to get education and information about the condition and how to manage it. There is also evidence to suggest that even if they do use general health services, they are likely to seek help much later than Caucasian people [20].

The use of Asian link workers and educators as part of the diabetes team can make a valuable contribution to meeting the needs of these vulnerable people [21]. With appropriate training and supervision, they can run group education sessions, teach simple practical skills like blood glucose monitoring, and work with specialists to interpret advice and feedback between the patient and their diabetes team. The Asian link worker usually has a good understanding of local cultural issues that can be potential barriers to concordance with diabetes care. They may know who has influence in the community and work with these people to promote diabetes services to those who need them.

The ongoing United Kingdom Asian Diabetes Study (UKADS) includes the use of link workers and specialist nurses with Asian language skills, working with practice nurses to demonstrate that a structured, culturally-sensitive care package tailored to the needs of the South Asian community will improve cardiovascular risk factors. The pilot study involving six inner city practices in Coventry and Birmingham showed significant improvements in blood pressure and total cholesterol levels [22].

People who are housebound, or who live in nursing and residential homes, may miss out on diabetes services [23]. In the UK, community nurses called district nurses are often the key HCPs in organizing diabetes care with housebound and residential care patients. They may perform much of the annual diabetes review, monitor blood glucose, give insulin injections and report problems to the general practitioner or refer to appropriate support (e.g. the community diabetes specialist nurse for insulin adjustment). Routine diabetes care, such as the provision of a healthy diet, monitoring of blood glucose, and arranging appointments for diabetes reviews and hospital care should be done by nursing home staff. However, they may not get opportunities for diabetes training as they are not usually employed by NHS organizations, and there may also be a rapid turnover of staff (so staff that have received some diabetes training may move to another home after a short period of time). Patients in these facilities often have quite complex needs, especially if they have other significant comorbidities, and they may need the skills of specialist diabetes staff. Nursing home staff need to know how to recognize when the patient has acute or chronic diabetes complications, and to know where and how to access appropriate diabetes HCPs.

SUMMARY

Most diabetes care has moved from the specialist hospital clinic setting to primary care. This has resulted in an increase in the number of different healthcare professionals involved in supporting the person with diabetes. There are many advantages in devolving the workload of diabetes care: local more easily accessible diabetes services, services shaped to the needs of the local population (e.g. delivered in languages common to the area), management of the diabetes epidemic, and more efficient use of specialist diabetes teams if routine diabetes care is managed elsewhere. However, there may be concerns about the skills and competencies of non-diabetes specialists, differences in referral procedures and communication, and repetition or omissions of care if there is not an efficient communication pathway between the healthcare professionals involved in an individual's diabetes management. As numbers of people with diabetes increase, diabetes will have an impact on all areas of healthcare, so all HCPs will need to develop diabetes management skills. Ensuring they possess appropriate skills, and use them effectively and synergistically, will be the challenge for those leading the development and maintenance of diabetes services.

REFERENCES

1. Bliss M. *The Discovery of Insulin*. Paul Harris, Edinburgh, 1982.
2. MacKinnon M. Through the looking glass. *Pract Diabetes Int* 1997; 14:14–16.
3. National Service Framework for *Diabetes: Standards*. Department of Health, London, December 2001.
4. Scottish Diabetes Framework (2002). Edinburgh (www.scotland.gov.uk).
5. National Service Framework for *Diabetes: Delivery Strategy*. Department of Health, London, November 2002.
6. Pierce M, Agarwal G, Ridout D. A survey of diabetes care in general practice in England and Wales. *Br J Gen Pract* 2000; 50:542–545.
7. Our Health, Our Care, Our Say: A New Direction for Community Services. Department of Health, London, 2006.
8. Donnan PT, MacDonald TM, Morris AD. Adherence to prescribed oral hypoglycaemic medication in a population of patients with Type 2 diabetes: a retrospective cohort study. *Diabet Med* 2002; 19: 279–284.
9. *Which?* Pharmacists get test of own medicine. (www.which.co.uk/news/2008/2009/pharmacies-get-test-of-own-medicine).
10. Skills for Health. Diabetes National Workforce Competence Framework. Guide Skills for Health: Bristol, 2004 (www.skillsforhealth.org.uk).
11. King H, Aubert RE, Herman WH. Global burden of diabetes 1995–2025: prevalence, numerical estmates, and projections. *Diabetes Care* 1998; 21:1414–1431.
12. Erskine PJ, Idris I, Daly H. Treatment satisfaction and metabolic outcome in patients with type 2 diabetes starting insulin: one to one vs group therapy. *Pract Diabetes Int* 2003; 20:243–246.

13. National Institute for Clinical Excellence (NICE). Guidance on the Use of Patient Education Models for Diabetes. Technical Appraisal No.60. NICE, London, 2003.

14. Structured patient education in diabetes: Report from the Patient Education Working Group. Department of Health, London, 2005.

15. DAFNE Study Group. Training in flexible, intensive insulin management to enable dietary freedom in people with type 1 diabetes: dose adjustment for normal eating (DAFNE) randomised controlled trial. *BMJ* 2002; 325:746–749.

16. Davies MJ, Heller S, Khunti K, Skinner TC. The DESMOND (Diabetes Education and Self Management for Ongoing and Newly Diagnosed) programme: from pilot phase to randomised control trial in a study of structured group education for people newly diagnosed with Type 2 diabetes mellitus: P333. *Diabet Med* 2005; 22:108.

17. Deakin TA, Cade JE, Williams R, Greenwood DC. Structured patient education: Diabetes X-PERT Programme makes a difference. *Diabet Med* 2006; 23:944–954.

18. Audit Commission. Testing Times: A review of diabetes services in England and Wales. Audit Commission, London, 2000.

19. Barnett AH, Dixon AN, Bellary S *et al.* Type 2 diabetes and cardiovascular risk in the UK South Asian community. *Diabetologia* 2006; 49:2234–2246.

20. Shakut N, de Bono DP, Cruikshank JK. Clinical features, risk factors, and referral delay in British patients of Indian and european origin with angina matched for age and extent of coronary atheroma. *BMJ* 1993; 307:717–718.

21. Curtis S, Beirne J, Jude E. Advantages of training Asian diabetes support workers for Asian families and diabetes health care professionals. *Pract Diabetes Int* 2003; 20:215–218.

22. O'Hare JP, Raymond NT, Mughal S *et al.* Evaluation of delivery of enhanced diabetes care to patients of South Asian ethnicity: the United Kingdom Asian Diabetes Study (UKADS). *Diabet Med* 2004; 21:1357–1365.

23. Sinclair AJ, Gadsby R. Diabetes in Care Homes. In: Sinclair AJ, Finucane P (eds). *Diabetes in Old Age*, 2nd edition. Wiley, Chichester, 2001.

Abbreviations

4S	Scandinavian Simvastatin Survival Study
ABCD	Appropriate Blood Control in Hypertensive and Normotensive DM
ACCORD	Action to Control Cardiovascular Risk in Diabetes
ACE-I	angiotensin-converting enzyme inhibitor
ACR	albumin/creatinine ratio
ACS	acute coronary syndrome
ADA	American Diabetes Association
ADOPT	A Diabetes Outcome Progression Trial
ADVANCE	Action in Diabetes and Vascular Disease: PreterAx and DiamicroN MR Controlled Evaluation
AGE	advanced glycosylation end-product
ALT	alanine transaminase
apoB	apolipoprotein B
ARB	angiotensin receptor blocker
AST	aspartate transaminase
AT1R	angiotensin 1 receptor
ATP	adenosine triphosphate
AVOID	Aliskiren in the Evaluation of Proteinuria in Diabetes
b.i.d.	twice daily
BMI	body mass index
BP	blood pressure
CABG	coronary artery bypass graft
CARDS	Collaborative Atorvastatin Diabetes Study
CB-1	cannabinoid receptor-1
CBG	capillary blood glucose
CEMACH	Confidential Enquiry into Maternal and Child Health
CGMS	continuous glucose monitoring system
CHD	coronary heart disease
CKD	chronic kidney disease
CLARITY-TIMI	Clopidogrel as Adjunctive Reperfusion Therapy – Thrombolysis in Myocardial Infarction
COC	combined oral contraceptive
COMMIT	Community Intervention Trial for Smoking Cessation
CRESCENDO	Comprehensive Rimonabant Evaluation Study of Cardiovascular ENDpoints and Outcomes
CRP	C-reactive protein
CURE	Clopidogrel in Unstable Angina to Prevent Recurrent Events
CVD	cardiovascular disease
DAFNE	Dose Adjustment for Normal Eating
DBP	diastolic blood pressure
DCCT	Diabetes Control and Complications Trial

DECODE	Diabetes Epidemiology: Collaborative analysis of Diagnostic criteria in Europe
DESMOND	Diabetes Education in Self-Management for Newly Diagnosed and Ongoing Diabetes
DIGAMI	Diabetes Mellitus Insulin-Glucose Infusion in Acute Myocardial Infarction
DM	diabetes mellitus
DPD	deoxypyridinoline
DPP	Diabetes Prevention Program
DPP-4	dipeptidyl peptidase-4
DPS	Diabetes Prevention Study
DSN	diabetes specialist nurse
EASD	European Association for the Study of Diabetes
ECG	electrocardiogram
EDIC	Epidemiology of Diabetes Interventions and Complications
eGFR	estimated glomerular filtration rate
EMEA	European Medicines Agency
EPHESUS	Eplerenone Post-Acute Myocardial Infarction Heart Failure Efficacy and Survival Study
ESR	erythrocyte sedimentation rate
ESRD	end-stage renal disease
FCT	fixed combination therapy
FDA	Food and Drug Administration
FPG	fasting plasma glucose
GDM	gestational diabetes mellitus
GFR	glomerular filtration rate
GIK	glucose, insulin and potassium
GIP	gastric inhibitory polypeptide
GLP-1	glucagon-like peptide-1
GMS	general medical services
GPsWI	GP with a special interest
GSH	glutathione
HCP	healthcare professional
HDL	high-density lipoprotein
HDL-C	high-density lipoprotein cholesterol
HEART2D	Hyperglycaemia and its Effects After Acute Myocardial Infarction on Cardiovascular Outcomes in Patients with Type 2 Diabetes Mellitus
HI-5	Hyperglycaemia: Intensive Insulin Infusion In Infarction
HOMA-B	homeostasis model assessment (β-cell function)
HOT	Hypertension Optimal Treatment
HPS	Heart Protection Study
HR	hazard ratio
hs-CRP	high-sensitivity C-reactive protein
ICD-10	International Statistical Classification of Diseases and Related Health Problems, 10th Revision
ICTP	carboxy-terminal telopeptide of type 1 collagen
IDNT	Irbesartan in Diabetic Nephropathy Trial
IFG	impaired fasting glucose
IGFBP-1	insulin-like growth factor-binding protein 1
IGT	impaired glucose tolerance
IHD	ischaemic heart disease
IL-6	interleukin-6

INNOVATION	Telmisartan (Micardis) in Incipient Diabetic Nephropathy study
IRMA-2	IRbesartan in patients with type 2 diabetes and MicroAlbuminaria
IT	information technology
JAK-STAT	Janus kinase signal transduction and translation system
LAM	lactation amenorrhoea
LAR	long-acting release
LDL-C	low-density lipoprotein-cholesterol
LEAD-3	Liraglutide Effect and Action in Diabetes-3
Look AHEAD	Action for Health in Diabetes
MAO	monoamine oxidase
MARVAL	MicroAlbuminuria Reduction with VALsartan
MDRD	Modification of Diet in Renal Disease
MI	myocardial infarction
MICRO-HOPE	MIcroalbuminuria Cardiovascular and Renal Outcomes
MMP	matrix metalloproteinase
MNT	medical nutritional therapy
MODY	maturity onset diabetes of the young
MR	magnetic resonance
MUR	Medicine Use Review
NADPH	nicotinamide adenine dinucleotide phosphate
NAVIGATOR	Nateglinide And Valsartan in Impaired Glucose Tolerance Outcomes Research
NICE	National Institute of Clinical Excellence
NIDDM	non-insulin-dependent mellitus
NO	nitric oxide
NPH	neutral protamine Hagedorn
O^{2-}	superoxide
OAD	oral antidiabetic
od	once daily
OGTT	oral glucose tolerance test
ONTARGET	ONgoing Telmisartan Alone and in combination with Ramipril Global Endpoint Trial
OR	odds ratio
ORIGIN	Outcome Reduction with an Initial Glargine Intervention
PACAP	pituitary adenylate cyclase-activating polypeptide
PAI-1	plasminogen activator inhibitor-1
PCI	percutaneous coronary intervention
PCOS	polycystic ovary syndrome
PIV	pressure-induced vasodilation
PKC	protein kinase C
PorGrow	Policy Options for Responding to the Growing Challenge of Obesity Research Project
PPARγ	peroxisome proliferators-activated receptor gamma
PPC	pre-pregnancy care
PREVEND	Prevention of REnal and Vascular ENd-stage Disease
PROactive	PROspective pioglitAzone Clinical Trial In macroVascular Events
PROVE-IT TIMI 22	Pravastatin or Atorvastatin Evaluation and Infection Therapy – Thrombolysis in Myocardial Infarction
QALY	quality adjusted life-year
RAAS	renin–angiotensin–aldosterone system
RAGE	receptor for advanced glycosylation end-product
RAS	renin–angiotensin system

RCT	randomized controlled trial
RECORD	Rosiglitazone Evaluated for Cardiac Outcomes and Regulation of Glycaemia in Diabetes
RENAAL	Reduction in Endpoints in Non-insulin dependent diabetes mellitus with the Angiotensin II Antagonist Losartan
RR	relative risk
RRR	relative risk ratio
SBP	systolic blood pressure
SCOUT	Sibutramine Cardiovascular OUTcomes
SERENADE	Study Evaluating Rimonabant Efficacy in Drug-Naive Diabetic patients
SMR	standardized mortality rate
SOS	Swedish Obese Subjects
SSRI	selective serotonin reuptake inhibitor
STIR	short tau inversion recovery
STOP-NIDDM	Study TO Prevent Non-Insulin-Dependent Mellitus
SU	sulphonylurea
SUR	sulphonylurea receptor
t.i.d.	three times daily
TFT	thyroid function test
TIMI	Thrombolysis in Myocardial Infarction
TNF-β	tumour necrosis factor alpha
TNT	Treating to New Targets
TRITON-TIMI 38	Trial to Assess Improvement in Therapeutic Outcomes by Optimizing Platelet Inhibition with Prasugrel–Thrombolysis in Myocardial Infarction
TZD	thiazolidinedione
UAE	urinary albumin excretion
UAER	urinary albumin excretion rate
UKADS	United Kingdom Asian Diabetes Study
UKPDS	United Kingdom Prospective Diabetes Study
UKPDS-PTM	United Kingdom Prospective Diabetes Study – post-trial monitoring
VADT	Veterans Affairs Diabetes Trial
WHO	World Health Organization
XENDOS	XENical in the prevention of Diabetes in Obese Subjects

Index